*Cardiology*

# Cardiology

## HUON H. GRAY
MD FRCP FESC FACC
*Consultant Cardiologist*

## KEITH D. DAWKINS
BSc MD FRCP FACC
*Consultant Cardiologist*

## IAIN A. SIMPSON
MD FRCP FACC
*Consultant Cardiologist*

## JOHN M. MORGAN
MA MD FRCP
*Consultant Cardiologist & Director of Cardiac Electrophysiology*

*Wessex Regional Cardiothoracic Unit*
*Southampton General Hospital*
*Southampton University Hospitals NHS Trust*
*Southampton SO16 6YD*
*UK*

**Fourth edition**

**With a foreword by**
**AUBREY LEATHAM**

**Blackwell**
Science

© 1967, 1974, 1991, 2002 by
Blackwell Science Ltd
Editorial Offices:
9600 Garsington Road
   Oxford OX4 2DQ UK
23 Ainslie Place, Edinburgh EH3 6AJ
350 Main Street, Malden
   MA 02148-5018, USA
54 University Street, Carlton
   Victoria 3053, Australia

Other Editorial Offices:
Blackwell Wissenschafts-Verlag GmbH
Kurfürstendamm 57
10707 Berlin, Germany

Blackwell Science KK
MG Kodenmacho Building
7–10 Kodenmacho Nihombashi
Chuo-ku, Tokyo 104, Japan

Iowa State University Press
A Blackwell Science Company
2121 S. State Avenue
Ames, Iowa 50014-8300, USA

First published 1967
Second edition 1974
Portugeuse translation 1980
Reprinted 1975, 1977 (twice), 1980
1982, 1983, 1984, 1985, 1986
Third edition 1991
Reprinted 1993
Fourth edition 2002
Reprinted 2002, 2005, 2006

Set by Best-set Typesetter Ltd.,
Hong Kong

Printed and bound by
Replika Press Pvt. Ltd, India

**DISTRIBUTORS**

   Marston Book Services Ltd
   PO Box 269
   Abingdon, Oxon OX14 4YN
   (*Orders*: Tel: 01235 465500
               Fax: 01235 465555)

USA
   Blackwell Science, Inc.
   Commerce Place
   350 Main Street
   Malden, MA 02148 5018
   (*Orders*: Tel: 800 759 6102
               781 388 8250
          Fax: 781 388 8255)

Australia
   Blackwell Science Pty Ltd
   54 University Street
   Carlton, Victoria 3053
   (*Orders*: Tel: 03 9347 0300
               Fax: 03 9347 5001)

A catalogue record for this title is
available from the British Library

ISBN-10: 0-86542-864-6
ISBN-13: 978-0-86542-864-5

Library of Congress
Cataloging-in-publication Data

Lecture notes on cardiology.—4th ed./
Huon H. Gray...[et al.].
p.; cm.
Rev. ed. of: Lecture notes on cardiolo-
gy/
Aubrey Leatham. 3rd ed. 1991.
ISBN 0-86542-864-6
1. Heart—Diseases. I. Gray, Huon
H. II. Leatham, Aubrey. Lecture
notes on cardiology.
[DNLM: 1. Heart Diseases. WG
L471 2001]
RC681.F54 2001
616.1'2—dc21

For further information on
Blackwell Publishing, visit our website:
www.blackwellpublishing.com

# Contents

# Foreword

The first edition was written near the start of modern surgical and medical cardiology in 1967 by M.V. Braimbridge, cardiac surgeon, and J.S. Fleming, cardiologist. The second edition came in 1974 and was reprinted nine times. It was the 'golden era' of British clinical cardiology, when Paul Wood and his colleagues had successfully co-ordinated cardiac physiology based on cardiac catheterization, with clinical groundwork laid by Mackenzie, the great sceptic, and Lewis, the scientist, and many others stimulated by these great men. Of Wood's colleagues at the Heart Hospital, Brigden coined the term 'cardiomyopathy' following the discovery of asymmetric hypertrophy by Teare at St George's, and auscultation was mapped out by means of phonocardiography by Leatham. Braimbridge was one of the first surgeons to understand and appreciate clinical cardiology and, therefore, particularly well placed to include the new surgical aspects which were revolutionizing the need for accurate diagnosis. Paediatric cardiology was then being developed by the adult cardiologists who were not then in great numbers because the specialty was small and frowned upon by the general physicians. Important contributions were made in cardiac radiology by Parkinson and in pathology by Reginald Hudson at the Heart Hospital, and later Michael Davies at St George's. All these sections of cardiology were pooled together by these two young authors in a slender synopsis with the catching title of *Lecture Notes on Cardiology* and was highly successful, being far in advance of the big textbooks except for that of Paul Wood.

In the third edition, published in 1991 and written by Leatham, Bull and Braimbridge, the physiological and clinical approach was maintained with the addition of many diagrams of the arterial and venous pulses and phonocardiograms to illustrate heart sounds and murmurs. An attempt was made to continue the accounts of surgical procedures and paediatric cardiology, summarized in some detail by Bull. These, however, are now specialities in their own right and have correctly been omitted from this next edition.

In this new fourth edition, a smooth readable text has been combined with 'boxes' of essential summarizing points. The text has been lengthened to include useful background information and essential evidence, but not made unwieldy by references to the source of the information. Useful chapters have been added such as 'Thrombosis in cardiovascular disease', valve disease is considered in less detail, and the account of congenital heart disease has been shortened and confined to adults.

Altogether this is now a short and readable text book of the essentials of cardiology and, in my opinion, vastly improved. The major feature is still the clinical approach and, as stated in the third edition, the objective of making an accurate diagnosis of cardiovascular disease (or equally important of its absence) at a single out-patient visit, by means of a careful history, physical examination and ECG (aided only if necessary by an exercise test and echo). What is essential to avoid is bypassing the busy clinical cardiologist with an isolated test such as an ECG or echo, reported on by a specialized technician who is ignorant of the general aspects of a case, or by a theoretical cardiologist in a back room making his report legally safe. The only hope for the nervous patient then is interception of the report by a wise general practitioner. A grasp of clinical cardiology as outlined in this excellent volume should prevent these bad practices in cardiology and avoid unnecessary investigations.

Aubrey Leatham

# Acknowledgements

The authors are grateful for the support of Novartis Pharmaceutical UK and Guidant Ltd who gave educational grants towards production of the illustrations, and to Dr Patrick Gallagher (Reader in Pathology, Southampton) who kindly supplied photographs of the pathological specimens.

# Abbreviations

| | |
|---|---|
| ACE | angiotensin-converting enzyme |
| ACTH | adrenocorticotrophic hormone |
| ADH | antidiuretic hormone |
| ADP | adenosine diphosphate |
| AF | atrial fibrillation |
| AICD | 'automatic' implantable cardiovertor defibrillator |
| ALS | advanced life support |
| ANP | atrial natriuretic peptide |
| APSAC | anisoylated plasminogen–streptokinase activator complex |
| aPTT | activated partial thromboplastin time |
| AR | aortic regurgitation |
| AS | aortic stenosis |
| ASD | atrial septal defect |
| ASO | antistreptolysin-O |
| AV | atrioventricular |
| AVN | atrioventricular node |
| BLS | basic life support |
| BMI | body mass index |
| BNP | brain natriuretic peptide |
| BP | blood pressure |
| CAA | Civil Aviation Authority |
| CABG | coronary artery bypass graft |
| cAMP | cyclic adenosine monophosphate |
| CCS | Canadian Cardiovascular Society |
| CCMAT | counterclockwise macro re-entrant atrial tachycardia |
| CHD | coronary heart disease |
| COPD | chronic obstructive pulmonary disease |
| CPAP | continuous positive airway pressure |
| CPK | creatine phosphokinase |
| CPR | cardiopulmonary resuscitation |
| CRP | C-reactive protein |
| CT | computerized tomography (scanning) |
| CTR | cardiothoracic ratio |
| CW | chest wall |
| Cx | circumflex |
| D & C | dilation and curettage |
| DC | direct current |
| DIC | disseminated intravascular coagulation |

| | |
|---|---|
| DVT | deep venous thrombosis |
| ECG | electrocardiogram |
| EDRF | endothelium derived relaxing factor |
| EMD | electromechanical dissociation |
| EMF | endomyocardial fibrosis |
| ESR | erythrocyte sedimentation rate |
| FTT | Fibrinolytic Therapy Trialists |
| GFR | glomerular filtration rate |
| HBD | hydroxybutyrate dehydrogenase |
| HCM | hypertrophic cardiomyopathy |
| HDL | high-density lipoprotein |
| HIV | human immunodeficiency virus |
| HOCM | hypertrophic obstructive cardiomyopathy |
| HOT | Hypertension Optimal Treatment (study) |
| HRT | hormone replacement therapy |
| INR | international normalized ratio |
| ISA | intrinsic sympathomimetic activity |
| ISIS | International Study of Infarct Survival |
| IVC | inferior vena cava |
| IVS | interventricular septum |
| JVP | jugular venous pressure |
| LA | left atrium |
| LAA | left atrial appendage |
| LAD | left anterior descending |
| LBBB | left bundle branch block |
| LDH | lactate dehydrogenase |
| LDL | low density lipoprotein |
| LMW | low molecular weight |
| LV | left ventricle |
| LVEDP | left ventricular end-diastolic pressure |
| LVH | left ventricular hypertrophy |
| LVOTO | left ventricular outflow tract obstruction |
| LVPW | left ventricular posterior wall |
| MIBI | methoxy-isobutyl isonitrile |
| MIC | minimum inhibitory concentration |
| MMD | minimal myocardial damage |
| MRI | magnetic resonance imaging |
| MR | mitral regurgitation |
| MS | mitral stenosis |
| MVA | mitral valve area |
| NIDDM | non-insulin-dependent diabetes mellitus |
| NIH | National Institutes of Health |
| NYHA | New York Heart Association |
| OCP | oral contraceptive pill |
| PA | posterior-anterior |
| PA | pulmonary artery |
| PAF | platelet activating factor |
| PDA | patent ductus arteriosus |

| | |
|---|---|
| PDA | posterior descending artery |
| PE | pulmonary embolism |
| PET | positron emission tomography |
| PFO | patent foramen ovale |
| PHT | pulmonary hypertension |
| PND | paroxysmal nocturnal dyspnoea |
| PR | pulmonary regurgitation |
| PTCA | percutaneous transluminal coronary angioplasty |
| PVR | pulmonary vascular resistance |
| RA | right atrium |
| RAA | renin-angiotensin-aldosterone |
| RBBB | right bundle branch block |
| RCA | right coronary artery |
| rt-PA | recombinant tissue-type plasminogen activator |
| RV | right ventricle |
| RVG | radionuclide ventriculography |
| SA | sinoatrial |
| SLE | systemic lupus erythematosus |
| SN | sinus node |
| SPECT | single photon emission computed tomography |
| SVC | superior vena cava |
| TGA | transposition of the great arteries |
| TIA | transient ischaemic attack |
| tPA | tissue plasminogen activator |
| TOE | transoesophageal echocardiography |
| TS | tricuspid stenosis |
| TTE | transthoracic echocardiography |
| VAD | ventricular assist device |
| VF | ventricular fibrillation |
| VSD | ventricular septal defect |
| VT | ventricular tachycardia |

# CHAPTER 1

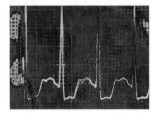

# Taking a Cardiovascular History

## Introduction

In an era when imaging and other diagnostic techniques have become more numerous and sophisticated, there is a tendency for the clinical assessment of the patient to seem less relevant. This is wrong, for the importance of the clinical examination cannot be overemphasized. However much information is gathered by other means, decisions about the correct management of patients still rely fundamentally on a good overall clinical assessment. It is bad practice to put patients through more than the minimum number of investigations needed to make a diagnosis and allow patient management to be planned, some of which may be uncomfortable and have associated risks. The good clinician selects investigations carefully and sparingly, always balancing the potential value of any information that may be obtained against the risks, cost and discomfort to the patient.

Establishing a good rapport and obtaining the confidence of a patient starts at the time of the clinical assessment and is extremely important later, when sometimes distressing information has to be discussed and difficult decisions made about potential treatment. The clinical assessment will often involve obtaining information from relatives or friends of the patient, who may be able to judge more objectively than the patient the extent of their limitations in daily activities.

The clinical assessment consists of obtaining a history to elicit symptoms, and performing a physical examination to observe signs, of cardiovascular disease. In this chapter broad principles will be covered but symptoms and signs relating to specific conditions will be detailed in the chapters relating to those conditions.

The art of good history taking involves allowing the patient to tell their story whilst, at the same time, through the questions asked, directing their attention to those aspects of their clinical presentation which are most likely to provide information that is relevant to making a diagnosis and determining treatment. Often a patient will unwittingly give vitally important clinical information almost as an aside remark, information that may never have come to light if the history taking consisted merely of asking numerous predetermined questions, or worse providing a questionnaire for the patient to complete. Taking time to obtain a clear history, in patients' own words and in their own time, is an important part of clinical training. As the clinician's expertise increases, this process can be achieved in relatively short periods of time. With experience, helpful information can also be gleaned from other sources, such as the patient's attitude, demeanor, emotional state and dress.

## Specific symptoms (see Boxes 1.1 and 1.2)

Because cardiac work is so closely related to

1

## Box 1.1 Symptoms of Cardiovascular Disease

The features most relevant when taking a history are:

- Dyspnoea, cough and haemoptysis
- Chest pain
- Syncope
- Palpitation
- Ankle swelling
- Fatigue
- Cyanosis
- Claudication

## Box 1.2 Symptom Details

The following information should be obtained about each symptom where relevant:

- Nature and severity
- Chronology
- Onset and duration
- Precipitating, aggravating and alleviating factors
- Associated symptoms
- Site and radiation of any pain

## Box 1.3 Causes of Dyspnoea

**Cardiac causes**

Acute
- Myocardial ischaemia or infarction
- Mitral regurgitation due to chordal rupture
- Onset of AF in mitral or aortic valve disease

Chronic
- Left ventricular dysfunction
- Mitral or aortic valve disease
- Atrial myxoma

**Non-cardiac**

Acute
- Pulmonary embolism
- Pneumothorax
- Asthma
- Hyperventilation syndrome

Chronic
- Obstructive or restrictive lung disease
- Pulmonary hypertension
- Chest wall abnormalities
- Anaemia
- Obesity and lack of fitness

exercise, many cardiac symptoms are worse during exertion, which should be enquired about specifically.

## Dyspnoea

Defined as an abnormal and uncomfortable awareness of breathing, dyspnoea is a common symptom of both cardiac and respiratory disease and is most commonly observed on exertion. This is unlike the breathlessness associated with anxiety where a heightened awareness of respiration progresses to hyperventilation, and where the sensation of dyspnoea is often worst at rest or in stressful situations. Hyperventilation also causes other symptoms (many of which are due to the fall in arterial $PCO_2$ and alkalosis), such as perioral and peripheral parasthesiae, clouding of consciousness, stabbing left inframammary chest pain and, in extreme cases, tetany. As the underlying cardiac condition progresses, the sensation of dyspnoea becomes present at ever lower levels of exertion and

ultimately occurs at rest. See Box 1.3 for causes of dyspnoea.

Dyspnoea due to cardiac disease arises due to pulmonary venous congestion. Left atrial pressure, and hence pulmonary venous pressure, is normally around 5 mmHg. When it rises, as will occur with mitral and aortic valve disease or left ventricular dysfunction, the pulmonary veins become distended and the bronchial walls congested and oedematous, causing an irritating non-productive cough and wheeze. As pulmonary venous pressure rises further and the plasma oncotic pressure (around 25 mmHg) is exceeded, so the lung tissue becomes stiffer due to interstitial oedema (increasing the muscular work required to inflate the lungs and the sensation of dyspnoea), a transudate collects in the alveoli and **pulmonary oedema** results. As this worsens frothy sputum is expectorated, which may be pink due to rupture of small bronchial vessels bleeding into the oedema fluid.

Cardiac dyspnoea is worst when lying flat

(**orthopnoea**), may wake the patient from sleep in the early hours of the morning (associated with sweating and anxiety—**paroxysmal nocturnal dyspnoea**), and tends to be relieved by sitting upright or standing. Systemic venous return to the right heart is increased in the recumbent position, especially in the early hours of the morning when blood volume is usually at its greatest, resulting in increased pulmonary blood flow and further increase in pulmonary venous pressure. However, if right ventricular contraction is severely impaired, as may occur with the dilated cardiomyopathies or right ventricular infarction, orthopnoea may be lessened because the right heart is unable to increase pulmonary blood flow in response to the increase in venous return.

Although cardiac dyspnoea may occur acutely, for example, due to left ventricular failure following acute myocardial infarction, it is more commonly of gradual onset and of a more chronic nature, slowly deteriorating over weeks or months. The sudden onset of dyspnoea should always make one consider alternative causes such as pneumothorax or pulmonary embolism.

See Box 1.4 for the **New York Heart Association (NYHA) classification**: the most commonly used classification to indicate the degree of disability from dyspnoea due to cardiac disease.

## Chest pain

Chest pain or choking discomfort, due to myocardial ischaemia (**angina**), typically has certain characteristics: a tight, constricting, band-like, or sometimes burning, retrosternal discomfort, occurring principally on exertion and relieved within minutes by rest or sublingual nitrates. Patients usually describe this as an uncomfortable rather than a truly painful sensation. The discomfort may radiate to either arm (most commonly the left), to the neck and jaw, or through to the back or abdomen. An attack is normally short-lived, lasting up to 20 min. Angina is sometimes atypical, causing neck, throat, jaw, back or abdominal discomfort without chest symptoms.

> **Box 1.4 NYHA Classification**
>
> Describes the degree of disability from dyspnoea due to cardiac disease:
> - Class 1—Patients with cardiac disease but without dyspnoea during normal activities
> - Class 2—Cardiac disease resulting in mild/moderate dyspnoea on normal exertion
> - Class 3—Marked dyspnoea on ordinary exertion
> - Class 4—Any exertion causes dyspnoea, or symptoms at rest

Angina is due to an imbalance between myocardial oxygen supply (coronary blood flow) and demand (myocardial oxygen consumption). The most common cause of angina is therefore coronary artery disease, but it may occur even with normal coronary arteries in conditions of severe left ventricular hypertrophy or dilatation where myocardial $O_2$ demand is high (see Chapter 8). Angina that occurs at rest or is rapidly worsening is termed 'unstable angina', and usually indicates critical coronary disease. Anginal pain lasting more than 30 min, and especially if associated with sweating, nausea and vomiting, should make one suspicious of myocardial infarction. Stabbing pain or episodes of pain lasting only seconds suggests a musculoskeletal cause.

Patients may describe exertional breathlessness rather than chest pain but, when pressed to be more precise, it is often the sensation of heaviness of the mid-chest (angina) that gives rise to a feeling of difficulty in expanding the chest. Breathlessness may, however, be due to the associated left ventricular dysfunction that occurs with myocardial ischaemia. Other symptoms that may be associated with myocardial ischaemia include belching, indigestion, nausea and dizziness, although their association with exertion is usually a consistent feature. Symptoms occurring above the mandible and below the umbilicus are very unlikely to be due to myocardial ischaemia. See Box 1.5 for the **Canadian Cardiovascular Society (CCS) classification**: the most commonly used

---

**Box 1.5  CCS Classification**

Describes the degree of disability caused by angina:
- Class 1—Angina only on strenuous or prolonged exertion
- Class 2—Slight limitation due to angina with normal activities
- Class 3—Marked limitation due to angina with ordinary activity
- Class 4—Unable to undertake any physical activity. Angina at rest

---

**Box 1.6  Non-Myocardial Causes of Chest Pain**

*Acute*
- **Oesophageal spasm**: very similar to angina but more prolonged and unrelated to exertion
- **Thoracic aortic dissection**: usually felt interscapular
- **Pneumonia**: usually pleuritic but may be more diffuse ache
- **Pneumothorax**: localized, intense, pleuritic
- **Pulmonary embolus**: either pleuritic and localized or dull central discomfort
- **Pericarditis**: varies with position and respiration

*Chronic*
- **Costochondritis** (Tietze's syndrome): localized, tender area of chest wall
- **Peptic ulceration**
- **Gall bladder disease**: usually abdominal symptoms also present
- **Pancreatic disease**
- **Cervical or thoracic spine disease**: related to movement

---

classification to describe the degree of disability caused by angina.

Almost any structure in the chest may also cause chest pain, but some of the more common are given in Box 1.6.

Usually a careful history will allow these causes to be differentiated. Perhaps the most common differentiation lies between cardiac pain and oesophageal spasm or reflux. The character of the pain caused by oesophageal spasm may be indistinguishable from angina and may be relieved by vasodilators, such as the nitrates. Oesophageal causes of pain often last longer than anginal episodes, are rarely related to exertion, and oesophageal reflux tends to be worse on bending or lying down. Functional or psychogenic chest pain (**Da Costa's syndrome**) may occur in patients with a fear of heart disease, for instance, due to a family history of myocardial infarction. It manifests as a dull persistent ache in the area of the cardiac apex lasting hours or days, and is often interspersed with more intense stabbing episodes. This pain may be associated with hyperventilation, palpitation and panic attacks. Chest pain is also well described in patients with mitral valve prolapse although the reason for this is not known.

## Syncope

Loss of consciousness may be caused by a number of cardiovascular causes but their final common pathway is a reduction in cerebral blood flow. A careful history will often suggest the underlying cause but there are a number of patients who have transient dizzy or syncopal episodes that defy cardiological and neurological diagnosis. See Box 1.7 for cardiovascular causes of syncope and presyncope.

Cardiac syncope is usually of rapid onset, without an aura, and is usually not associated with convulsions or incontinence. Recovery is typically rapid (unlike the slower recovery of neurological causes which may cause post-syncopal confusion), and may be associated with profound vasodilatation as blood supply is restored to arterioles that have become vasodilated by the accumulation of local metabolites. A gradual reduction of consciousness is more suggestive of vasodepressor syncope or postural hypotension.

## Palpitation

This is a common symptom and is defined as an unpleasant awareness of the heart beating. At the outset it is important to determine exactly what sensation the patient is describing. It may be an awareness of the heart beating more forcefully than usual, more rapidly, more slowly, erratically or a combination of these.

## Box 1.7 Cardiovascular Causes of Syncope and Presyncope

- **Aortic stenosis (AS)**: usually exertional, or at rest with the onset of AF (atrial fibrillation) or heart block
- **Left ventricular outflow tract obstruction (LVOTO)**: as occurs with hypertrophic obstructive cardiomyopathy (HOCM). Syncope may be due to associated arrhythmias as well as LVOTO
- **Tachyarrhythmias**: may be associated with awareness of palpitation
- **Heart block**: patient may be aware of bradycardia or pauses
- **Hypotensive drugs**: symptoms often postural
- **Vasovagal syndrome**: often occurs in painful situations, after standing up or prolonged standing, with emotional stress. Attacks often occur for many years
- **Carotid sinus syndrome**: sensitivity of carotid sinus to neck movement or palpation results in vagal stimulation, causing bradycardia and hypotension
- **Myocardial ischaemia**: rarely causes syncope in the absence of other cardiac disease (e.g. AS) except if left main stem coronary artery is stenosed
- **Severe pulmonary hypertension**: usually exertional. Comparable mechanism to hypertension or AS. Fixed obstruction to circulatory blood flow
- **Acute pulmonary embolism**: only when massive embolism produces circulatory obstruction
- **Subclavian steal syndrome**: due to severe subclavian artery stenosis or occlusion. Occurs with ipsilateral arm movement
- **Cerebrovascular disease**: often causes dizzy spells (transient ischaemic episodes), and mainly in the elderly
- **Atrial myxoma**: rare. May be posturally related. Produces intermittent mitral valve obstruction

fibrillation, or slower, as in an awareness of ectopic beats.

- With ectopics the patient may be aware of the prematurely occurring 'extra beat' (ectopic), the compensatory pause after the ectopic which may give the sensation of a 'missed beat', or of the post-ectopic beat which is accentuated and felt as a 'more forceful' beat because, occurring later, it has a larger stroke volume than the preceding sinus or ectopic beats.

Palpitation associated with a slow rate may be due to atrioventricular block or sinus node disease. Rapid palpitations usually start and stop suddenly, and imply an atrial, AV nodal or ventricular tachycardia. A gradual termination of the palpitation is more in keeping with a sinus tachycardia.

## Oedema

An elevation in right heart pressure increases systemic venous pressure in the inferior and superior vena cavae, and this will be greatest in the most dependent parts of the body, most usually the feet and ankles, but will be the sacral region in those confined to bed. Oedema occurs when plasma oncotic pressure is exceeded by the raised intravascular pressure, a situation which is exacerbated in hypoalbuminaemic states.

- Elevation of right heart pressure may be secondary to left heart disease (left ventricular failure, mitral or aortic valve disease) or may be due to right heart failure as a consequence of pulmonary hypertension, right ventricular or constrictive pericardial disease.
- Oedema due to superior vena cava obstruction (usually caused by malignancy) is obviously confined to the head, neck and arms.
- A history of periorbital oedema is characteristic of renal disease (nephrotic and nephritic syndromes).
- Unilateral oedema of a limb implies local vascular or lymphatic obstruction, as occurs following deep venous thrombosis or chronic venous insufficiency due to varicose veins.
- Other causes of oedema include the cyclical oedema that may occur perimenstrually and

- An awareness of a forceful beat may suggest an increased stroke volume (e.g. aortic or mitral regurgitation) or may just represent an individual's heightened awareness of their heart.
- Rapid palpitation suggests a tachycardia.
- An erratic palpitation may be fast, as in atrial

angioneurotic oedema that occurs as an allergic reaction to various stimuli, including seafood.

## Fatigue

This is a non-specific but common symptom in cardiac disease. It may arise due to a low cardiac output or an inability to raise cardiac output sufficiently on exercise. Drug therapy may cause fatigue, either directly as in the case of β-blockers, or indirectly such as that due to hypokalaemia caused by diuretic therapy.

## Cyanosis

As well as being a sign which should be sought on examination, patients may complain of a bluish discoloration of the skin and mucous membranes, and thus cyanosis may also be a presenting symptom. The blue discoloration arises as a result of the presence of increased amounts of deoxygenated haemoglobin in the blood perfusing the tissues. Cyanosis can be divided into 'central' and 'peripheral', terms which indicate the cause of the cyanosis rather than where it is observed.

• **Central cyanosis** is characterized by decreased arterial oxygen saturation, due to central venous–arterial admixture of blood in conditions causing right-to-left shunting, or due to pulmonary disease causing impaired arterial oxygen uptake. Right-to-left shunting may be intracardiac in origin (**cyanotic congenital heart disease involving absence of or defects in ventricular or atrial septa**) or may be extracardiac (**pulmonary arteriovenous malformations**). Central cyanosis is best observed by examining the oral mucous membranes and is clinically apparent when >40 g/L of deoxygenated (reduced) haemoglobin is present. Cyanosis of central origin is usually not improved by giving higher concentrations of inspired $O_2$, whereas peripheral cyanosis may be. In darker skinned individuals, cyanosis may not be observed until greater levels of reduced haemoglobin are present. More rarely cyanosis may be due to the presence of abnormal haemoglobin pigments, such as methaemoglobin.

• **Peripheral cyanosis** is usually due to cutaneous vasoconstriction, either because of exposure to cold or to Raynaud's phenomenon. Cyanosis is most readily seen when cardiac output is reduced for any reason. Whereas cyanosis of central origin usually worsens on exercise, peripheral cyanosis is usually unchanged if cardiac output is poor, or may improve with reflex vasodilatation if the principal abnormality is vasoconstriction.

When there is a central cause for the cyanosis, peripheral cyanosis must also be present, whereas cyanosis due to a peripheral cause will not result in cyanosis of the mucous membranes.

## Claudication

This aching discomfort in the legs, usually the calves, occurs after varying amounts of exercise and is due to skeletal muscle ischaemia as a consequence of peripheral vascular disease. Since this is almost always atheromatous, the presence of claudication should alert one to the probability that the patient also has underlying coronary artery disease.

## Additional history

A full medical history should be obtained from the patient; Box 1.8 details what this should include.

### Box 1.8 Patient History

A full medical history for the patient should include:
• **Systems review**: for urinary, menstrual and gastrointestinal symptoms
• **Drug history**: specific cardiovascular drugs, contraceptive pill, other medication (e.g. treatment for indigestion)
• **Past medical history**: for tuberculosis, rheumatic fever, diabetes mellitus, hypertension, stroke, venereal or tropical diseases, thyroid disease, asthma, previous operations
• **Social history**: exercise, occupation, smoking, alcohol consumption, family/partner
• **Family history**: for any cardiovascular or other possibly genetically linked disease

# CHAPTER 2

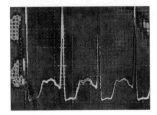

# Examination of the Cardiovascular System

## Introduction

The examination of a patient should be thorough but when applied in routine and busy clinical practice must also be undertaken quickly. The goal of the examination is to obtain clinical information that advances diagnosis and is not merely an exercise in repeating a set series of tasks. The examiner should have a clear understanding of why a particular part of the examination may be relevant to that patient and how to interpret the physical signs when present.

There are various ways by which the cardiovascular system can be examined, the pattern of which is less important than consistency and thoroughness. Below (Table 2.1) is a suggested approach to eliciting cardiovascular signs and the observations that should be made.

## General approach (see Tables 2.1 and 2.2)

On approaching the patient, the examiner should make an appropriate introduction and attempt to put the patient at ease. The patient should be asked to lie semi-recumbent (30–40°) and the examiner should ensure that it is possible to examine the patient's chest, abdomen and legs without the interference of clothing, whilst maintaining the patient's dignity using bedclothes and removable garments. The

examiner should already be making general observations about things such as the patient's demeanour, any obvious confusion and degree of co-operation. Once the patient is comfortably positioned, specific observations should be made such as the pattern of respiration, the presence of any distress and the patient's general appearance and body habitus. For example, it may be obvious that the patient has features of **Marfan's syndrome** (tall with arm-span greater than height, arachnodactyly, and skeletal deformities such as pectus carinatum and kyphoscoliosis), or may look thyrotoxic or dysmorphic (e.g. **Down's syndrome**). The patient may be morbidly obese or cachectic, may have malar flushing (**mitral valve disease, systemic lupus erythematosus**) or look generally unwell.

## Examination of the head and neck (see Tables 2.1 and 2.2)

### Hands and arms
The patient should be asked to raise their arms, outstretched with palms downwards, and the fingers should be examined for nail clubbing, splinter haemorrhages, Janeway lesions, peripheral cyanosis (see Chapter 1), or xanthomata (**hypercholesterolaemia**) over extensor tendons. Observe any tar staining suggesting past cigarette consumption and therefore the possibility of coronary and peripheral vascular

## EXAMINATION PROCESS

1 *General approach*
   Introduce yourself
   Position the patient
   Ensure patient's comfort
   Make general observations—dyspnoea, distress, build, body habitus

2 *Examination of arms, head and neck*

| | |
|---|---|
| Hands | Clubbing, splinter haemorrhages, cyanosis, tar staining |
| Arms | Radial and brachial pulses, scars, blood pressure, xanthomata |
| Face | Malar flush |
| Eyes | Anaemia, jaundice, corneal arcus, fundoscopy, xanthelasmata |
| Mouth | Palate, dentition, cyanosis |
| Neck | Thyroid, carotid pulse, jugular venous pulse |

3 *Cardiac examination*

| | |
|---|---|
| Inspect anterior chest wall | General appearance, scars |
| Palpate precordium | Cardiac impulses, thrills, apex beat |
| Auscultate | Heart sounds (S1, S2, added sounds) |
| | Systole (murmurs) |
| | Diastole (murmurs) |

4 *Examination of the chest*

| | |
|---|---|
| Inspect posterior chest wall | General appearance, scars |
| Palpate | Lung expansion |
| Percuss | Pleural effusion |
| Auscultate | Bronchial breathing, crepitations |

5 *Examination of the abdomen*

| | |
|---|---|
| Palpate | Liver, spleen, kidneys, aorta |
| Percuss | Ascites |
| Auscultate | Bowel sounds, bruits |

6 *Examination of the legs*

| | |
|---|---|
| Pulses | Presence, femoro-radial synchrony, bruits |
| Oedema | |
| Toes | Splinter haemorrhages, clubbing |

Table 2.1 Summary of the examination process.

disease. Palpate both radial pulses to confirm their presence, and use one to assess the heart rate and rhythm (**regularity**). Palpate the elbows for xanthomatous eruptions, inspect the antecubital fossa for evidence of scars (**previous cardiac catheterization**) and palpate the brachial pulse for its **presence and character**. Taking the blood pressure is a vital part of the cardiovascular examination and care should be taken to ensure that the sphygmo-manometer cuff is inflated to well above systolic blood pressure before slowly deflating (see Chapter 4). A discrepancy of >10mmHg between the two arms should raise the possibility of obstruction (**intimal dissection, stenoses**) in the aorta, innominate, subclavian or brachial arteries. If aortic coarctation is suspected, measure the blood pressure in the leg for comparison.

### Head

Make general observations (**malar flush, dysmorphic features, cushingoid or**

## NON-CARDIAC PHYSICAL SIGNS

| Sign | Causes | Comments |
| --- | --- | --- |
| Finger clubbing | Infective endocarditis<br>Cyanotic heart disease<br>Suppurative lung disease<br>Bronchial carcinoma<br>Gastrointestinal disease<br>Idiopathic | Usually seen as finger clubbing but may occur in the toes |
| Splinter haemorrhages (subungual) | Infective endocarditis<br>Local trauma | Less likely to be traumatic if seen near nail bed rather than nail tips |
| Janeway lesions | Infective endocarditis | Slightly raised, non-tender haemorrhagic lesions on the palms of hands and soles of feet |
| Peripheral cyanosis | Vasoconstriction<br>Low cardiac output | Vasoconstriction due to cold or Raynaud's phenomenon |
| Central cyanosis | Venous-arterial admixture of blood | Intracardiac and extracardiac shunts |
| Malar flush | Mitral stenosis<br>SLE | Mechanism uncertain. SLE associated with valvular disease and sterile endocarditis |
| Facial dysmorphism | Down's syndrome<br>Turner's syndrome<br>Noonan's syndrome | Associated with various congenital cardiac abnormalities |
| Cushingoid fascies | Hyperadrenalism | Hypertension, oedema |
| Paget's skull or long bones | Paget's disease | High cardiac output heart failure |
| Myopathic fascies | Myopathies and muscular dystrophies | Various types (dystrophia myotonica, Friedrich's ataxia, Duchenne's, Becker's, facio-scapulohumeral) associated with cardiomyopathies |
| Acromegalic fascies | Acromegaly | Associated with cardiomyopathies |
| Thyrotoxic appearance | Hyperthyroidism | Sinus tachycardia, palpitations, atrial fibrillation, high cardiac output cardiomyopathy if severe |
| Hypothyroid appearance | Hypothyroidism | Sinus bradycardia, dilated cardiomyopathy, coronary disease due to associated hypercholesterolaemia |
| Corneal arcus | Hyperlipidaemia<br>Ageing | Significant if present in those <60 years |
| Cataracts | Age<br>Congenital rubella | Rubella associated with patent ductus, ASD, or pulmonary stenosis |

*continued on p. 10*

| NON-CARDIAC PHYSICAL SIGNS (cont.) | | |
|---|---|---|
| Sign | Causes | Comments |
| Lens dislocation | Marfan's syndrome | Associated with aortopathy and mitral valve prolapse |
| Kayser–Fleischer ring | Wilson's disease | Copper overload and rare cause of cardiomyopathy |
| Argyll Robertson pupil | Syphilis | May have associated aortopathy |
| Roth spots | Infective endocarditis | Retinal haemorrhages near the discs and with white spots in centre |
| Angioid streaks and blue sclerae | Pseudoxanthoma elasticum | Pink retinal streaks and/or blue scleral discolouration. Associated with aortopathy and/or coronary lesions |

ASD, atrial septal defect; SLE, systemic lupus erythematosus.

Table 2.2 Non-cardiac physical signs in cardiovascular disease.

acromegalic, exophthalmic) and then examine the eyes. Observe the skin bordering the medial aspect of the eyes for xanthelasmata (hypercholesterolaemia), inspect the conjunctivae (anaemia, jaundice) and anterior eyes (corneal arcus, cataracts, lens dislocation and rarities such as blue sclera, Kayser–Fleischer ring and Argyll Robertson pupils) and then use an ophthalmoscope to examine the fundi (diabetic or hypertensive retinopathy, Roth spots, angioid streaks). Examine the mouth for the presence of mucosal cyanosis (central cyanosis), state of the dentition (poor dentition predisposes towards bacterial endocarditis), and presence of high-arched palate (Marfan's syndrome). Facial oedema and engorgement of the neck veins may be present in cases of obstruction to the superior vena cava (SVC).

## Neck

Palpate the thyroid and if a goitre is suspected auscultate the thyroid for bruits, then examine the carotid pulse and jugular venous waveform.

*Carotid pulse* (see Figs 2.1 and 2.2)

Using the thumb, palpate the carotid arteries separately on both sides to confirm their presence and also to assess the character of the pulse. The normal waveform consists of an upstroke, a peak, and a decline which is less steep than the upstroke and is interrupted soon after the peak by the incisura (dicrotic notch) which coincides with closure of the aortic valve. Various abnormalities may be detected.

The pulse may be slow rising due to aortic stenosis or subaortic obstruction (subaortic membrane or hypertrophic obstructive cardiomyopathy), with a peak which occurs later and is more sustained than usual, and is often associated with a thrill (palpable bruit). A notch may occur on the upstroke (anacrotic notch) and may be so prominent as to produce two distinct peaks (anacrotic pulse). In elderly patients, the carotid artery wall may be so inelastic that the upstroke may be normal even in the presence of significant aortic stenosis.

The pulse may be low volume due to a low cardiac output, for whatever reason, or high volume (hyperdynamic) due to any high cardiac output state (fever, pregnancy, anaemia, hyperthyroidism).

## ARTERIAL PULSE WAVES

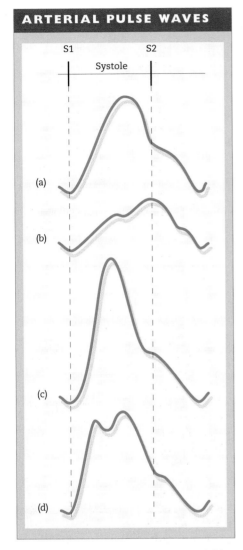

Fig. 2.1 The arterial pulse waves. (a) Normal. (b) Slow rising. (c) Sharp ('water hammer'). (d) Bisferiens. S1, first heart sound; S2, second heart sound.

A **collapsing (water hammer or Corrigan's) pulse** has a rapid upstroke and then abrupt collapse, and is typically due to aortic regurgitation. When severe this may be associated with a number of eponymous clinical signs, such as pistol shot femoral pulses (**Traube's sign**), an audible diastolic murmur over the femoral artery when it is compressed (**Duroziez' sign**), and visible pulsation of the nail capillaries (**Quincke's sign**), retinal vessels (**Becker's sign**) and uvula (**Mueller's sign**).

A **bisferiens** pulse has two systolic peaks (percussion and tidal waves) separated by a mid-systolic dip. This occurs in conditions where a large stroke volume is ejected rapidly from the left ventricle (**aortic regurgitation or combined aortic stenosis and regurgitation**), and disappears as heart failure develops. Contrary to general teaching, it is not usually clinically detectable in hypertrophic cardiomyopathy except by using the Valsalva manoeuvre, though it may be seen on intra-arterial pressure recordings, where it is due to early left ventricular ejection being halted as the left ventricular outflow tract obstruction (**septal hypertrophy**) occurs, and is followed by a reflected (**tidal**) wave.

A **dicrotic** pulse occurs when the dicrotic notch is exaggerated, as may occur when a low stroke volume is ejected into an elastic aorta under lower than usual pressure, in conditions such as cardiac tamponade, severe heart failure and hypovolaemic shock. It is rarely seen if the systolic pressure exceeds 120 mmHg. The normal carotid systolic wave is reduced but the dicrotic notch is preserved, giving a double peak to the palpated pulse, one systolic and one early diastolic. This should not be confused with a bisferiens pulse where both peaks are systolic.

**Pulsus alternans** consists of alternating strong and weak pulse waves on consecutive beats and is a sign of severe left ventricular dysfunction. The alternating intensity can also be heard on sphygmomanometry. It is clinically detectable if systolic pressures differ by >20 mmHg between beats and is best assessed in held mid-respiration, to avoid the effects of the respiratory cycle on stroke volume.

**Pulsus bigeminus** is due to an ectopic beat, usually ventricular, occurring after each sinus beat. The ectopic beat is weaker than the preceding sinus beat, and occurs prematurely (in contradistinction to pulsus alternans where the weaker beat occurs when the beat would normally be expected). The sinus beat following the

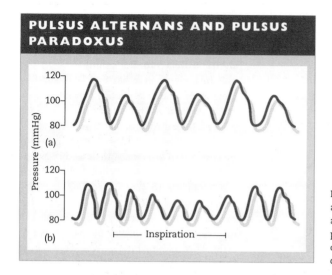

**PULSUS ALTERNANS AND PULSUS PARADOXUS**

Fig. 2.2 (a) Pulsus alternans — alternate large and small amplitude pulses. (b) Pulsus paradoxus — marked diminution of pulse amplitude during inspiration.

ectopic may be stronger than usual due to **post-ectopic accentuation**.

**Pulsus paradoxus** is an exaggeration of a normal phenomenon. Systolic pressure normally falls slightly on inspiration due to the effects of negative intrathoracic pressure on the aorta and on left ventricular stroke volume, but if this fall is >10 mmHg during quiet respiration then it is considered abnormal, and when >25 mmHg is often detectable even by palpation. It is characteristic of pericardial tamponade, is seen in approximately 50% of patients with pericardial constriction, and may also be seen in conditions with wide swings in intrathoracic pressure (**asthma, emphysema**), or less commonly in hypovolaemic shock, pulmonary embolism, pregnancy and severe obesity. A reverse paradox, a rise in systolic pressure with inspiration, may occur in hypertrophic obstructive cardiomyopathy.

Having palpated the carotids, they should next be auscultated. When an artery becomes >50% stenosed, the sound of blood passing through the stenotic segment in systole may be heard (**bruit**). When aortic valve disease is present, it is usually impossible to distinguish between a radiated systolic murmur and intrinsic arterial stenosis, and carotid ultrasound scanning may be required.

### Jugular venous pulse

Both internal jugular veins lie deep to the sternocleidomastoid muscles. The right internal jugular drains directly into the SVC whereas the left drains first into the innominate vein and thereafter into the SVC, with the SVC draining directly into the right atrium. The jugular venous column of blood therefore allows a clinical assessment of right atrial pressure to be made at the bedside. Careful observation of the jugular venous pulse should be made, but clinically it can often be difficult to see visually what is classically described below, and students should not be disheartened if the more subtle observations remain obscure. However, understanding the jugular venous pressure (JVP) and waveform assist greatly in an understanding of cardiac physiology.

**JVP:** the normal JVP is <4 cm $H_2O$ above the manubriosternal joint (sternal angle) when the patient is lying semi-recumbent (30–40°), and so the upper end of the column of systemic venous blood will either be below or only just be visible above the level of the sternal notch. The top of the venous column may be seen more easily if the patient reclines closer to the horizontal, and some recommend using hepatojugular reflux. This is a potentially uncomfortable manoeuvre whereby firm pressure is exerted by the examiner's hand in the patient's right hypochondrium for 10–30 s. This manoeuvre will tend to raise the JVP transiently by up to 3 cm $H_2O$, sometimes making it visible when at normal or low pressure. More simply, confirmation that the JVP is low may be undertaken by exerting moderate pressure on the base of the patient's neck using the ulnar edge of the examiner's hand. By doing this, venous drainage from the jugular vein is obstructed and the vein above the level of compression will be seen to fill from above and become engorged. By releasing compression the examiner should be able to see clearly that the venous column disappears rapidly by normal drainage into the SVC, thus confirming a normal pressure.

The JVP is elevated in conditions causing a rise in right atrial pressure (**right heart failure, reduced right ventricular diastolic compliance, pericardial disease, hypervolaemia, pulmonary hypertension**), or if the SVC is compressed (**usually due to mediastinal tumour involvement**). When the JVP is very high it may be difficult to see the top of the column of venous blood but may be easier if the patient is asked to sit vertically. Pulsation may be seen near the angle of the jaw or the ear lobes may be seen to pulsate. When the patient is obese, or in men with short, thick necks, it may be difficult to see the engorged jugular vein even when it is dilated. The JVP normally falls with inspiration as a result of an increase in negative intrathoracic pressure, augmenting venous return. Paradoxically, an abnormal rise in JVP on inspiration (**Kussmaul's sign**) occurs when the right heart cannot accommodate the additional venous return. Classically, this occurs in pericardial constriction but may also occur in pericardial tamponade.

**Jugular venous waveform** (Fig. 2.3): in normal sinus rhythm the waveform consists of two main parts, the 'a' and 'v' waves.

The '**a**' **wave** coincides with right atrial contraction and consists of a rise to a peak followed by a decline ('**x**' **descent**), occurring just before the first heart sound (S1) (**closure of the tricuspid and mitral valves**).

A small '**c**' **wave** occurs on the 'x' descent and coincides with carotid pulsation, but is of little importance and is usually undetectable at the bedside.

The SVC opens directly into the right atrium without any intervening valve, and so contraction of the right atrium causes a transient increase in SVC and jugular venous pressure. The 'a' wave is prominent when there is resistance to right atrial emptying (right ventricular hypertrophy, right ventricular restriction, pulmonary hypertension, tricuspid stenosis (TS)). It is described as a '**cannon wave**' when the right atrium contracts against a closed tricuspid valve, as occurs intermittently in atrioventricular dissociation (complete heart block). The 'a' wave is absent in atrial fibrillation since coordinated atrial contraction does not occur. The 'x' descent occurs as a result of the right atrium relaxing (atrial diastole) at the end of its contraction together with the effects of right ventricular contraction (RV systole) which tends to pull the right atrioventricular ring and closed tricuspid valve downwards. The 'x' descent will therefore be rapid in conditions where the 'a' wave is increased in association with an enlarged right ventricle due to volume overload, as typically occurs with an atrial septal defect and significant left-to-right shunting.

The '**v**' **wave** upstroke coincides with the later half of atrial diastole, as the right atrium becomes more distended with venous blood. It is followed by the '**y**' **descent** which coincides with opening of the tricuspid valve and consequent passive emptying of the right atrium into the right ventricle at the start of atrial systole. It occurs after the second heart sound (S2). Later in diastole, atrial contraction occurs again ('a' wave) and the cycle is repeated.

In mild to moderate tricuspid incompetence, blood regurgitates into the right atrium in ventricular systole (atrial diastole) and results in accentuation of the 'v' wave. In severe tricuspid incompetence, this accentuation occurs early in atrial diastole causing the normally invisible 'c' wave to become prominent, the 'x' descent to be abolished and resulting in the so-called 'cv' wave. The 'y' descent is typically rapid in pericardial constriction but also occurs in tricuspid

## JUGULAR VENOUS PULSE WAVEFORMS

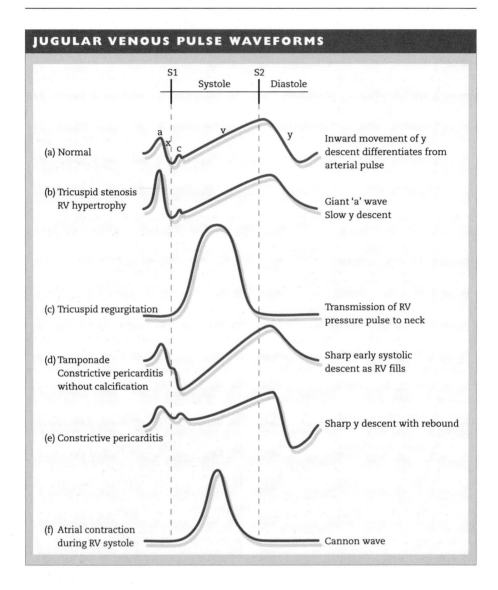

**Fig. 2.3** Jugular venous pulse waveforms in relation to S1 and S2.

regurgitation and any condition associated with right ventricular dilatation and dysfunction. The descent is typically slow in tricuspid stenosis.

The jugular venous pulse can usually be differentiated from carotid pulsation because of its double waveform (if in sinus rhythm), the ability of the examiner to abolish venous pulsation with light-to-moderate external compression and the fact that venous pressure alters visibly with phases of the respiratory cycle and position of the patient.

### Cardiac examination

**Inspection** (see Table 2.3)
Assess the respiratory rate and observe any thoracic deformities, such as pectus excavatum (**depressed sternum**), which may displace the

## PRECORDIAL INSPECTION AND AUSCULTATION

| Action | Observation | Association |
|--------|-------------|-------------|
| Inspection | Kyphoscoliosis or pectus carinatum | Marfan's syndrome |
| | Ankylosing spondylitis (kyphosis) | Aortic regurgitation |
| | Wide-spaced nipples | Turner's syndrome |
| | | Noonan's syndrome |
| | Median sternotomy scar | Approach for most modern cardiac operations |
| | Lateral thoracotomy scar | Old mitral valvotomy or present approach for coarctation, patent ductus or descending thoracic aortic aneurysm surgery |
| | Respiratory rate | Normal 16–20 per min at rest |
| Palpation | Apex beat displaced | Left ventricular dilatation or aneurysm |
| | Apical heave (lift) | Left ventricular hypertrophy or dilatation |
| | Tapping apex | Mitral stenosis |
| | Double apical impulse | Hypertrophic obstructive cardiomyopathy |
| | Left parasternal heave | Right ventricular dilatation |
| | Hyperdynamic precordium | Severe mitral or aortic regurgitation, large left-to-right shunts, fever, hyperthyroidism |
| | Pulsation right 2nd ICS | Dilated aorta |
| | Pulsation left 3rd ICS | Dilated main pulmonary artery |
| | Knocking sensation | Mechanical prosthetic heart valve |

ICS, intercostal space.

Table 2.3 Findings on precordial inspection and auscultation.

cardiac apex to the left and give the false impression of cardiomegaly, or cause 'innocent' ejection flow murmurs due to mild compression of the right ventricular outflow tract. Pectus carinatum (**pigeon chest**) and kyphoscoliosis may be associated with Marfan's syndrome. The presence of a median sternotomy scar suggests previous surgery on the heart (**valvular or coronary bypass grafting**) or ascending aorta (**aneurysms, aortic dissection**). Large ventricular or aortic **aneurysms** may produce visible pulsations, and either superior or inferior **vena cava obstruction** may produce prominent venous collateral channels, of the chest wall.

## Palpation (see Table 2.3)
The widespread use of chest radiographs and more specialized cardiac investigations have meant that percussion of the precordium is now rarely undertaken. Firstly, determine the **position** of the apex beat using the tips of the fingers, and then palpate it using the palm of the hand to assess its **character**. The apex beat usually consists of the left ventricular impulse, and normally lies slightly medial and superior to the fifth intercostal space in the mid-clavicular line. It is often impalpable in the supine position, especially in older individuals, but may more easily be felt if the patient is turned towards the left side. The apex beat consists of a brief outward motion, followed by a more sustained inward one. With moderate or severe left ventricular hypertrophy, the outward thrust persists throughout ejection (**left ventricular heave or lift**), although this is even more obviously detected when the left ventricle is dilated or aneurysmal, where the lift is over a larger area and is displaced laterally. The apical impulse reduces as stroke volume declines. In significant mitral stenosis (MS), the apex beat is described

as 'tapping' in nature (the tapping being due to accentuated mitral valve closure), or may have a double impulse in hypertrophic obstructive cardiomyopathy. Palpation of the rest of the precordium using the palm or ulnar border of the hand is intended to detect such things as a left parasternal heave, generally hyperdynamic precordium or abnormal pulsations in specific areas. Mechanical prosthetic cardiac valves create sounds which can often also be felt on palpation of the chest wall.

## Auscultation

Auscultation of the heart is the skill which students find the most difficult to acquire and there is no substitute for experience. The more times, and the greater the variety of cardiac conditions in which auscultation is undertaken, the more comfortable and accurate the examiner becomes. Theory is important but without the ability to put it into clinical practice it is of little value. Before describing the signs that occur in cardiac disease, it is helpful to describe the normal cardiac cycle and the events that occur.

### Cardiac cycle (see Fig. 2.4)

Atrial emptying of blood into the ventricles starts when the atrioventricular (**mitral and tricuspid**) valves open and for most of this period blood flows passively from the atria across the valves. A later phase of active atrial contraction (**atrial systole**) occurs, during which approximately the last 20% of atrial emptying and ventricular filling takes place. The opening of normal atrioventricular valves is clinically inaudible.

At the end of atrial contraction the atria start to relax (atrial diastole), intra-atrial pressure starts to fall and ventricular diastolic pressure then exceeds atrial pressure. Because of this reversal in pressure gradient the atrioventricular (AV) valves close. Closure of the AV valves generate S1, which is made up of mitral (M1) and tricuspid (T1) components, and mitral closure

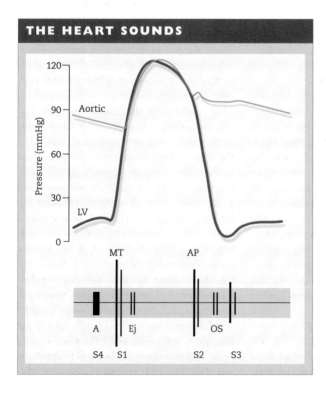

**THE HEART SOUNDS**

Fig. 2.4 The heart sounds and their relation to the LV and aortic pressure pulses (RV pulse occurs 10–20 ms later). Left-sided events precede right except for RA contraction (sinus node in RA). Events within the pink-shaded area are inaudible when normal but may become audible when pathological. S4 and A, atrial sounds (right and left); S1, first sound – mitral (M) and tricuspid (T) components; Ej, ejection sounds (pulmonary and aortic); S2, second sound – aortic (A) and pulmonary (P) components; OS, opening snaps of mitral and tricuspid valves; S3, third sounds (left and right). Only those sounds spreading beyond the shaded area are audible in a normal subject.

occurs fractionally before tricuspid. Almost immediately, ventricular contraction (**ventricular systole**) starts.

Just before the onset of left ventricular systole, pressure in the left ventricle is low (5–10 mmHg) but very rapidly increases in early systole until it exceeds aortic diastolic pressure (approximately 80 mmHg) and, once it does so, the aortic valve opens. This short phase in early systole, when left ventricular pressure is rising but the aortic valve is still closed, is termed '**isovolumic contraction**' because the volume of blood in the left ventricle is not changing. Opening of a bicuspid, as opposed to the more usual tricuspid, aortic valve may result in an audible ejection click even in the absence of any stenosis. Once the aortic valve is open, left ventricular stroke volume (approximately 45 mL/m$^2$) is quickly ejected and aortic pressure rises to a peak (equal to systolic blood pressure, around 110–140 mmHg).

When the left ventricle starts to relax, ventricular and aortic pressures fall and the aortic valve closes, creating the aortic component (A2) of the second sound (S2). This precedes the pulmonary component (P2) by a short period. Ventricular diastole starts at S2 and for a short period of time diastolic ventricular pressure, whilst falling, is still higher than atrial pressure. This short period of time, when both atrioventricular (**mitral, tricuspid**) and ventriculoarterial (**aortic, pulmonary**) valves are closed, is termed **isovolumic relaxation** because ventricular volumes remain constant. These principles also apply to right ventricular function except that right ventricular pressure is considerably lower, at around 20% of left ventricular, and events in the cardiac cycle usually occur a short time after corresponding events in the left heart.

### Principles of auscultation

The stethoscope has two components, the bell and the diaphragm. Low frequency sounds are best heard with the bell and high frequencies with the diaphragm. When using the bell, just enough pressure should be applied to form skin contact around its circumference. Greater pressure stretches the underlying skin and makes it more like a diaphragm.

**Respiration:** inspiration increases the amount of lung tissue around the heart and as such, if unopposed by other factors, would tend to muffle all cardiac sounds and murmurs. However, inspiration also augments negative intrathoracic pressure and increases systemic venous return. For a few cardiac cycles this results in increased right heart volumes and pressure, and delays pulmonary valve closure (P2) which causes increased splitting of S2. Right heart murmurs (**tricuspid stenosis and regurgitation, pulmonary stenosis and regurgitation**) and added sounds tend to be accentuated by the inspiratory effect on venous return, but offset by the 'muffling' effect of an increase in lung volume. Overall, right-sided murmurs and added sounds are either accentuated or not diminished on inspiration. On the other hand, for the first few cardiac cycles after inspiration, left heart volumes are unchanged and left-sided murmurs and added sounds will be diminished because of the muffling effect of increased lung volume. On full expiration this muffling effect is reduced, and left heart murmurs and added sounds become accentuated.

**Valsalva manoeuvre:** this is forced expiration against a closed glottis followed by a release from straining, and can be employed to affect the intensity and timing of some murmurs and added sounds. It consists of four sequential phases:

• **phase 1** is associated with an increase in blood pressure;

• **phase 2** with a fall in systemic venous return and blood pressure, and a reflex tachycardia;

• **phase 3** starts as the straining phase ends and expiration is allowed to occur, and is associated with a further small fall in systemic venous return and blood pressure;

• **phase 4** follows during which there is a considerable increase in blood pressure (overshoot) and a reflex bradycardia.

**Effects of posture and exercise:** sudden lying down from a standing position or leg raising will increase systemic venous return. Initially this augments right ventricular stroke volume, and a few cardiac cycles later also results in an increase in left ventricular stroke volume. Sudden changes from a standing to a squatting position initially increase systemic venous return and systemic vascular resistance simultaneously, increasing both stroke volume and blood pressure. Handgrip exercise (**isometric exertion**) increase systemic vascular resistance, heart rate and cardiac output. Treadmill or bicycle exercise normally results in a gradual increase in heart rate and blood pressure.

### General comments

Areas of the precordium are often described as 'mitral', 'tricuspid', 'aortic' and 'pulmonary'. This tends to imply that murmurs originating from these valves are always best heard in these defined areas. This is often not the case and it is probably a better discipline to describe the anatomical position on the chest wall where a particular murmur is best heard, such as lower left sternal edge, upper right sternal edge or cardiac apex. Such an approach encourages the examiner to decide the origin of the murmur by its characteristics and not by imprecise surface landmarks. Placing the patient in different positions (supine, semi-recumbent, leaning forward or lateral decubitus) is designed to maximize the chances of gaining as much auscultatory information as possible and, after an initial learning phase, the examiner should be flexible in

Table 2.4  Auscultation of cardiac murmurs.

approach, selecting a position and determining the radiation of any murmur so as best to identify its origin. Such an approach can only come with practice.

### Starting auscultation (see Table 2.4)

Try to ensure surrounding quiet when auscultating and initially listen briefly over the precordium with the diaphragm and bell and the patient in the semi-recumbent (40°) position; this allows an initial impression to be gained. To accentuate sounds and murmurs originating from the aortic and pulmonary, and possibly the tricuspid, valves the patient should lean forwards, and for the mitral valve should be asked to turn on to their left side. In each position the appropriate phase of respiration (inspiration or expiration) should be used to maximize the information gained. Once a murmur has been identified, its **radiation** should be determined. Mitral regurgitation may radiate posteriorly towards the axilla or anteriorly towards the sternum depending on the principal valve leaflet affected, and aortic stenosis generally radiates towards the upper right sternal edge and carotids. Timing of events in relation to the cardiac cycle can be helped by knowing that S1 approximately coincides with the carotid pulse.

### Heart sounds (see Table 2.5 and Fig. 2.5)

These are vibrations of varying intensity (**loudness**), frequency (**pitch**) and quality (**timbre**). S1 marks the start of ventricular systole and S2 the start of ventricular diastole.

## CARDIAC MURMURS AUSCULTATION

| Murmur | Patient position | Phase of respiration | Bell or diaphragm |
|---|---|---|---|
| Aortic | Sitting forwards | Expiration | Diaphragm |
| Mitral | Lying on left side | Expiration | MS = Bell, MR = Diaphragm |
| Pulmonary | Sitting forwards | Inspiration | PS = Diaphragm, PR = Bell or diaphragm depending on PA pressure |
| Tricuspid | Sitting forwards | Inspiration | TS = Bell, TR = Diaphragm |

MR, mitral regurgitation; MS, mitral stenosis; PA, pulmonary artery; PR, pulmonary regurgitation; PS, pulmonary stenosis; TR, tricuspid regurgitation; TS, tricuspid stenosis.

## HEART SOUNDS

| Heart sound | Increased | Decreased |
|---|---|---|
| S1 | MS or TS | Severe MS or TS when valve immobile |
| Ejection clicks | Bicuspid aortic valve<br>PS<br>Mechanical aortic prosthetic valves | Severe AS or PS when valve immobile |
| Mid and late systolic sounds | Mitral valve prolapse | |
| S2 | | |
|   Intensity | Systemic hypertension (A2)<br>Pulmonary hypertension (P2) | Severe aortic or pulmonary stenosis with immobile valve |
|   Splitting | Increased in inspiration, and in right bundle branch block<br>Fixed split in atrial septal defect | Decreased in expiration, pulmonary hypertension<br>Reversed split in left bundle branch block, right ventricular pacing |
| Early diastolic sounds | | |
|   Opening snap | Mitral or tricuspid stenosis | Severe MS or TS with immobile valve |
|   Other | Mechanical aortic valves<br>Pericardial constriction<br>Atrial myxoma | |
| Mid and late diastolic sounds | | |
|   S3 | Youth<br>Ventricular dysfunction | |
|   S4 | Elderly<br>LV fibrosis or hypertrophy | |

AS, aortic stenosis; LV, left ventricle; MS, mitral stenosis; PS, pulmonary stenosis; TS, tricuspid stenosis.

Table 2.5 Heart sounds.

**S1:** this high-pitched sound consists of mitral and tricuspid components and is due to abrupt restraint of the papillary muscles of the respective valve. It is best heard at the lower left sternal edge. M1 is dominant and occurs just before T1, which is often inaudible. M1 is accentuated in mitral stenosis when the valve still retains some mobility. Tricuspid stenosis is rare but similarly will accentuate T1.

**Early systolic sounds:** aortic and pulmonary **ejection clicks** are high frequency and are usually due to congenital abnormalities, such as a bicuspid aortic valve or pulmonary stenosis. They coincide with the fully opened position of the valve and the valve must retain some mobility for the sound to be heard. Timing of these clicks is simulated by mechanical aortic prosthetic valves (ball and cage or tilting disc varieties) which make audible opening sounds.

**Mid to late systolic sounds:** the most commonly heard of these is the **mitral click** of mitral valve prolapse, caused by the sudden cessation of movement of the prolapsing component of the mitral valve.

**S2:** (Fig. 2.6) this high-pitched sound consists of aortic and pulmonary components, with the

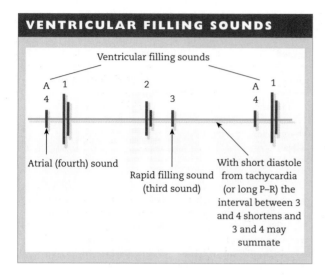

**Fig. 2.5** Ventricular filling sounds.

aortic component (A2) being louder and occurring earlier than the pulmonary (P2). A2 is heard widely but is usually loudest at the upper right sternal edge, whereas P2 is loudest at the upper left sternal border. Each coincides with its respective valve closure, which in turn coincides with the dicrotic notch on the pressure downstroke of its respective great vessel (aorta or pulmonary artery). Splitting of A2 and P2 is audible in normal individuals and may be increased (**inspiration, right bundle branch block**), decreased (**expiration, pulmonary hypertension**), fixed (**atrial septal defect**) or may move in a reverse direction (reverse splitting) in which splitting decreases on inspiration (**complete left bundle branch block, right ventricular pacing**). Either of the components of the second sound may be absent if the respective valve is immobile (aortic stenosis, pulmonary stenosis), or accentuated (systemic hypertension (A2), pulmonary hypertension (P2)).

**Early diastolic sounds:** the most common of these is the **opening snap** of MS. Normal left atrial pressure is low (around 5 mmHg) and even in severe MS may only rise to levels of 15–25 mmHg. Levels significantly above this predispose towards pulmonary oedema. Thus, even in severe MS, the pressure gradient be-

tween the left atrium and left ventricle (LV) during diastolic emptying is small in absolute terms. Hence, the diastolic murmur and opening snap of MS are low-pitched sounds, best heard in expiration using the bell of the stethoscope positioned at the apex with the patient turned to the left. The opening snap is generated by the opening movement of the anterior leaflet of the mitral valve being abruptly halted in early diastole, the thickened valve being unable to open fully. A shuddering sound is generated which is accentuated by the elevated left atrial pressure. For an opening snap to be present the valve must retain some mobility, and hence it may disappear as the stenotic process becomes severe. The higher the left atrial pressure, the more severe the MS and the earlier the opening snap occurs after the second sound. The gap between S2 and the opening snap can therefore be used as an indicator of the severity of the MS.

Other rarer early diastolic sounds include a 'pericardial knock' (**pericardial constriction**) and a 'tumour plop' (**atrial myxoma**). An opening early diastolic sound will be heard when a mechanical mitral valve prosthesis (ball and cage or tilting disc) is present.

**Mid and late diastolic sounds:** added sounds occurring after very early diastole coincide with the three phases of diastolic ventricu-

## THE SECOND HEART SOUND

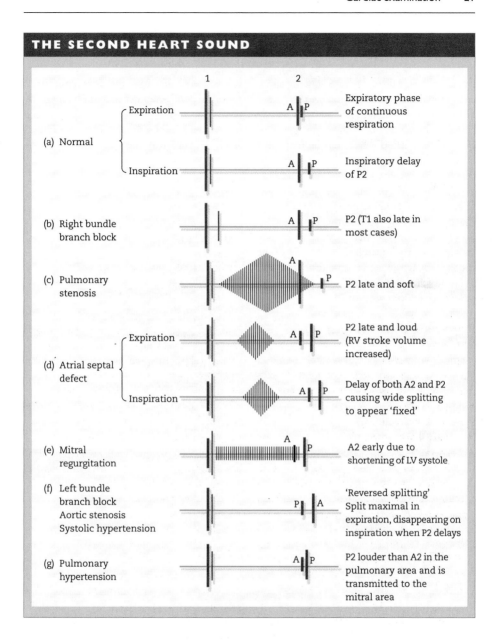

Fig. 2.6 S2 as heard in the pulmonary area.

lar filling. The first phase is the so-called 'passive' one when the ventricles fill as a result of a complex interaction of ventricular relaxation (causing an effect like suction) and the positive pressure gradient that exists between atria and ventricles. Rapid filling in this phase is associated with a **third sound** (S3). The second phase (**diastasis**) is short and relatively unimportant in terms of its contribution to ventricular filling. The third phase coincides with atrial contraction and when ventricular filling is rapid during this period a **fourth sound** (S4) may be heard.

All diastolic added sounds are best heard with the bell of the stethoscope and may originate in either of the ventricles. Children and young adults may have a physiological S3 but not an S4, and in the elderly an S4 may be present, especially after exercise. An S3 in adults is usually pathological (ventricular dysfunction) and an S4 is usually associated with a fibrotic (coronary artery disease) or hypertrophic (hypertension) ventricle. Since these sounds reflect rapid rises in ventricular filling pressure, their presence implies an unobstructed atrioventricular valve on the corresponding side of the heart. When present an S3 or S4 will create a **triple or gallop rhythm**. When both S3 and S4 occur the rhythm is described as **quadruple** and as the heart rate increases S3 and S4 may merge to form a **summation sound**.

*Murmurs* (see Table 2.6 and Fig. 2.7)

*Introduction*

Murmurs represent the audible flow of blood between vascular structures, and are characterized according to the seven features in Box 2.1.

Some may be innocent, due to flow turbulence, but when pathological usually imply that a pressure gradient exists between the chamber from which blood is flowing to the chamber or vessel to which it is directed. When the pressure gradient is large the murmur will be high pitched and best heard with the diaphragm of the stethoscope. Examples of these include the systolic

> **Box 2.1 Characterization of Murmurs**
>
> • **Intensity (loudness)**: graded 1–6 (murmurs of grades 4–6 are usually palpable as well as audible)
> • **Quality**: descriptive terms such as blowing, harsh, musical, etc.
> • **Frequency (pitch)**: graded high to low
> • **Duration**: short to long
> • **Configuration**: for systolic murmurs this is crescendo, decrescendo, crescendo-decrescendo (diamond shaped), plateau (even) and variable (uneven). Diastolic murmurs are usually decrescendo
> • **Timing**: in relation to the cardiac cycle
> • **Radiation**: direction in which the murmur radiates

Table 2.6 Cardiac murmurs.

## CARDIAC MURMURS

| Murmur | Cause |
|---|---|
| Ejection (mid) systolic | AS, PS, HOCM or innocent flow turbulence |
| Holosystolic | MR or TR, VSD |
| Late systolic | MV prolapse |
| Systolic arterial | Increased flow, arterial tortuosity or innocent turbulence, arteriosclerosis, coarctation of aorta |
| Early diastolic | AR or PR |
| Mid-diastolic | MS or TS, high diastolic flow |
| Late diastolic | MS in sinus rhythm, Austin Flint murmur of severe AR |
| Continuous | Patent ductus arteriosus |
| | Ruptured aortic sinus of Valsalva |
| | Aortopulmonary collaterals |
| | Arteriovenous fistulae |
| | Anomalous origin of coronary arteries |
| | Pulmonary arteriovenous malformations |

AR, aortic regurgitation; AS, aortic stenosis; HOCM, hypertrophic obstructive cardiomyopathy; MR, mitral regurgitation; MS, mitral stenosis; MV, mitral valve; PR, pulmonary regurgitation; PS, pulmonary stenosis; TR, tricuspid regurgitation; TS, tricuspid stenosis; VSD, ventricular septal defect.

## MURMURS AND PRESSURE WAVEFORMS

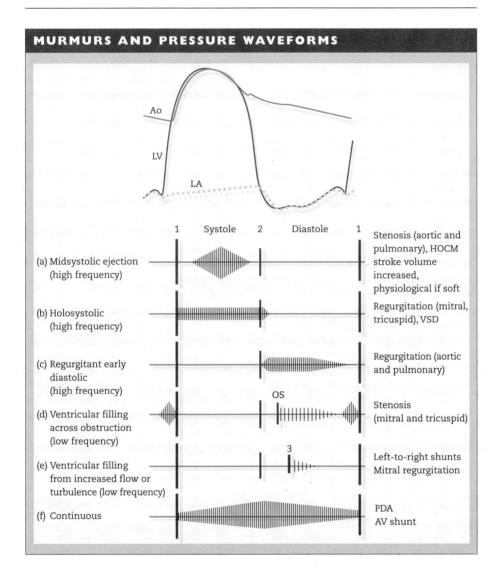

Fig. 2.7 Murmurs and their relation to the pressure pulses.

murmurs of **aortic stenosis, mitral regurgitation and ventricular septal defect**, and the diastolic murmur of **aortic regurgitation** (AR). Conversely, when the pressure gradient is relatively small, the murmur is lower pitched and best heard with the bell of the stethoscope. Examples of these include the diastolic murmurs of **mitral stenosis and tricuspid stenosis**. The pitch of the murmurs associated with pulmonary stenosis (systolic) or regurgitation (diastolic) will depend on the level of right ventricular and pulmonary artery pressures.

A murmur will disappear when the pressure in the two chambers has equalized and flow between them therefore ceases. For example, in severe AR a large volume of blood will reflux from the aorta into the LV from the time when the aortic valve attempts to close (A2). By mid-diastole the combination of this gross regurgitant flow, and forward flow through the mitral valve, may raise left ventricular pressure to the point where it is equal to the lowered aortic diastolic pressure (a consequence of the AR). At this point, further filling of the LV ceases and the aortic regurgitant murmur disappears. In this situation therefore, a short diastolic murmur suggests severe valvular disease. By contrast, in severe MS left atrial pressure will remain higher than left ventricular pressure throughout diastole and hence a long diastolic murmur exists. Here it is a long, rather than short, diastolic murmur that is suggestive of a severe valve problem.

Timing the murmur in relation to the cardiac cycle is crucial and forms the basis of its classification as: (i) **systolic** (starting at or after S1 and ending at or before the corresponding S2 on its side of origin); (ii) **diastolic** (starting at or after S2 and ending before the corresponding S1 on its side of origin); or (iii) **continuous** (starting in systole and continuing without interruption into all or part of diastole). Pericardial rubs will be included here although they are not strictly murmurs.

*Systolic murmurs*

**Ejection (mid) systolic** murmurs do not start at the very beginning of ventricular systole (S1) because contraction occurs before the aortic or pulmonary valves (**termed semilunar valves**) open, during which no movement of blood occurs (isovolumetric phase of systole). Once the semilunar valves open, the murmur gradually increases in intensity and then declines, ending just before A2 or P2. Causes include **aortic and pulmonary stenosis, ventricular outflow tract obstruction** (e.g. HOCM), **high flow situations** (flow across the pulmonary valve in left-to-right shunting, fever, pregnancy, thyrotoxicosis) or **innocent flow murmurs** (vibratory mid-systolic murmurs especially in those with narrow anteroposterior chest diameter).

**Holosystolic** murmurs start at the beginning of ventricular systole (S1) and end at or very soon after S2. In other words, they occupy the whole (Gr. *Holos*=entire) of systole. The term holosystolic is preferable to pansystolic because the latter tends to imply pan-intensity (same intensity throughout systole), and whilst murmurs caused by **mitral or tricuspid regurgitation or ventriculoseptal defects** are typically holosystolic, they are not always pan-intensity. Indeed, the murmur of mitral regurgitation, which is the one most commonly termed 'pansystolic', may sometimes occur mainly in early systole (severe MR), or in mid to late systole depending on factors determined by the prolapsing valve leaflet, and in these cases is neither holosystolic nor pan-intensity.

**Late systolic** murmurs begin in mid- to late systole and end at or very soon after S2. The most typical example of this is the murmur of mitral valve prolapse, which often starts after a mid- to late systolic click.

**Systolic arterial** murmurs may occur in normal arteries in the presence of increased flow or vessel tortuosity, or in abnormal arteries due to narrowing. They are usually diamond-shaped and are often heard innocently in the supraclavicular fossa in children and young adults, when they can frequently be made to disappear by extension of the shoulders. In older subjects they usually indicate atherosclerosis. **Aortic coarctation** produces a systolic murmur best heard in the interscapular region.

*Diastolic murmurs*

**Early diastolic** murmurs begin immediately after S2 and are usually decrescendo in configuration. The most common cause is AR. **Pulmonary regurgitation** is less common but may occur in severe MS (**Graham Steell murmur**) when secondary pulmonary hypertension has developed.

**Mid-diastolic** murmurs begin a clear interval after S2 and the most common example is the decrescendo low-pitched 'rumbling' diastolic murmur of MS with atrial fibrillation. In sinus rhythm a mitral stenotic murmur often has a late diastolic (presystolic) crescendo accentuation due to the onset of atrial contraction, giving an overall decrescendo-crescendo pattern. TS produces similar murmurs but is rare. Mid-diastolic murmurs may occur in the presence of an unobstructed atrioventricular valve due to high blood flow across it (e.g. **mitral regurgitation or ventriculoseptal defect causing high diastolic flow across the mitral valve, and tricuspid regurgitation or large atrioseptal defect causing high diastolic flow across the tricuspid valve**).

**Late diastolic** murmurs occur immediately before S1 and follow atrial contraction. Consequently, they occur rarely in patients with atrial fibrillation, in which atrial contraction is lost. Typically, they are mitral in origin and usually due to MS in sinus rhythm (see above). However, mitral late diastolic murmurs may occur in severe AR when the large volume of refluxing blood causes such a rise in left ventricular diastolic pressure that partial closure of the mitral valve occurs before the onset atrial contraction. When atrial contraction then occurs it is against a partially closed mitral orifice, resulting in a late diastolic murmur (**Austin Flint murmur**).

*Continuous murmurs*

These begin in systole and continue through S2 into all or part of diastole. They are uncommon and usually best heard with the diaphragm of the stethoscope. Examples include **patent ductus arteriosus, ruptured aortic sinus of Valsalva, aortopulmonary collaterals in pulmonary atresia, the anomalous origin of a coronary artery from the pulmonary trunk, arteriovenous fistulae including iatrogenic shunts created for haemodialysis, and pulmonary arteriovenous malformations.**

*Pericardial rubs*

These are 'scratchy' sounds produced by inflamed visceral and parietal layers of pericardium rubbing on one another (pericarditis — see Chapter 13). They are frequently heard after **cardiac surgery**, and commonly occur with **viral pericarditis** or following **myocardial infarction**. Rubs usually have systolic and diastolic components and are most easily heard using the diaphragm of the stethoscope. They may be positional, sometimes disappearing when the patient leans forwards.

## Examination of the lungs

The posterior chest wall should be inspected, particularly for thoracotomy scars which might suggest previous cardiothoracic surgery. Left posterolateral surgical approaches, as opposed to the more common median sternotomy (**valvular, coronary or ascending aortic surgery**), are used for operations on the distal aortic arch (**coarctation**) or descending thoracic aorta (**aneurysms, aortic dissection**), and were used in the past for surgical mitral valvotomy (**MS**).

Lung expansion should be assessed by palpation, observing any discrepancy between the two sides. Dullness on percussion of the lung bases may suggest pleural effusions, which are not uncommon in advanced heart failure or in the early post-operative period following cardiac surgery.

On auscultation, crepitations or fine crackles may be heard, due to fluid in the bronchioles that arises when pulmonary venous pressure is elevated above plasma oncotic pressure. This generally implies left-sided cardiac disease (**mitral or aortic valve disease, left ventricular dysfunction**). Crepitations tend to be heard mainly in late expiration at the lung bases, but as pulmonary oedema worsens they are heard more extensively and may be associated with a wheeze due to peribronchial oedema causing bronchoconstriction. Reduced breath sounds and bronchial breathing may be heard in association with a pleural effusion. Because the pleural veins drain into the systemic as well as the pulmonary venous circulation, venous hypertension in one system will not result in pleural fluid collection as frequently as hypertension in both. Hence, pleural effusions due to cardiac disease are most commonly seen in congestive (right and left) heart failure.

## Examination of the abdomen

Apart from any general abdominal abnormalities that might be sought as a consequence of

## Box 2.2  Abdominal Examination

- **Liver**: for enlargement and tenderness (right heart failure, tricuspid regurgitation, pericardial constriction) and pulsatility (tricuspid regurgitation)
- **Ascites**: (right heart failure)
- **Spleen**: for enlargement (infective endocarditis, infiltrative disorders)
- **Kidneys**: because renal failure and renovascular causes of hypertension are relevant to the cardiovascular system. The kidneys may be enlarged (polycystic disease), there may be renal arterial bruits (atherosclerosis, fibromuscular dysplasia, aortic dissection) or the patient may have undergone renal transplantation
- **Abdominal aorta**: should be palpated (aortic aneurysm) and auscultated for bruits (atherosclerosis) and the abdomen inspected for scars suggesting abdominal aortic or ilio-femoral arterial surgery

the patient's history, the liver, presence of ascites, spleen, kidneys and abdominal aorta should be examined because of their particular relevance to the cardiovascular system; see Box 2.2 for details.

## Examination of the legs

This is the final part of the cardiovascular examination and the following should be specifically assessed.

**Femoral pulses** should be palpated to confirm their presence and, if absent or reduced, should suggest **atherosclerosis** or, less commonly, **aortic coarctation**. If coarctation is suspected, the presence of any **radio-femoral delay** should be sought by comparing the radial and femoral pulses simultaneously. The femorals should also be auscultated for **systolic bruits**, which are most commonly due to atherosclerotic disease. Femoral arterial abnormalities are of relevance if the patient is to undergo cardiac catheterization, which is most commonly undertaken via a femoral approach. Also, femoral arterial (false) aneurysms may occur following catheterization and may be palpable and cause a bruit.

**Peripheral pulses** (popliteal and foot) should be palpated, their weakness or absence suggesting **peripheral vascular disease**.

**Peripheral oedema** is usually pitting in nature and occurs in **right heart failure** and **deep venous thrombosis**, as a side-effect of using **calcium antagonist drugs** (especially nifedipine) and where the long saphenous vein has been harvested for **coronary artery bypass graft surgery**. Other causes include the effects of gravity in patients who are relatively immobile, varicose veins, hypoproteinaemia or lymphatic obstruction.

**Toes** should be examined for the presence of **clubbing** and **splinter haemorrhages**, both of which have the same associations as with their respective finger abnormalities.

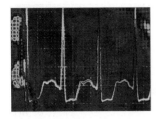

# CHAPTER 3

# *Imaging*

## Introduction

Imaging has become a major part of modern cardiac diagnosis and includes a wide range of investigative procedures, the optimum choice depending on clinical circumstances. See Box 3.1 for a summary of cardiac imaging techniques. It is important to understand the strengths and limitations of these various imaging techniques.

> **Box 3.1 Cardiac Imaging Techniques**
>
> - Chest radiograph
> - TTE
> - TOE
> - Cardiac catheterization
> - Coronary arteriography
> - CT scanning
> - MRI
> - Radionuclide ventriculography
> - Myocardial perfusion nuclear scanning
> - Positron emission tomography

## The chest radiograph

Although the chest radiograph remains valuable, much of its importance has been superseded by cross-sectional imaging techniques such as two-dimensional echocardiography and magnetic resonance imaging (MRI). Nevertheless, a good quality chest radiograph can be very helpful for diagnosis and for serial monitoring of the effects of treatment.

### The cardiac silhouette

An example of a normal posterior-anterior (PA) chest radiograph is shown in Fig. 3.1. The cardiovascular structures that make up the cardiac silhouette are illustrated. It is important to recognize that the right ventricle does not contribute to the cardiac silhouette of a PA radiograph, but is readily seen on a lateral film immediately behind the sternum (Fig. 3.2). Interpretation of the chest radiograph should include an assessment of overall heart size, evidence of specific chamber enlargement, and any changes in the lung fields. The overall heart size should be less than 50% of the cardiothoracic diameter and should be measured from the widest point of the cardiac silhouette. Enlargement of the left ventricle (LV) produces a more spacious, rounded appearance to the lower left heart border but the evidence of left ventricular enlargement may be quite subtle. The radiographic appearances of left atrial dilatation include a double shadow at the right heart border, filling in and later bulging of the bay below the main pulmonary artery due to enlargement of

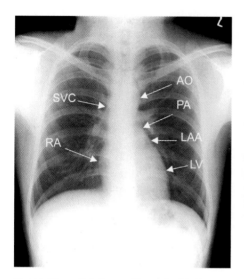

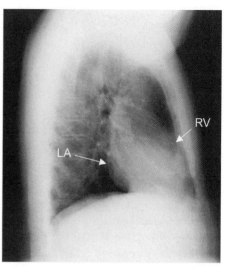

Fig. 3.1 Normal PA chest radiograph with the structures of the cardiac silhouette illustrated. SVC, superior vena cava; RA, right atrium; LV, left ventricle; LAA, left atrial appendage; PA, pulmonary artery; AO, aorta.

Fig. 3.2 Normal lateral chest radiograph with the structures of the cardiac silhouette illustrated. LA, left atrium; RV, right ventricle.

the left atrial appendage (LAA), and an increase in the angle of the carina at the tracheal bifurcation. Left atrial dilatation is often associated with enlargement of the main pulmonary arteries due to secondary pulmonary arterial hypertension. This combination causes straightening of the left heart border, a sign often associated with significant mitral valve disease.

Right ventricular enlargement can only be appreciated from a lateral chest radiograph where the cardiac shadow is more fully apposed to the sternum. The lateral chest radiograph is also useful for identifying the presence of pericardial calcification or calcification of the mitral and aortic valves, which can be easily missed on a standard PA chest radiograph. Valvar calcification is readily appreciated by echocardiography but pericardial calcification is much more difficult to appreciate and a lateral chest radiograph can be particularly helpful in selected cases.

## The lung fields

There are no valves between the pulmonary veins and the left atrium (LA), and therefore an increase in the left atrial pressure will cause distension of the pulmonary veins and an increase in the pulmonary capillary pressure. This will result in upper lobe venous distension and subsequently pulmonary oedema (Fig. 3.3) (recognized by diffuse bilateral opacification of the lung fields), and lymphatic distension, the so-called Kerley B lines. Cardiomegaly is present and there may be associated small pleural effusions.

Pulmonary oedema can also result from noncardiac causes, such as hypoalbuminaemia and the so-called 'shock lung' (adult respiratory distress) syndrome, or the appearances may be mimicked by other conditions such as bronchopneumonia, pulmonary fibrosis or lymphangitis carcinomatosis. Thus, pulmonary oedema on a chest radiograph does not always imply left heart failure, and when it is due to a cardiac cause it is often difficult to determine the underlying cardiac pathology from a plain film. Serial chest radiograph appearances may be useful for monitoring the progress of disease and the success of therapeutic interventions.

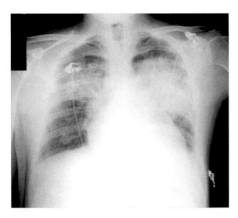

Fig. 3.3 Chest radiograph of pulmonary oedema.

## Echocardiography

The introduction of echocardiography has revolutionized non-invasive cardiac diagnosis by providing high-resolution, real-time, two-dimensional images of cardiac structure and function. Not only is the investigation painless but it can be repeated as often as necessary, so it is ideally suited to serial assessment of patients with a wide range of cardiac disorders. There are a number of different imaging modalities that combine to provide a comprehensive cardiac ultrasound examination:

- M-mode echocardiography;
- two-dimensional echocardiography;
- Doppler ultrasound;
- colour Doppler flow mapping.

### M-mode echocardiography

Ultrasonic waves will be reflected from any tissue interface and this reflected signal can be used to build up a picture of cardiac structures. If a single beam of pulsed ultrasound is used and the reflected signal recorded on moving paper, then a picture can be constructed from one line through the heart extending from the chest wall through to the posterior heart structures such as the LA and the posterior pericardium deep within the chest. This is known as M-mode echocardiography and, by angling the ultra-sound transducer in different directions from the base of the heart towards the apex, M-mode echocardiographic images can be obtained at the level of the aortic valve with the LA behind, at the level of the mitral valve, and at a level which transects the right and left ventricles (Fig. 3.4). The structural information is displayed over time so a number of cardiac cycles can be displayed on a single tracing. M-mode echocardiography has largely been superseded by two-dimensional imaging but remains useful for measuring chamber dimensions, most usefully made for clinical purposes at end-diastole and at peak systole. A reasonably accurate assessment of left ventricular function can be obtained by visualizing the contraction of the ventricular myocardium and from the change in ventricular dimension during systole.

### Two-dimensional echocardiography

The limitations of M-mode echocardiography should be immediately apparent. Imaging a single point within the heart is less than ideal, particularly as abnormalities of both structure and function can often be quite complex especially in patients with congenital heart disease. Two-dimensional imaging of the heart can be obtained by two basic methods. Firstly, a number of ultrasound elements (often up to 64 individual elements) can be mounted within a single transducer. Each element transmits an ultrasound pulse sequentially building up a cross-sectional image of the heart. Alternately, a single ultrasound crystal can be mechanically swept across the heart to produce the same effect. The resulting two-dimensional image (Fig. 3.5) is constructed from a series of individual M-mode lines. Information can be gathered rapidly enough to allow as many as 25 frames per second to be constructed, thereby providing a real-time image of the heart. It allows a comprehensive appreciation of the cardiac structures in a dynamic format and is useful for assessing global and regional myocardial function, chamber dimensions and valve pathology. Echocardiography images the cardiac structures with a high level of accuracy, and some

## M-MODE ECHO

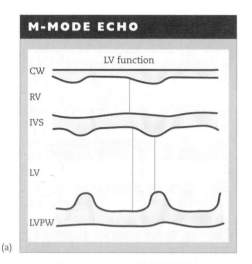

(a)

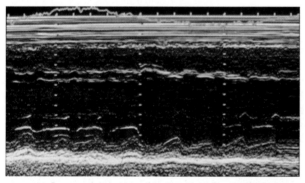

(b)

Fig. 3.4 (a) Schematic representation of M-mode echo at level of left ventricle. (b) Clinical image in a patient with left ventricular dysfunction. CW, chest wall; RV, right ventricle; IVS, interventricular septum; LV, left ventricle, LVPW, left ventricular posterior wall.

information can be obtained about myocardial function from the images of the heart at different points in the cardiac cycle. Much less information is available about the functional significance of valve disease or congenital heart lesions.

### Doppler ultrasound

Doppler ultrasound is a further ultrasound technique which allows ultrasound evaluation of blood flow velocity within the heart and great vessels rather than just the structural information provided by echocardiography.

The Doppler effect is well known to all of us, even though we may not recognize it. As a train or car approaches, the pitch of the noise it creates increases and, when it is going away from the observer, it decreases. This is because the sound waves are compressed in one direction and stretched out in the other direction, resulting from the motion of the train or car. The faster it is moving, the more the pitch of the sound is altered. Because the change in frequency is proportional to the velocity of the moving structure, in this case the blood stream, then the velocity of blood can be accurately measured. Doppler ultrasound can be performed using pulsed or continuous wave Doppler. Pulsed wave Doppler has one major limitation, which is the maximum velocity that it is able to estimate. In the normal heart, velocities are usually around 1 m/s, well within the resolution of pulsed wave Doppler, but in heart disease and particularly valve disease, velocities may exceed 6 m/s and pulsed wave Doppler is unable to measure the maximum velocity value. This

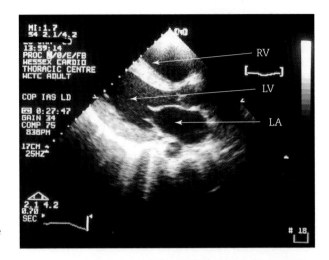

**Fig. 3.5** Two-dimensional echocardiographic image in the long axis of the heart.

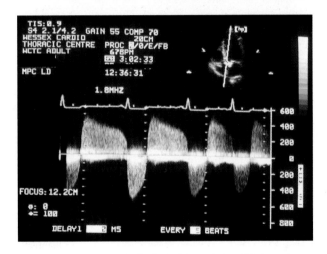

**Fig. 3.6** Spectral display of Doppler ultrasound information with the velocity on the Y-axis and time on the X-axis. The intensity of the spectral display indicates the strength of the signal. Direction away from the transducer is indicated by the signal shown below the zero velocity line (as seen in systole) rather than toward the transducer indicated as signal above the zero velocity line (as seen in diastole).

can be overcome by using continuous wave Doppler but at the expense of spatial resolution, so that it may not be apparent which point in the heart is generating the high velocity signal. This is not usually problematic as it is often clear from the two-dimensional echocardiogram where the significant pathology lies, for example, a thickened, calcified aortic valve.

Doppler ultrasound information is displayed in a format as illustrated in Fig. 3.6. This **spectral** display indicates the velocity value on the *y*-axis and time on the *x*-axis, the phase of the cardiac cycle apparent from the displayed electrocardiogram. The intensity of the signal is pro-portional to the number of blood cells travelling at that particular velocity. Because it is also possible to determine the direction of blood flow from Doppler ultrasound, the spectral signal can be displayed above the zero-velocity line, when blood flow is directed towards the ultrasound transducer, and below it when blood flow is away from the transducer.

## Colour Doppler flow mapping

By colour encoding pulsed wave Doppler information for both direction of blood flow and for velocity, and overlaying this display onto the two-dimensional structural echocardiogram, a composite image which includes structural and flow velocity information can be produced, blood flow towards the transducer being displayed as increasing intensities of red, and flow away from the transducer as increasing intensities of blue. The higher the velocity the more intense the colour. Green is added when there are a range of velocity values, such as occurs in high velocity, turbulent jets associated with valve stenosis or regurgitation. Such high velocity turbulent jets produce characteristic multi-coloured, mosaic patterns on a colour flow map easily distinguishable from normal (Fig. 3.7).

## Clinical applications

Echocardiography and Doppler ultrasound techniques have gained widespread clinical application in modern cardiac diagnosis. They are of particular value in the assessment of ventricular function, valvular heart disease and congenital heart disease, providing a comprehensive assessment of cardiac structure and function. Echocardiography tends to be more useful in assessing ventricular function, whereas spectral Doppler techniques may provide more quantitative information in patients with valvular heart disease.

### Assessment of ventricular function

Echocardiography can provide accurate, quantitative assessment of ventricular function, both

in patients with global dysfunction such as dilated cardiomyopathy, or regional ventricular dysfunction associated with myocardial infarction. Appreciation of the global nature of the myocardial dysfunction is much more apparent on two-dimensional imaging and it is also superior to M-mode imaging for assessing ventricular dysfunction in patients with regional defects where more of the LV can be imaged simultaneously. In myocardial infarction M-mode echocardiography may miss the segment of infarction and underestimate the true extent of the left ventricular dysfunction. Similarly, in a patient with a limited infarct, if the M-mode cursor passes through that portion of the myocardium, the overall ventricular function may appear worse and a truer representation of ventricular function will only be obtained with two-dimensional imaging.

### Valvular heart disease

It is in the area of valvular heart disease that echocardiography and Doppler techniques have had their greatest impact on adult cardiology. Prior to their introduction, much of the information now gained by cardiac ultrasound could only be obtained by cardiac catheterization. The role of echocardiography and Doppler ultrasound in the assessment of valvular heart disease falls into two main categories: (i) confirmation of diagnosis; and (ii) quantification of the severity of individual valve lesions.

Quantification of the severity of valve pathology, particularly valve stenosis, by Doppler ultrasound relates to the principle that velocity increases through a narrowed orifice and that this increase in velocity is directly proportional to the severity of the obstruction. It is possible to estimate fairly accurately the pressure gradient across a stenotic valve from the following modified Bernoulli equation

$$\Delta P = 4V^2$$

where $\Delta P$ is the pressure gradient in mmHg across the stenotic valve, and V is the maximum velocity measured by continuous wave Doppler.

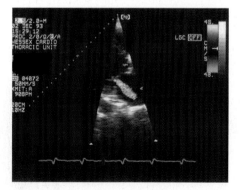

Fig. 3.7 Colour Doppler flow map image of mitral regurgitation.

## Mitral stenosis

The diagnosis of mitral stenosis (MS) is usually suspected clinically but echocardiography confirms the presence of a thickened, often calcified valve with reduced opening on both M-mode echocardiography and two-dimensional imaging. Quantification of the severity of MS is more difficult to define using echocardiography alone. Spectral Doppler can accurately estimate the severity of MS from the increase in velocity across the mitral valve and the reduced rate at which this velocity returns to the baseline (Fig. 3.8). The rate at which mitral velocity decreases during diastole can be measured in milliseconds as the **mitral pressure half-time**. This is the time taken for the initial peak velocity of mitral flow to fall to a velocity value that is half the initial mitral pressure drop, calculated by the modified Bernoulli formula shown above. Mitral pressure half-time is particularly valuable because it is not significantly affected by changes in cardiac output and therefore provides an accurate reflection of the actual degree of stenosis rather than simply the gradient across the valve, which is dependent on blood flow across it. As a result it is possible to estimate the mitral valve area (MVA) in $cm^2$ from the mitral pressure half-time using the formula MVA = 220/pressure half-time.

## Aortic stenosis

The presence of a thickened, calcified valve is usually seen on echocardiography but the degree of obstruction may not be clear from imaging alone. Doppler ultrasound can estimate the severity of aortic stenosis (AS) from the increase in velocity through the stenotic aortic valve. Figure 3.9 illustrates the appearance on Doppler ultrasound from a normal aortic valve and from a patient with severe AS. As with MS, the modified Bernoulli equation can be used to estimate the pressure gradient across the aortic valve. Colour Doppler flow mapping provides little if any useful additional information in the majority of patients with AS.

## Valve regurgitation

Doppler ultrasound is extremely sensitive in

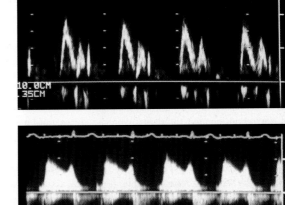

Fig. 3.8 (a) Spectral Doppler of normal mitral flow and (b) mitral stenosis. In the normal flow, the peak velocity is only 0.8 m/s and falls towards zero rapidly with a late diastolic increase due to atrial contraction, whereas in mitral stenosis the initial peak velocity is higher, almost 2 m/s, and reduces more slowly sustaining a high velocity throughout diastole prior to the secondary increase associated with atrial contraction.

(a)

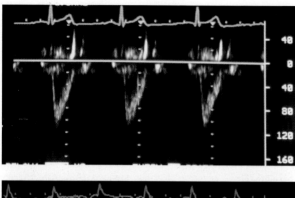

(b)

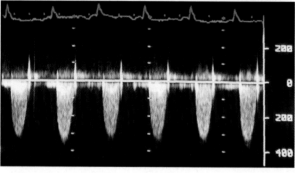

Fig. 3.9 (a) Spectral Doppler of normal aortic flow and (b) aortic stenosis. Note that the normal peak velocity is around 1 m/s compared to almost 4 m/s in the patient with significant aortic stenosis.

detecting valve regurgitation and even trivial valve lesions can be easily detected. In fact, a small degree of regurgitation can even be detected in normal individuals through the tricuspid and pulmonary valves, and occasionally through the mitral valve, particularly in children. This is not apparent clinically and is of no clinical significance, though the relationship of this 'physiological' regurgitation and the need for antibiotic prophylaxis for endocarditis remains to be established. Currently, antibiotic prophylaxis is not recommended for these patients. Both mitral (Figs 3.7 and 3.10) and aortic regurgitation (AR) (Figs 3.6 and 3.11) are readily apparent on spectral Doppler and colour Doppler flow mapping. When using colour Doppler flow mapping, it is important not to assume that the size of the colour flow jet directly reflects the severity of regurgitation as it can be affected by many instrumentation and haemodynamic factors.

## Limitations of echocardiography

Although echocardiography has revolutionized the evaluation of cardiac anatomy and function, it does have a number of limitations. Ultrasound does not penetrate air filled cavities such as lung tissue, and this limits the available windows on the precordium for echocardiographic imaging. In addition, there is a considerable learning curve in acquiring high-quality echo images as well as some subjectivity in their interpretation. Doppler ultrasound can underestimate the true velocity of flow through a stenotic or regurgitant valve if the ultrasound beam is at a significant angle to blood flow or if the narrow jet is not interrogated by the Doppler signal. Overestimation of flow velocity is much less common but the instantaneous valve gradient obtained by Doppler ultrasound may be significantly higher than the gradient obtained by comparing peak pressures after withdrawing a catheter across the valve (peak-to-peak gradient) at cardiac catheterization. Measurements taken at different times and/or under different physiological conditions will often vary significantly.

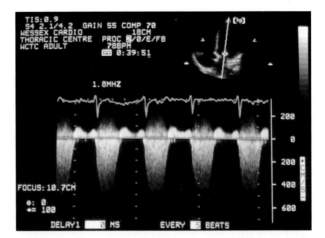

**Fig. 3.10** Spectral Doppler recording of mitral regurgitation. Note the high velocity pansystolic jet below the zero velocity line.

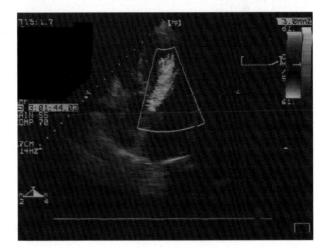

**Fig. 3.11** Colour Doppler flow map image of aortic regurgitation.

## Transoesophageal echocardiography (see Box 3.2)

Transoesophageal echocardiography (TOE) overcomes many of the limitations of transthoracic imaging, particularly the problems of acoustic penetration through lung tissue, but at the expense of being a more invasive technique. The procedure, which is similar to endoscopy, is usually performed under intravenous sedation and with topical pharyngeal local anaesthetic. As with transthoracic echocardiography (TTE), transoesophageal imaging combines two-dimensional, real-time imaging of cardiac structures with flow velocity information from spectral Doppler ultrasound and spatial velocity information from the addition of colour Doppler flow mapping.

Transoesophageal images are considerably clearer than their transthoracic counterparts due to higher frequency transducers and the fact that the ultrasound does not have to penetrate the chest wall structures. The best images are obtained from structures that lie close to the oesophagus: the LA, pulmonary veins, mitral and aortic valves and the interatrial septum. The right atrium (RA) is generally well seen but the tricuspid valve, right ventricle, pulmonary valve and the right ventricular outflow tract are quite distant from the oesophagus and are often seen better from the transthoracic approach. So sensitive is the transoesophageal technique that it can also identify very sluggish blood flow as a smoke-like contrast effect within the affected cardiac chamber, most often the LA. Commonly, the underlying cause is MS though it is also seen in a dilated LA secondary to left ventricular dysfunction, particularly dilated cardiomyopathy.

## Source of cardiac embolism

In the vast majority of patients with a cerebrovascular accident or transient ischaemic attack (TIA), the heart is not implicated. However, in young patients in whom one may not antici-

pate cerebrovascular disease, or in those who have TIA in more than one cerebral arterial territory, the search for a source of embolism may be indicated. TTE is generally unhelpful in the investigation of these patients unless they have overt heart disease such as MS or severe left ventricular dysfunction due to dilated cardiomyopathy. Even here, TTE may detect the major cardiac pathology but it will still be insensitive to the presence of thrombus within the LV, or atrium, particularly the LAA which often harbours thrombus but is rarely seen using conventional transthoracic imaging. TOE (Fig. 3.12) is therefore essential in this group of patients in whom a source of embolism is sought.

A patent foramen ovale between the right and left atria is a common finding on TOE being present in as many as 25% of normal individuals. The importance of this finding in patients with TIA or stroke is uncertain, but the ability to shunt across the foramen from right to left can allow venous thrombus to pass into the left side of the heart and hence cause systemic embolization. This is rare, but in patients with no other source of embolism this possibility should be considered, particularly if the patient has high right heart pressures or a tendency to venous thrombosis. Because transoesophageal imaging can visualize virtually all the thoracic aorta, it can demonstrate the presence of aortic atheroma. This is a potential source of embolism particularly if the atheroma is mobile and pedunculated.

---

**Box 3.2  Indications for TOE**

- Poor transthoracic echo images
- Cardiac source of embolism
- Suspected thoracic aortic dissection
- Aortic regurgitation
- Assessment for mitral reconstructive surgery
- Hypotension following cardiac surgery
- Mitral regurgitation
- Intracardiac tumours
- Infective endocarditis
- Adult congenital heart disease
- Prosthetic valve function

---

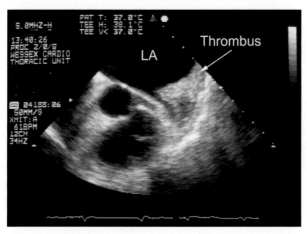

**Fig. 3.12** Transoesophageal echo image of thrombus in the left atrial appendage. LA, left atrium.

## Suspected aortic dissection

TOE can visualize virtually all of the thoracic aorta, the first third of the aortic arch being partially obscured by the left main bronchus passing between the aorta and the oesophagus. Dissection confined to this part of the aorta is rare and most commonly occurs in the ascending aorta or at the upper descending aorta just distal to the origin of the left subclavian artery, both areas well visualized on TOE. Aortic dissection is seen as an intimal flap within the aorta, dividing it into a true and a false lumen (Fig. 3.13). The major advantage of TOE is the rapidity of diagnosis, in that it takes only a few minutes to perform the investigation once a transthoracic echocardiogram has been completed. Additionally, the investigation can be performed within the confines of the intensive care unit and does not require the patient to be moved from a specialist care area into the scanner. If the clinical suspicion of aortic dissection involving the ascending aorta is high, or has been seen using TTE, transoesophageal imaging can even be performed in the anaesthetic room as the patient is being prepared for surgery.

## Mitral valve surgery

Mitral reconstructive surgery rather than mitral valve replacement is now commonly used for patients with isolated mitral regurgitation. TOE has two main roles to play in the evaluation of these patients. Firstly, preoperative TOE can provide high-resolution images of the structural abnormalities of the mitral valve. This is usually prolapse of one or both of the mitral leaflets with or without chordal rupture and TOE can precisely define the valve morphology, the severity of regurgitation and the suitability for mitral valve repair surgery (Fig. 3.14). Secondly, TOE is now commonly used within the operating theatre to evaluate the success of mitral valve reconstruction immediately following surgery, so that if significant regurgitation remains, the patient can undergo mitral valve replacement at the same operation.

## Transoesophageal echocardiography in the intensive care unit

Pre- and particularly post-operative patients who are lying prone and who are ventilated are notoriously difficult to image using conventional TTE. Additionally, precordial dressings over a sternotomy scar further limit the accessibility of transthoracic imaging. In comparison, TOE is extremely easy to perform in a ventilated patient providing high-resolution, dynamic imaging of cardiac anatomy and function.

## Contrast echocardiography

Contrast echocardiography has been a standard part of echocardiographic examination for

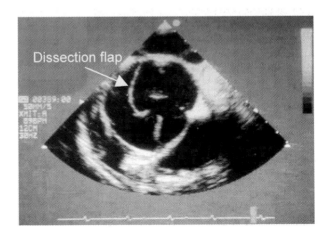

**Fig. 3.13** Transoesophageal echo image of a patient with dissection of the ascending aorta.

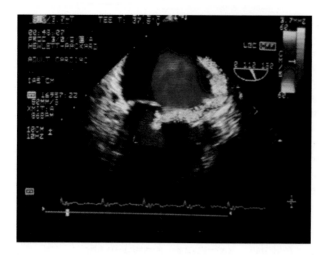

**Fig. 3.14** Transoesophageal echo image of a patient with mitral valve prolapse and significant mitral regurgitation prior to mitral valve repair. Note the jet of regurgitation swirling around the lateral wall of the left atrium.

many years, but since the introduction of colour Doppler flow mapping it has been less commonly used. An intravenous injection of agitated normal saline or commercially available contrast agents, will cause echo reflections from the microbubbles in the right heart chambers. These microbubbles do not normally pass through the pulmonary circulation, so any opacification of the left heart structures implies the presence of a shunt. It is useful in patients with congenital heart disease or embolic stroke, and in commercial or recreational divers it can establish the presence of a patent foramen ovale by detecting the presence of right-to-left shunting during a Valsalva manoeuvre at the time of contrast injection.

More recently, new contrast agents which cross the pulmonary circulation and allow opacification of left heart structures from an intravenous injection, have led to a resurgence in contrast echocardiographic imaging. Although still at an early stage in development, the ability to image myocardial perfusion with contrast enhanced echocardiography is likely further to improve the non-invasive assessment of the functional significance of coronary artery lesions and may allow a simple, non-invasive method for identifying viable myocardium in patients with coronary artery disease and significant left ventricular dysfunction who would gain particular benefit from coronary revascularization.

## Stress echocardiography

Exercise or pharmacological stress can be combined with echocardiographic assessment of regional and global LV function in an attempt to improve the sensitivity and specificity for the detection of significant coronary artery disease. The left and right ventricles are divided into 16 segments with each segment being visually assigned a number based on the presence of wall motion abnormalities, where normal= 1, hypokinesis=2, akinesis=3, dyskinesis=4. A wall motion score index achieved by dividing the total by the number of segments provides a semi-quantitative assessment of global left ventricular function. Individual segments are examined at rest and during stress to identify new wall motion abnormalities, implying the presence of ischaemia in that particular territory.

• Anterior wall motion abnormalities usually imply significant disease in the left anterior descending (LAD) artery.

• Lateral wall motion abnormalities relate to the circumflex coronary artery and inferior.

• Right ventricular abnormalities indicate disease in the right coronary artery (RCA) though there is significant overlap particularly in the myocardial territories supplied by the circumflex and right coronary arteries.

## Three-dimensional echocardiography

Three-dimensional reconstruction of two-dimensional echocardiographic imaging, whether derived from transthoracic or TOE imaging, is now possible. The potential advantages of three-dimensional imaging are obvious in areas such as complex congenital heart disease but it also allows a better dynamic appreciation of cardiac structure in a variety of cardiac conditions including valve pathology and left ventricular dysfunction. It can also allow structural and functional images to be viewed from any direction, allowing the cardiac surgeon to view complex cardiac pathology from a similar perspective to that observed in the operating theatre.

## Cardiac catheterization and coronary angiography (see Boxes 3.3 and 3.4)

Although the vast majority of patients undergo cardiac catheterization to determine the presence and severity of coronary artery disease, it remains an important investigation for those patients in whom non-invasive information is inadequate, for example, in patients with valvular heart disease who are poor echo subjects. Also, in the assessment of left ventricular dysfunction or the severity of valve disease, clinical evaluation and the non-invasive investigations are not always concordant and cardiac catheterization may be necessary to establish more precise diagnostic information.

Although the indications for invasive cardiac investigation are wide and varied they fall into three basic categories:
1 haemodynamic assessment;
2 angiography; and
3 coronary arteriography.

> **Box 3.3 Indications for Coronary Angiography**
>
> - Diagnosis of coronary artery disease
> - Angina uncontrolled by medication
> - Assessment of suitability for coronary intervention
> - Recurrence of angina following coronary angioplasty or bypass grafting
> - Strongly positive exercise test and/or poor blood pressure response to exercise
> - Preoperative assessment in patients undergoing surgery for valvular heart disease

> **Box 3.4 Indications for Cardiac Catheterization**
>
> - Assessment of left ventricular function
> - Haemodynamic assessment of valvular heart disease
> - Aortic trauma
> - Massive pulmonary embolism
> - Constrictive pericarditis
> - Post myocardial infarction ventricular septal defect
> - Acute ischaemic mitral regurgitation
> - Congenital heart lesions

Haemodynamic assessment and angiography can be performed on both the right and left side of the circulation, whereas coronary arteriography is obviously performed only from the systemic circulation. All these procedures carry minimal risk in experienced hands but it should be remembered that no invasive procedure is entirely free from risk, and this is an important factor when patients are being considered for cardiac catheterization.

### Right heart catheterization
Right heart catheterization is the safest of the cardiac catheterization procedures as the systemic circulation is not entered unless the patient has a congenital communication between the systemic and pulmonary circulations, such as an atrial septal defect. It is usually performed either via the femoral vein, via a cephalic or brachial vein in the antecubital fossa or by subclavian vein puncture.

Femoral vein cannulation is performed by the Seldinger technique of direct venous puncture under local anaesthetic. Right heart catheters are available in a variety of different shapes. They are designed to allow passage through the right heart into the pulmonary arteries and to allow both pressure measurements and blood samples to be obtained. Blood samples are used to measure the oxygen saturation of the blood at each catheter position. On the right side of the heart, blood is normally desaturated of oxygen ($\approx 70\%$) in comparison to that of the systemic circulation ($\approx 99\%$). A single end hole catheter with a curved tip is ideal for right heart catheterization, though a balloon tipped Swan–Ganz catheter may be necessary to enter the PA in the presence of significant right heart dilatation and severe pulmonary hypertension. The fluid-filled catheter is connected to a pressure transducer via a three-way tap to allow both pressure measurement and blood sampling to be performed easily. Pressures and blood samples are usually obtained from the following positions with the aid of radiograph screening:

• inferior and superior venae cavae;
• right atrium;
• right ventricle;
• main pulmonary artery;
• left pulmonary artery;
• right pulmonary artery;
• pulmonary capillary wedge.

The pulmonary capillary wedge position relates to the point at which the catheter is 'wedged' in a distal PA. Because there are no valves between this position and the LA, the pulmonary capillary wedge pressure is an indirect measurement of left atrial pressure. If a blood sample is taken at this point, it should be fully oxygen saturated as pulmonary capillary blood is withdrawn, in comparison to the desaturated blood samples obtained from the other venous positions. Oxygen saturation measurements should be similar at each catheter position with the exception of the pulmonary capillary wedge position, as described above. If there is an increase in oxygen saturation at any position in the pulmonary circulation, this implies there has been transfer or 'shunting' of systemic circula-

tion blood into the pulmonary circulation. 'Shunting' of blood is usually from the left (heart) to right (heart) due to the higher pressures in the systemic as opposed to the pulmonary circulation. The position of this oxygen 'step-up' can be identified from the catheter position on radiograph screening and the pressure waveform. The amount of systemic blood entering the pulmonary circulation can be calculated from the degree of oxygen 'step-up'. Because a shunt from left to right will cause more blood to flow through the pulmonary circulation compared to the systemic circulation, the size of the shunt is traditionally expressed as a ratio of pulmonary to systemic flow, the so-called Qp : Qs ratio. The formula for calculation of the Qp : Qs ratio from the oxygen saturation results is as follows:

$$Q_p : Q_s \text{ ratio} = \frac{\text{Arterial saturation} - \text{Mixed venous saturation}}{\text{Pulmonary venous saturation} - \text{Pulmonary artery saturation}}$$

The mixed venous saturation reflects the oxygen saturation in the venous system proximal to the point of shunting and is usually estimated from an average of two SVC samples and one IVC sample. For example, if the systemic arterial saturation was 99%, the mixed venous saturation was 69%, pulmonary venous saturation was 99% and the PA saturation was 89%, the Qp : Qs ratio would be 3 : 1.

The right atrial pressure is low (0–5 mmHg), and has an 'a' wave and a 'v' wave resulting from atrial systole and atrial filling duing ventricular systole. The right ventricular systolic pressure is usually between 15 and 25 mmHg and should be the same as the systolic pressure in the PA, as the pulmonary valve is open at this time. The diastolic pressure in the right ventricle is matched by the right atrial pressure, because the tricuspid valve is open and there is equilibration of atrial and ventricular pressures during diastole. PA diastolic pressure is usually between 5 and 15 mmHg, and in the absence of lung disease is similar to the pulmonary capillary wedge pressure. Because the pulmonary wedge pressure is an indirect measurement of left atrial pressure, it has an 'a' wave and a 'v' wave similar to the right atrial pressure, with a mean pressure between 5 and 10 mmHg.

## Common abnormalities from right heart pressure tracings

The most common abnormality of right heart catheterization encountered in adult practice is the presence of pulmonary hypertension. This is usually secondary to left heart abnormalities, particularly mitral valve disease or left ventricular dysfunction. It is also a common association with primary lung disease or with severe pulmonary embolism. Here, the waveforms do not change but the actual pressure measurements increase. Initially, the PA and right ventricular systolic pressure increases, but if the right ventricle begins to fail under the increased afterload, right ventricular diastolic and hence, right atrial pressure rises. Dilatation of the right ventricle can cause functional tricuspid regurgitation with a resultant large 'v' wave in the right atrial tracing.

Obstruction to flow at any point in the right heart will cause a difference in pressure between the two sides of the obstruction. For instance, in pulmonary valve stenosis, the right ventricular systolic pressure will be higher than the PA systolic pressure, reflecting an obstruction at the level of the pulmonary valve. However, right heart obstruction is rare in adult practice. The most common obstruction is mild residual pulmonary valve stenosis as a consequence of congenital pulmonary valve stenosis. Pulmonary and/or tricuspid valve stenosis from rheumatic heart disease or carcinoid syndrome are extremely rare.

## Left heart catheterization

Entry to the systemic circulation for the purposes of left heart catheterization is performed from either the femoral artery or the right brachial artery, or more uncommonly the right radial or left brachial artery. Left heart catheterization is a safe procedure in experienced hands, with a mortality of less than 0.2% of cases. Other serious complications of left heart catheterization such as stroke, myocardial infarction or malignant arrhythmias are also uncommon.

Femoral artery cannulation is generally performed from the right side though in the presence of a diminished right femoral pulse, left femoral cannulation may be performed. The technique is similar to that described above for right heart catheterization, with an arterial sheath, usually 6 or 7 French in size, being inserted into the femoral artery. As with right heart catheterization, the sheath is removed at the end of the procedure and haemostasis is secured either by direct compression of the femoral artery over the site of arterial puncture, or by the use of a percutaneous femoral artery closure device such as a collagen plug or a direct suturing device. If compression is used, it must be maintained for at least 10 min because of the comparatively high arterial pressure, and the patient is maintained on bed rest following the procedure for at least 6 hours, and usually overnight if larger arterial sheaths are used. Left heart catheterization via the brachial approach requires cut-down onto the artery, with direct suture repair at the end of the procedure.

Left heart catheterization usually involves combined angiography (aortography and/or left ventricular angiography) and coronary arteriography. Direct access to the arterial circulation allows pressure measurement within the aorta and, if a catheter is passed retrogradely across the aortic valve, left ventricular pressure. Using this method, any systolic pressure difference between the LA and the aorta indicates a degree of obstruction to flow as a result of AS, with the degree of pressure difference representing a measure of its severity (Fig. 3.15). Although a pressure gradient of 50 mmHg or greater is indicative of significant AS likely to merit surgical intervention, one should be careful to interpret the pressure gradient in the context of left ventricular function, as patients with severe AS and poor left ventricular function may be unable to generate a such a high pressure gradient. This potential error can be overcome by assessing left ventricular function by echocardiography, or at the time of left heart catheterization using

## PRESSURE GRADIENT ACROSS THE AORTIC VALVE

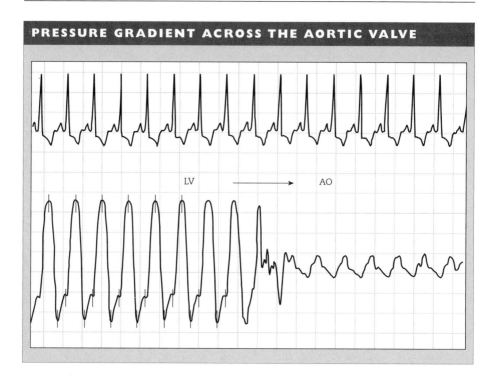

LV ⟶ AO

**Fig. 3.15** Withdrawal pressure tracing from left ventricle to aorta in aortic stenosis demonstrating pressure gradient across the aortic valve.

left ventricular angiography. In addition, cardiac output can be measured and combined with the aortic pressure gradient to provide an assessment of the functional area of the aortic valve, with an area of $0.8\,cm^2$ or less indicating the presence of significant AS. Pressure gradients can be measured within the LV itself as a result of hypertrophy, particularly in patients with hypertrophic cardiomyopathy. Supravalve AS is rare but produces a pressure gradient within the ascending aorta immediately above the aortic valve, and coarctation of the aorta can similarly produce a pressure gradient usually located at the distal aortic arch and upper part of the descending thoracic aorta.

## Cardiac output

There are three main methods of measuring cardiac output at cardiac catheterization:

1 dilution techniques—thermodilution and dye dilution;
2 Fick cardiac output estimation; and
3 angiographic cardiac output.

In day-to-day clinical practice thermodilution or Fick cardiac outputs are the most commonly used.

### Dilution techniques

Thermodilution is probably the most commonly used method of cardiac output estimation and one of the most reliable. A known volume (usually 10 cc) of cold saline (or dextrose) is rapidly injected into the RA via the proximal port of a Swan–Ganz catheter. A temperature probe at the distal end of the catheter situated in the PA monitors the change in temperature and a computer generated curve of changing temperature against time can be used to calculate cardiac output. In essence, the more rapidly the temperature drops and returns to baseline in the PA, the greater the cardiac output. A similar effect can be obtained by injecting a known amount of dye (indocyanine green) into a peripheral vein and sampling from a systemic artery, to produce a dye-dilution curve based on the appearance and disappearance of the dye against time rather than a temperature change as with the thermodilution technique.

## Fick cardiac output

By measuring the oxygen saturation in systemic arterial (aorta) and venous (vena cavae) blood, the amount of oxygen consumed by tissue metabolism can be calculated. If the rate of tissue oxygen consumption (a reflection of metabolic rate) is known, then the amount of blood passing through the tissue (cardiac output) can be calculated. The most difficult aspect of the Fick technique is the accurate estimation of oxygen consumption. Traditionally, this is done by measuring expired gases over a period of time, but this is rarely undertaken and most centres use an 'assumed' value for oxygen consumption, calculated from age, sex and body surface area, and assuming a basal metabolic rate. The Fick technique is subject to a number of inaccuracies but has generally been regarded as more useful at very low cardiac outputs, in atrial fibrillation or in the presence of significant tricuspid regurgitation, where thermodilution techniques can be unreliable.

## Angiographic cardiac output

Stroke volume can be estimated from a left ventricular angiogram, taking end diastolic and end systolic images, and estimating volumes from these images assuming a geometric shape to the LV. Cardiac output is then calculated from the product of stroke volume and heart rate. Significant errors can arise in patients with segmental abnormalities of left ventricular function, as commonly occurs in coronary artery disease. The technique is rarely used in preference to the other techniques described above, unless there is significant valvular heart disease with aortic or mitral regurgitation where errors can occur with the Fick technique.

## Angiography

Injection of radio-opaque dye into the circula-

tion allows real-time dynamic appreciation of cardiovascular structures and the relationship of blood flow in a variety of pathophysiological situations. The two most common angiographic investigations in adult cardiology are left ventricular angiography and aortography, both performed via left heart catheterization as described above. A multihole catheter, usually of a 'pig-tail' design, is used to allow rapid injection of contrast without displacement of the catheter. Between 30 and 50 mL of contrast is typically injected over around 2 s for most angiography in the systemic arterial circulation.

## Left ventricular angiography

Injection of contrast medium into the LV allows assessment of both global and regional left ventricular function, and left ventricular ejection fraction can be calculated from end systolic and diastolic images (Fig. 3.16). Left ventricular angiography is usually performed in the right anterior oblique projection, though for a more thorough assessment of regional wall abnormalities, a further angiogram in the orthogonal left anterior oblique projection may also be used. The ejection fraction, an estimate of the percentage of the end diastolic volume ejected with each beat, is a useful measurement of overall left ventricular function but, in patients with coronary artery disease, regional abnormalities are more common. The function of individual myocardial segments is often graded as normal, hypokinetic, akinetic or dyskinetic (aneurysmal). This regional assessment allows comparison of wall motion abnormalities with the extent and distribution of coronary artery disease, assessed at coronary arteriography.

In addition to the assessment of myocardial function in coronary artery disease, left ventricular angiography can provide information on primary muscle abnormalities, such as dilated cardiomyopathy where there is a dilated LV with globally poor function in the absence of coronary artery disease, or hypertrophic cardiomyopathy where obliteration of the left ventricular cavity can occur during systolic contraction.

Left ventricular angiography is also useful for the assessment and quantification of mitral re-

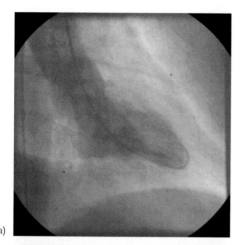

(a)

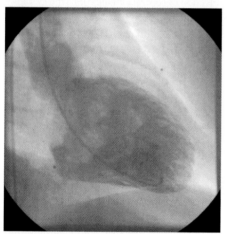

(b)

**Fig. 3.16** (a) End systolic and (b) end diastolic frames from a normal left ventricular angiogram.

gurgitation. Injection of contrast into the LV with regurgitation through the mitral valve during systole opacifies the left atrial cavity to a varying degree, depending on the severity of regurgitation. Although much information on the severity of mitral regurgitation can be obtained clinically and from non-invasive imaging techniques, left ventricular angiography remains an important confirmatory investigation. While doming of a stenotic aortic valve may be apparent during left ventricular angiography, this is a poor discriminator of severity in isolation and is never used as an accurate quantitative assessment of the severity of AS.

## Aortography

Aortography is generally used for the assessment of aortic root pathology or AR. The presence and extent of aortic root dilatation can be accurately visualized, and in patients with suspected aortic dissection an intimal flap may be seen. However, the superb resolution of modern imaging techniques such as TOE, CT scanning and MRI have largely superseded aortography in these conditions. The inherently volumetric nature of contrast angiography preserves a role for aortography in the quantification of AR. As with left ventricular angiography and mitral regurgitation, aortography allows assessment of the severity of regurgitation through the aortic valve. Again, much information on regurgitation severity can be obtained clinically and from the other available and less invasive imaging techniques, but aortography remains a valuable confirmatory and diagnostic investigation in doubtful or difficult cases.

## Pulmonary angiography

In adult cardiology, pulmonary angiography is almost exclusively used for the diagnosis of acute massive pulmonary embolism, though even here imaging techniques such as helical CT scanning are gradually replacing it. Acute massive pulmonary embolism implies there is partial or complete obstruction of one or both of the main branch pulmonary arteries. It is performed using a 'pig-tail' or NIH (National Institutes of Health) multihole catheter with injection of contrast directly into the main and branch pulmonary arteries. Relatively small emboli can be visualized in the peripheral branch pulmonary arteries using this technique but it is only indicated in circumstances where hypoxia or haemodynamic compromise demand early intervention. Despite the fact that pulmonary embolism is commonly associated with thrombus in the pelvic veins, it is rare to find difficulty advancing the catheter safely via a percutaneous femoral venous approach or displacing further thrombus in the process. Having advanced the catheter up the inferior vena cava, through the RA, across the tricuspid valve, through the right ventricle into the main PA across the pulmonary valve, it is possible directly to measure PA pressure and inject 40–50 mL of contrast.

Right ventricular and pulmonary angiography is occasionally used in the assessment of adult congenital heart disease particularly if previous surgical reconstruction of the right ventricular outflow tract has been performed. In addition, right ventricular angiography may be indicated in patients with ventricular arrhythmias where right ventricular dysplasia is the suspected arrhythmic substrate, but again other imaging techniques such as MRI and CT scanning now provide similar information.

## Coronary arteriography

Coronary arteriography, although invasive, is a low-risk procedure with a combined risk of death and stroke of around 0.2% in elective patients, although the risk becomes higher in patients with myocardial ischaemia or poor left ventricular function at the time of the procedure, or those with severe valvular disease. The procedure is usually performed in conjunction with left heart catheterization as described above. Direct access to the arterial circulation is achieved under local anaesthesia via either the femoral (Judkins) or brachial (Sones) approach, the former being used much more commonly. With the introduction of high-resolution, digital radiograph imaging systems, the size of the femoral catheters has been reduced so that is it now common to perform coronary arteriography using 6 French or even 5 French catheters. The catheters themselves are manufactured from polyurethane or polyethylene and are single use, disposable and preshaped to allow easier intubation of the ostium of the left and right coronary arteries. Once positioned within the ostium of the coronary artery, 5–10 mL of radiograph contrast medium is injected by hand through the catheter to opacify the coronary artery with the images acquired as a radiograph loop that can be stored and replayed for further analysis. Several views of each coronary artery are obtained by manoeuvring the radiograph camera around the patient to acquire images from different angulations. This allows assessment of the course of all the major epicardial coronary arteries.

The severity of stenoses within the coronary vessels can be assessed visually by an experienced operator or quantitative angiography can be used to provide computer assessment of lesion severity, in comparison with a normal segment of artery. The severity of coronary lesions is described using the percentage stenosis, with >50% usually being regarded as significant. Figure 3.17 demonstrates a normal coronary angiogram of the left and right coronary arteries. The first segment of the left coronary artery, the left main stem, is a common trunk which arises from the aortic sinus of the left coronary cusp of the aortic valve and soon divides into its two main branches, the LAD artery and the circumflex (Cx) coronary artery. The LAD traverses the front of the heart in the interventricular groove, and supplies the majority of the anterior surface of the heart and approximately the anterior two-thirds of the interventricular septum (IVS). The Cx traverses the left lateral aspect of the heart in the atrioventricular groove and supplies the lateral wall of the heart and is usually the smallest of the three main coronary vessels. The RCA has a separate origin from the aortic sinus of the right coronary cusp of the aortic valve. It follows the atrioventricular groove on the right and supplies the inferior surface of the heart and the right ventricle. In around 90% of patients, the RCA is described as 'dominant' because it supplies the artery to the AV node and gives off the posterior descending artery (PDA) which runs in the posterior interventricular groove and supplies the posterior one-third of the IVS. In the remaining 10%, the PDA arises from the Cx artery (left dominant anatomy). The RCA supplies the whole of the inferior left ventricular myocardium but in some cases the circumflex coronary artery is the dominant vessel and the RCA is relatively small and non-dominant.

An example of a severe lesion in the RCA is shown in Fig. 3.18. Coronary artery disease is often classified as 1-vessel, 2-vessel or 3-vessel

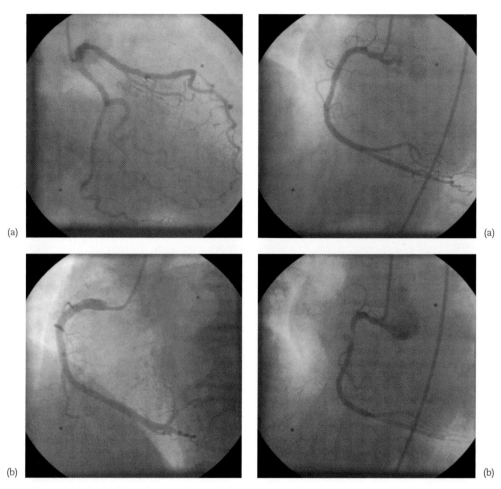

(a)

(a)

(b)

(b)

Fig. 3.17 (a) Normal coronary angiogram left and (b) right coronary arteries.

Fig. 3.18 (a) Normal right coronary artery and (b) one with a severe narrowing in the proximal segment of the vessel.

disease, depending on the distribution of significant lesions in the three major coronary vessels. This classification is useful as patients with multivessel disease have a poorer prognosis, and the recommendations for treatment are often based on the extent and severity of coronary artery disease and left ventricular function as well as on symptomatic grounds.

### Endomyocardial biopsy

Biopsy of the ventricular myocardium is occasionally performed at the time of cardiac catheterization, either to assist the diagnosis of cardiomyopathy, particularly infiltrative myopathies such as cardiac amyloid, or in patients who have undergone cardiac transplantation where regular biopsies are required to monitor tissue rejection. Biopsy is performed through a long outer sheath inserted into the right or left ventricle, with the biotome introduced through the sheath to obtain a small piece of endomyocardium. Several biopsies are usually taken and although the risks are small they include ventricular arrhythmias, chest pain, pericardial effusion and cardiac perforation with tamponade.

## CT scanning and MRI

Cross-sectional imaging of the heart using either CT scanning or MRI has gained an increasingly important role in cardiac imaging particularly with the introduction of helical, ultra-fast CT scanning. Using ECG-gating to allow for cardiac motion during the cardiac cycle, high-resolution cross-sectional images of the heart can be obtained. CT scanning and MRI are not affected by body habitus unlike TTE, although it may not be possible physically to fit grossly obese patients into the scanner. Static images are produced, usually in the axial, sagittal or coronal views, though off-axis imaging can also be performed, usually to enhance imaging of the great vessels. Three-dimensional reconstruction can be performed to provide a better appreciation of the spatial relationship between cardiac structures, and a cine-loop format of images constructed throughout the cardiac cycle can provide dynamic appreciation of cardiac function and flow. Centres may not have access to both ultra-fast CT and MRI scanning but much of the clinical information provided by these two techniques is comparable and both techniques are rarely required in an individual patient. However, each has its strengths and limitations which merit brief discussion.

### Magnetic resonance imaging

MRI uses extremely powerful magnets (usually 0.5–1.5 Tesla) which have to be located in a protected environment for safety reasons, excluding ferro-magnetic objects and credit cards which are easily damaged. The strong magnetic field 'lines up' the body's protons and a radio-frequency signal applied to the required cross-section allows construction of an image from the received signal. Different RF pulse sequences can be used to highlight or enhance certain types of tissue or blood flow. Conventional ECG-gated images, or spin-echo imaging, produce a static cross-sectional image with cardiac tissues displayed at varying intensity and blood, which produces no signal and is displayed as black (Fig. 3.19). In the cine-loop format, or

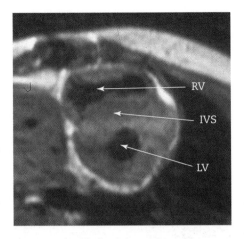

Fig. 3.19 MRI of the heart in a patient with hypertrophic cardiomyopathy showing the left ventricle (LV) in cross-section with marked thickening of the interventricular septum (IVS). Note that blood within the ventricle is displayed as black, with no signal.

gradient echo imaging, which displays dynamic cardiac motion and flow throughout the cardiac cycle, blood has a high signal and is displayed as white with cardiac tissues shown at lower intensity (Fig. 3.20). Image quality can be adversely affected by the presence of cardiac arrhythmias because of the need for ECG-gating. The presence of vascular clips in the brain and cardiac pacemakers are absolute contraindications to performing MRI. Prosthetic heart valves, cardiovascular clips and sternal wires are not contraindications to performing MRI but may cause significant artefacts, usually seen as black holes in the image, when using the flow-enhanced cine-loop imaging techniques. Flow velocities within the heart and great vessels can be measured accurately by some magnetic resonance scanners, though this information is often more readily obtained by echocardiography and Doppler ultrasound techniques.

### CT scanning

CT scanning uses ionizing radiation to construct cross-sectional imaging of the heart. Ultra-fast, helical CT scanning now provides high-resolution imaging much more rapidly with

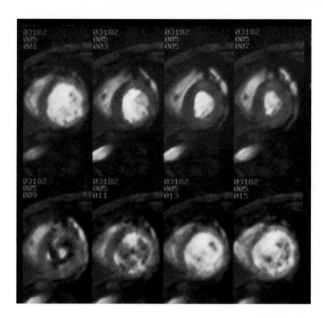

**Fig. 3.20** Cine-loop flow-enhanced MRI showing a cross-section of the left ventricle at different time periods throughout the cardiac cycle from diastole in the top left-hand image through systole and diastole to the bottom right-hand image. Note that with flow enhanced MRI blood produces a high intensity signal.

the total scan being performed within a single breath hold, to minimize respiratory artefact. CT scanning detects the presence of calcification much better than MRI and, for example, may be more useful in patients with pericardial disease where calcification may occur without much pericardial thickening or effusion. CT scanning can also be performed in patients in whom MRI is contraindicated (see Box 3.5).

### Aortic disease
CT scanning and MRI can provide images of the whole of the thoracic and abdominal aorta which may be helpful in patients with extensive aortic dissection. In a haemodynamically unstable patient, TOE may be a more appropriate investigation as it can be performed in the intensive care unit or anaesthetic room. However, in a stable patient or one in whom immediate surgical intervention is not necessary, CT or MRI may be a better investigation as it can often provide additional information, particularly if the dissection extends beyond the thoracic aorta.

### Pericardial disease
Pericardial effusion is readily identified by echocardiography but evaluation of pericardial

> **Box 3.5 Common Clinical Indications for Cardiac CT and MRI**
>
> - Aortic disease (aortopathy, dissection)
> - Pericardial disease
> - Pulmonary hypertension/pulmonary embolism
> - Adult congenital heart disease
> - Cardiomyopathy particularly hypertrophic and infiltrative
> - Paracardiac tumours and masses

thickening and/or calcification is notoriously difficult and both CT scanning and MRI can be useful. CT scanning has the advantage of more readily identifying the presence of calcification (Fig. 3.21). Tumour involvement of the pericardium, usually from carcinoma of the lung or breast, can also be delineated whereas this can easily be missed by echocardiography.

### Pulmonary hypertension/pulmonary embolism
Pulmonary hypertension has a wide spectrum of aetiology and CT/MRI can be helpful in diagnosis when this is either primarily cardiac or

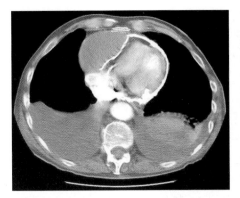

Fig. 3.21 Helical CT scan from a patient with pericardial disease. The calcified pericardium is clearly seen as a white band surrounding the heart.

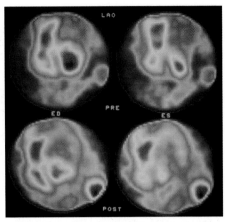

Fig. 3.22 End diastolic and end systolic image from a radionuclide ventriculogram using technetium-99 m imaging. The patient has a left ventricular aneurysm, and the diastolic and systolic images are shown before (top) and after (bottom) surgical resection.

respiratory in origin. Many cardiac causes such as chronic left ventricular failure or mitral valve disease may be apparent using echocardiography, but CT scanning is particularly valuable when evaluating a respiratory aetiology or in patients with suspected primary pulmonary hypertension, where it is not only helpful in excluding many pathologies, but it can also demonstrate the effects of pulmonary hypertension on the pulmonary vasculature and right heart.

Ultra-fast, helical CT scanning is now proving valuable for the diagnosis of pulmonary embolism, both acute and chronic. The high resolution of the pulmonary vasculature from the central main pulmonary vessels into the periphery of the lung allows accurate diagnosis of even relatively small pulmonary embolism and may soon supersede the established use of radionuclide V/Q scanning.

## Nuclear cardiology

There are a number of nuclear techniques both established and developing that play a role in cardiac diagnosis. They fall into four main categories:
1 blood pool imaging;
2 infarct imaging;
3 myocardial perfusion imaging; and
4 positron emission tomography.

### Blood pool imaging
The basis of blood pool imaging is to 'tag' red blood cells with a radionuclide isotope so that imaging can be performed as the labelled red cells initially pass through the cardiac chambers, so-called 'first pass' imaging, or once the labelled blood cells are in equilibrium with the rest of the circulation. Because the value of this technique is in the investigation of global and regional ventricular function, it is often known as radionuclide ventriculography (RVG). Technetium-99 m is the radioactive tracer used for red blood cell labelling. Gamma camera imaging over the heart allows acquisition of images throughout the cardiac cycle so that end-systolic and end-diastolic images (Fig. 3.22) can be used to measure ejection fraction from the difference between the number of nuclear 'counts' obtained as:

Ejection fraction %

$$= \frac{\text{End diastolic counts} - \text{End systolic counts}}{\text{End diastolic counts}} \times 100$$

Although this technique has the advantage over echocardiography of being unaffected by factors such as ultrasound penetration and body habitus, as echocardiographic and MRI techniques have continued to advance, the need of nuclear blood pool imaging has reduced. It is now more usually regarded as a second line investigation for assessment of ventricular function where other imaging techniques are either difficult, unavailable or contraindicated.

## Imaging of myocardial infarcts

Technetium pyrophosphate is a radionuclide tracer used for bone scan imaging. Myocardial cell death allows this agent access to intracellular calcium in areas of myocardial necrosis and can potentially be used to diagnose, localize and assess the extent of myocardial infarction. However, this is almost never used in clinical practice for several reasons.

• A substantial area of myocardial damage is required for a positive scan, residual blood flow to the necrotic area is required in order to allow delivery of the tracer, and the optimal scan time is 24 hours after the onset of infarction, by which time the major potential advantages of thrombolytic and other reperfusion techniques have disappeared.

• Also, newer biochemical markers of myocardial damage such as Troponin T and Troponin I more easily and rapidly provide information on myocardial damage. As such, although myocardial infarct imaging is possible using nuclear imaging techniques, it is largely of historical interest.

## Myocardial perfusion imaging

Unlike infarct imaging, myocardial perfusion imaging is a well established and widely used clinical imaging technique. There are a number of different isotopes that can be used, most commonly thallium-201 or technectium-99 m 2-methoxy-isobutyl isonitrile (MIBI). Different imaging techniques are used, including multiple, single plane imaging to tomographic imaging using a single photon emission computed tomography (SPECT), but the basic technique is identical. These isotopes accumulate in viable myocardium with normal perfusion. Ischaemic muscle or infarct territory do not demonstrate isotope accumulation to the same extent and are indicated on the scan as areas of reduced isotope uptake. In order to induce ischaemia, scans are performed under stress conditions, either exercise induced or pharmacological stress using infusion of either dobutamine, arbutamine, adenosine or dipyridamole. Scans are then later repeated under resting conditions in order to detect areas of 'reversible ischaemia' (see Chapter 8). 'Non-reversible' defects which occur at both rest and during stress usually reflect the presence of myocardial infarction, though it is possible that an area of infarction may also be surrounded by or adjacent to another area of myocardium demonstrating reversible ischaemia.

Myocardial perfusion scanning can be used in a variety of ways. It can provide a useful adjunct to conventional exercise testing improving both the sensitivity and specificity for the detection of significant coronary artery disease. It should be recognized that around 20% of patients will still have either falsely negative or falsely positive scans and coronary angiography may still be required to confirm or refute the diagnosis of coronary artery disease. Myocardial perfusion imaging can also be used in patients with known coronary artery disease to detect the area of myocardium causing ischaemic symptoms, and/or to provide some estimate of the extent of myocardium at jeopardy from the disease in individual coronary vessels as an aid to making decisions about coronary intervention by angioplasty or coronary artery bypass surgery.

## Positron emission tomography

PET scanning is not widely available as it requires the presence of a linear accelerator to generate the appropriate isotopes, often glucose- or oxygen-related analogues, which have such a short high-life that they need to be generated in the immediate proximity of the scanner. PET scanning is a method of performing radioactive tagging of intracellular metabolites within the myocardium so that imaging is obtained dependent solely on the presence of living or viable muscle. The ability to provide information on true myocardial viability, irrespective of myocardial perfusion, or muscle function is of considerable clinical potential. Patients with an occluded coronary artery and consequent reduced or absent muscle function may still have viable myocardium which will recover once myocardial perfusion is restored either by thrombolysis, angioplasty or coronary artery bypass surgery. PET scanning is the current 'gold standard' for determining the presence of viable myocardium in non-functioning segments of the heart but its expense precludes its use from routine clinical practice at present.

# Hypertension

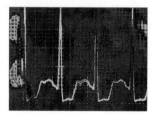

## Introduction

In Western societies, blood pressure (BP) rises with age and the distribution of BP readings within societies is a continuous variable, making it somewhat arbitrary where the normal range is defined as ending and an abnormally elevated range (hypertension) begins. The importance of defining hypertension arises out of the morbidity associated with its natural history if uncontrolled. Patients are usually asymptomatic and a diagnosis of hypertension carries with it a likelihood of drug treatment for life and implications regarding life assurance risk analysis, so its definition is important. BP varies enormously depending on circumstances, rising with exercise, emotion and stress and falling during sleep. Multiple readings on at least three occasions over 4–6 weeks should therefore be taken before the diagnosis of hypertension is made. Home measurements can be undertaken by patients with the use of proprietary sphygmomanometers so as to increase the number of readings available for analysis. Because 24-hour ambulatory BP has been shown to correlate better with subsequent end-organ damage than measurements made by physicians, and is a better predictor of cardiovascular outcome, this technique is employed where doubt remains concerning the diagnosis, and in the assessment of response to treatment. Much of what follows is based on recommendations made by the British Hypertension Society (1999).

## Measuring blood pressure

The patient should be allowed to rest in a quiet room for 5–10 min. Stimulants such as tea, coffee and caffeine-containing soft drinks should be avoided in the preceding hour. The usual sphygmomanometer cuff is 12.5 cm wide and should cover at least two-thirds of the upper arm, because narrower cuffs with less coverage may give spuriously high readings. In obese patients, it may be necessary to use a wide thigh cuff on the upper arm instead of the standard cuff. The patient should be seated with the arm at the level of the heart. Palpate the radial pulse on the ipsilateral side and inflate the sphygmomanometer cuff gradually to a systolic pressure 20 mmHg above the point where the radial pulse is felt to disappear. Auscultate over the brachial artery and allow the cuff to deflate at approximately 2 mmHg/s, recording the point at which the first pulsation is heard (first Korotkoff sound), which is the systolic BP, and the point at which the pulsatile sound disappears (fifth Korotkoff sound), which is now universally taken to represent diastolic pressure, rather than where the sound becomes muffled (fourth Korotkoff), which was used in the past in some definitions. Measure the BP at least twice, and ensure there is no difference between arms. If there is a difference, use the arm with the higher pressures for future readings. On each occasion try to take the BP twice, separated by as long a period as possible (at least 5–10 min).

Intra-arterial cannulation allows the direct measurement of BP to be made but is rarely undertaken outside research studies. All adults should have their BP measured routinely at least every 5 years until the age of 80. If found to be borderline, measurements should be every 3–12 months.

## Primary hypertension

This has also been termed 'essential' or 'idiopathic' hypertension and accounts for 95% of all cases of hypertension. Its aetiology has been the subject of considerable research over the last 75 years. BP is related to the product of cardiac output and vascular resistance, so for BP to rise either cardiac output must be increased or peripheral vascular resistance must be elevated, or both. Although the mechanisms involved in generating hypertension must involve these changes, hypertension as a clinical condition is usually diagnosed some years after any tendency towards it has started. By this time, many secondary compensatory physiological mechanisms have been initiated so these fundamental abnormalities of cardiac output or peripheral resistance may not be clearly identifiable. In early established hypertension, cardiac output is usually normal or only slightly increased and peripheral resistance is normal. In the later stages of hypertension, cardiac output tends to fall and vascular resistance increase. Also, the presence of hypertension will cause arterial and arteriolar wall thickening, perhaps partly mediated by factors known to stimulate vascular hypertrophy and vasoconstriction (insulin, catecholamines, angiotensin, growth hormone), creating secondary reasons why an elevation of BP will be perpetuated. The presence of these complex compensatory mechanisms and secondary consequences of established hypertension has made research into its aetiology difficult and observations made open to a variety of interpretations. It is likely to be due to a complex interplay between factors, which may be different between individuals.

Some of the factors that have been suggested as being relevant to the mechanisms resulting in hypertension are as follows.

*Genetic.* Western blacks are more predisposed to hypertension, have generally higher levels and have greater morbidity and mortality due to their hypertension than whites, suggesting possible genetic differences. Some have postulated abnormalities in the region of the angiotensinogen gene but the mechanisms are probably polygenic.

*Geographic and environmental.* Marked population differences exist with economically less developed races, such as certain South American Indians, having significantly lower BP which rises less with age than in Western societies.

*Fetal.* These may exert an influence because low birth weight appears to predispose to hypertension later in life, perhaps due to a lower number of nephrons and ability to excrete a sodium load in low birth-weight babies.

*Sex.* Hypertension is less common in premenopausal women than in men suggesting hormonal influences.

*Sodium.* Much evidence supports a role for sodium in the genesis of hypertension, perhaps due to a genetic or acquired inability to excrete a sodium load efficiently. Some have argued for the presence of a natriuretic hormone (de Wardener) which inhibits cell sodium pump (sodium-potassium ATPase) activity and has a pressor effect. Population studies, such as the INTERSALT Study (1988), have shown a correlation between average sodium intake and BP, and that reductions in BP can be achieved by restricting salt consumption.

*Renin-angiotensin system.* Renin stimulates the production of angiotensin (a pressor agent) and aldosterone (which promotes sodium and consequent water retention). Some studies have shown a proportion of patients with primary hypertension to have elevated renin levels, but the majority have been normal or low, a finding which has been attributed to the homeostatic effects of negative feedback because volume overload and an increase in BP would both be expected to suppress renin production.

*Sympathetic hyperactivity.* This may be seen in young hypertensives. Catecholamines will stimulate renin production, constrict arterioles and veins, and increase cardiac output.

*Insulin resistance/hyperinsulinaemia.* The association of primary hypertension with insulin resistance has been noted for years, especially in obese subjects. Insulin is a pressor agent itself and increases levels of catecholamines and renal sodium reabsorption.

*Endothelial cell dysfunction.* Hypertensives may have reduced vasodilatory responses to nitric oxide, and endothelium contains local vasoconstrictor substances, such as endothelin-1, although their relevance to hypertension is uncertain.

## Natural history

Individuals with hypertension are usually asymptomatic, an elevated BP being detected during medicals for screening, employment or life assurance purposes. Symptoms commonly attributed to hypertension (headache, dizziness, tinnitus, fainting) are just as common in the normotensive population. In particular, the presence of headaches has been found to correlate poorly with the level of BP. Organ damage, principally cardiac, cerebral and renal, is related to the severity of the hypertension. The principal organ changes seen include the following.

*Cardiac.* Left ventricular hypertrophy results in increased wall stiffness to diastolic filling and a prominent 'a' wave (atrial systole) on echocardiography. Left ventricular failure (systolic and diastolic dysfunction) may ensue, often with a ventricle that is not dilated. Treatment with most antihypertensive agents, and especially the angiotensin-converting enzyme (ACE) inhibitors, have been shown to reduce left ventricular hypertrophy if BP is reduced. Coronary artery disease is common in hypertensives, and this together with left ventricular dysfunction probably accounts for their higher cardiac mortality. The risk of cardiac events (death, myocardial infarction, heart failure, ventricular arrhythmias) is reduced if BP is lowered. When diastolic pressure is lowered below 80 mmHg the risk starts to increase again, the so-called J-shaped curve, although this observation is disputed. An increase in cardiac events at lower diastolic pressures may be due to lower coronary perfusion pressure which, in the presence of a thickened myocardium and increased arteriolar resistance due to the hypertensive process, may result in cardiac ischaemia, especially nocturnally when BP is likely to be at its lowest.

*Renal.* The gradual development of renal impairment and failure is frequently seen in long-standing hypertension, especially where control has been poor, and is more common in black individuals. Loss of urinary concentrating ability may cause nocturia to develop. Microalbuminuria progresses to more severe proteinuria and creatinine clearance declines. Eventually, end-stage renal failure may occur and dialysis may be necessary. In accelerated severe hypertension (see below in chapter) acute renal failure is common and is a major cause of mortality if the hypertension is left inadequately treated. Such an occurrence is a medical emergency.

*Cerebral.* Strokes and transient ischaemic attacks are more common in hypertensives. During a stroke, BP may increase acutely and caution must be taken in lowering it too rapidly or too vigorously. Cerebral vascular resistance will be increased due to the long-standing effects of hypertension, as well as to the possible acute effects of cerebral oedema, and too great a reduction in cerebral arterial perfusion pressure may increase cerebral ischaemia.

An indication of end-organ damage can be gained by examining the fundi for changes associated with hypertension (see Box 4.1 and Fig. 4.1). Grades 3 and 4 are more commonly seen in accelerated severe hypertension, whereas grades 1 and 2 correlate more closely with other target organ damage in chronic hypertension.

## Assessment

All patients with suspected or established hypertension should have a thorough history taken and a full examination, but only a few

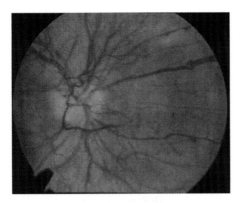

Fig 4.1 Fundal changes of Grade 4 hypertensive retinopathy.

## Box 4.1 Retinopathy Associated with Hypertension

• **Grade 1**: mild narrowing or sclerosis of the retinal arteriolar lumen producing a 'silver wiring' effect
• **Grade 2**: moderate to marked sclerosis of the arterioles, visible as arteriovenous 'nipping'
• **Grade 3**: progressive retinal changes resulting in oedema, 'cotton wool' spots and haemorrhages
• **Grade 4**: all of the above with papilloedema (see Fig. 4.1)

routine investigations are necessary (see Box 4.2); in the majority even these will be normal.

Some patients will need more complex investigations and specialist referral, such as those with:
• accelerated (malignant) hypertension (see below in text);
• suspected secondary hypertension (see below in text);
• therapeutic problems or failures;
• special circumstances (e.g. pregnancy).

### Indications for treatment

From numerous trials, it has become clear that the morbidity and mortality associated with hypertension progressively rise as its severity increases, with systolic elevations carrying at least as much risk as diastolic. Also, the benefits achieved by lowering BP are greatest for those with the highest pressures. Meta-analysis of trials involving a total of over 420 000 patients has shown a continuous and independent association of BP with both stroke and coronary heart disease. Prolonged elevation of diastolic pressure by >10 mmHg appears to increase the risk of stroke by 56% and coronary heart disease by 37%. Once the diastolic pressure rises above 95–100 mmHg, the risks of future cerebral and cardiac events are significant, and drug therapy should be given if satisfactory control cannot be achieved by lifestyle changes. Treatment is clearly not required for those with diastolics less than 80–85 mmHg where the risk is acceptably low. Between these two levels, 85–95 mmHg, borderline and mild hypertension may still double the relative risk of future adverse events, though the frequency of these events will still be low in absolute terms. Around 60% of hypertensives fall into these categories, amounting to a large number of individuals, and it has been debated how cost-effective it is as a population health strategy to treat all these individuals.

The massive Framingham study and other

## Box 4.2 Investigations for Hypertension

| Test | Reason |
| --- | --- |
| • Urinalysis for blood and protein, blood electrolytes and creatinine | May indicate renal disease either causing or caused by the hypertension, or rarely may suggest adrenal (secondary) hypertension |
| • Blood glucose | To exclude diabetes or glucose intolerance |
| • Serum total and high-density lipoprotein (HDL) cholesterol | To help assess future cardiovascular risk |
| • ECG | May suggest left ventricular hypertrophy |

epidemiological data have demonstrated a number of independent risk factors for the development of premature vascular disease (see Box 4.3).

It has been calculated that a man aged 55 years, with a systolic BP of 160 mmHg, may have a risk of a vascular event over the next 10 years of around 14%, whereas the same man with the same BP, but with all the risk factors in Box 4.3, will have a 60% risk. The higher the overall risk the more vigorous one should be at lowering BP, and in patients with mild hypertension the lower the BP threshold at which treatment should be considered. Algorithms have been published (see Joint British recommendations on prevention of coronary heart disease in clinical practice, in Further Reading) for the calculation of future cardiovascular risk based on levels of BP, cholesterol and the presence or otherwise of diabetes.

As a general guide, almost all treated patients should have diastolic pressures <85–90 mmHg and systolics <140–149 mmHg, and in diabetics the target should be <140/80. In practice this ideal is often not achievable.

## Mild or borderline hypertension

The decision regarding treatment of those with systolic blood pressures of 140–149 mmHg and/or diastolic pressures of 90–99 mmHg can be difficult, not least because such levels are so common. Not all patients will have a high overall cardiovascular risk, especially in the younger age group. The British Hypertension Society guidelines suggest that if lifestyle changes are ineffective, drug treatment is indicated in this group under the following circumstances:

- if evidence of target organ damage is present (retinopathy, proteinuria, left ventricular hypertrophy);
- if diabetes mellitus is present;
- if there are established cardiovascular complications (previous stroke or known ischaemic heart disease);
- if the 10-year coronary heart disease risk is 15% or more.

## Hypertension in the elderly

Both men and women are living longer and >50% of those above the age of 60 years will have isolated systolic hypertension (systolic BP 160 mmHg and diastolic 90 mmHg). Because cardiovascular risk rises with age, elderly patients with these levels of BP are more likely to require treatment than younger ones. Lowering BP has been shown to decrease the incidence of heart failure, may reduce dementia and may help preserve cognitive function, and trial data have shown that this treatment benefit extends up to at least the age of 80 years. There are little trial data on patients older than 80 years, but if treatment has been started at an earlier age it should be continued in these elderly patients.

## Secondary hypertension

Defined causes of hypertension account for around 5% of cases and may be grouped as follows.

*Renal parenchymal disease (3%).* Any cause of renal failure (glomerulonephritis, pyelonephritis, obstructive causes) that involves parenchymal damage will tend to cause hypertension, and hypertension itself will cause renal damage.

*Renovascular disease (1%).* This encompasses conditions affecting renal blood supply and can be broadly divided into **atherosclerosis**, which affects mainly the proximal third of the renal artery and is most common in older patients, and **fibrodysplasia** which mainly affects the distal two-thirds and is most common in younger individuals, especially women. Re-

---

### Box 4.3 Independent Risk Factors in the Development of Premature Vascular Disease

- Advancing age
- Elevated serum total cholesterol
- Reduced levels of serum high-density lipoprotein (HDL) cholesterol
- Elevated serum glucose
- Cigarette smoking
- Left ventricular hypertrophy on electrocardiographic voltage criteria

duced renal blood supply stimulates ipsilateral production of renin and hence elevation of BP. It should be suspected if the hypertension is abrupt in onset, refractory to treatment generally but appears to normalize with ACE inhibitors, is severe or accelerated, and if an abdominal bruit is detected.

*Endocrine (1%).* Consider **primary aldosteronism (Conn's syndrome)** when hypokalaemia is associated with hypertension. High aldosterone and low renin levels result in sodium and water overload. Usually due to a solitary benign adenoma or bilateral adrenal hyperplasia. Diagnosis is helped by computerized tomographic (CT) or magnetic resonance (MR) scanning, and treatment is by tumour resection or use of the aldosterone antagonist, spironolactone.

**Cushing's syndrome** is due to bilateral adrenal hyperplasia caused by an adrenocorticotrophic hormone (ACTH) secreting pituitary adenoma in two-thirds of cases, and a primary adrenal tumour in one-third. Suspect if hypertension is associated with obesity, thin skin, muscle weakness and osteoporosis. Diagnosis is by 24-hour urinary cortisol and dexamethasone suppression test, then pituitary and adrenal CT or MR scanning if cortisols are abnormal.

**Congenital adrenal hyperplasia** is a rare cause of hypertension in childhood.

**Phaeochromocytoma** is due to cathecholamine secreting tumour of chromaffin cells of neural origin, 90% arising in the adrenals. Approximately 10% occur elsewhere in the sympathetic chain, 10% of all tumours are malignant and 10% of adrenal adenomas are bilateral. Suspect phaeochromocytoma if BP fluctuates widely, is associated with tachycardia, sweating, or sometimes pulmonary oedema due to cardiac failure. Diagnosis is by 24-hour or spot urine measurement of total metanephrine (cathecholamine metabolite), although levels may be affected by certain antihypertensive drugs, especially labetalol. If metanephrines are equivocal measure plasma norepinephrine (noradrenaline) after a dose of clonidine (adrenergic inhibitor). Once diagnosed, attempt to locate the secreting tumour using CT, MR or ra-

dioisotope scanning. Optimum treatment is to resect the tumour if possible.

*Coarctation of the aorta* (see Chapter 15). Most commonly affects the aorta at or just distal to the left subclavian artery and results in hypertension in the arms and lower pressures in the legs, with weak or absent femoral arterial pulses. Systemic arterial vasoconstriction occurs due to stimulation of the renin-angiotensin system (due to low renal arterial perfusion pressure) and sympathetic hyperactivity. Diagnosis is by CT or MR scanning and/or contrast aortography. Hypertension may often persist even after successful surgical resection, especially if the hypertension has been longstanding preoperatively.

*Pregnancy related.* Gestational hypertension occurs in up to 10% of first pregnancies, is more common in younger mothers, is thought to be due to poor uteroplacental blood flow and generally occurs in the last trimester or early in the post-partum period. It is associated with proteinuria, increased serum urate levels and when severe causes the syndrome of pre-eclampsia. Delivery of the fetus results in resolution of the hypertension. Pregnancy may also worsen pre-existing primary hypertension and this 'acute-on-chronic' variety is more common in older, multigravid mothers and reveals itself usually before 20 weeks' gestation. Antihypertensive drugs should be avoided in pregnancy where possible and the hypertension should be treated by bed rest and fetal monitoring, with delivery where appropriate. However, when drug therapy has to be used methyldopa and labetalol are possible choices.

*Drug induced.* The most common medication associated with hypertension is the oral contraceptive pill (OCP), with around 5% of women developing hypertension within 5 years of starting. Older women (>35 years) are more predisposed, as are women who have had hypertension in pregnancy. BP will fall to normal in 50% within 3–6 months of stopping the OCP. It is uncertain whether the hypertension is caused by the OCP or whether taking it merely reveals an underlying predisposition. Post-menopausal use of oestrogens is cardioprotective and does not increase BP. Other drugs associated with hypertension include ciclosporin, erythropoietin and cocaine.

## Accelerated hypertension

Also known as malignant hypertension, this condition arises when the BP rises rapidly to diastolic levels above 130–140 mmHg. It occurs in <1% of patients with primary hypertension, but more commonly in cases of secondary hypertension, especially phaeochromocytomas and conditions causing rapidly progressive renal failure. Retinal haemorrhages and exudates are common and papilloedema will ensue. Initially the cerebral vessels constrict with increasing hypertension (autoregulation) but, in accelerated cases, the vessels eventually cannot withstand the rapidly rising pressure and they dilate, resulting in cerebral hyperperfusion and cerebral oedema (hypertensive encephalopathy), with symptoms of headache, irritability and alterations in consciousness. If left untreated, accelerated hypertension results in progressive renal damage, hyperaldosteronism due to renal ischaemia, microangiopathic haemolytic anaemia and disseminated intravascular coagulation (DIC). In these advanced cases, the mortality rate is high.

## Management of hypertension

### Potential benefits of treatment
Trials have been conducted over long time periods to assess the benefits of treatment and, hence, most data relate to the use of the earlier antihypertensive agents and, in particular, β-blockers and diuretics. Meta-analysis of the larger treatment trials suggest an overall 40% reduction in stroke and 16% reduction in coronary events.

### Lifestyle modifications
All hypertensive patients and individuals with a strong family history of hypertension should be advised regarding lifestyle changes, such as re-

ducing obesity, salt intake (total <5 g/day), saturated fat intake and alcohol consumption (men <21 units, women <14 units per week), increasing intake of fruit and vegetables (at least 7 portions/day), avoiding smoking, and taking regular physical exercise; all of these have been shown to contribute to a lowering of BP and may reduce the need for medication. For those with mild or borderline hypertension and no complications, the effects of these changes can be monitored during the initial 4–6 month evaluation.

### Drug therapy
When drug therapy is felt necessary, use the lowest dose initially and increase incrementally depending on the response to treatment, allowing at least 4 weeks to see the effect, unless more urgent reduction in BP is needed. In general, medication should be taken in the morning rather than at night, to try to avoid exacerbating the usual early morning drop in BP which may be a contributing factor towards the observation of a higher incidence of cardiovascular events during the hours 5.00–8.00 am. Most physicians still tend to prescribe diuretics or β-blockers as first-line therapy because these are the agents with the most research data supporting benefit. The importance of systolic hypertension is strongly emphasized, as it is at least as important as diastolic BP as a predictor of cardiovascular risk.

### Diuretics
All diuretics will lower BP acutely by salt and water loss, but over 4–6 weeks equilibrium is restored and BP returns towards previous levels. However, the thiazides have a direct vasodilatory effect on arterioles which results in a sustained hypotensive effect. Thiazides reduce serum potassium and tend to increase blood glucose, urate, insulin, cholesterol and calcium. Nearly 25% of men suffer impotence as a side-effect. For treatment of hypertension use the longer acting thiazides, such as hydrochlorothiazide (12.5–50 mg/day) or bendrofluazide (2.5–5.0 mg/day), perhaps with the addition of a potassium sparing agent such as amiloride,

unless an ACE inhibitor is also being used. Indapamide is a sulphonamide diuretic with actions similar to thiazides but with little effect on glucose or cholesterol. Thiazides are particularly the drug of first choice in elderly patients.

## Adrenergic inhibitors

These may act centrally on the vasomotor centre in the brain stem, peripherally on neuronal catecholamine release, or by blocking α- or β-receptors, or both. Examples of each of these agents are given in Table 4.1, with those agents in brackets rarely being used nowadays. In vascular smooth muscle, alpha stimulation causes vasoconstriction and beta stimulation causes relaxation. In the vasomotor centre, sympathetic outflow is inhibited by alpha stimulation. The effects of β-blockers centrally are less certain.

β-blockers are widely used antihypertensives. All seem about equally effective at lowering BP but some have greater selectivity towards cardiac β-receptors (see Table 4.1) than others which are non-cardioselective. Also, some β-blockers have some intrinsic sympathomimetic activity (ISA) (pindolol, oxprenolol, acebutalol and celiprolol), a characteristic that results in less fall in heart rate, cardiac output and renin for a similar change in BP when compared to β-blockers

without ISA. β-blockers may worsen bronchospasm, claudication and untreated congestive cardiac failure and are relatively contraindicated in these conditions. Symptoms of hypoglycaemia in diabetics may be blunted and glucose control may be worsened due to interference with insulin sensitivity. Side-effects may include fatigue, insomnia, nightmares, hallucinations, depression and impotence. They are relatively ineffective in the elderly hypertensive.

## Direct vasodilators

These lower BP by reducing peripheral vascular resistance. The most common examples of this group of drugs are the oral agents hydralazine, prazosin and minoxidil and the intravenous agents diazoxide and nitroprusside. All tend to cause a reflex tachycardia, hydralazine may be associated with a lupus syndrome if used in high doses, and minoxidil commonly results in hirsutism.

## Calcium antagonists

These are now commonly used antihypertensives. The choice of agent depends partly on their different effects with regard to slowing the heart rate (negative chronotropism), reducing myocardial contractility (negative inotropism) and their propensity to cause side-effects such as flushing, peripheral oedema and constipation. Examples of the oldest agents are

Table 4.1 Adrenergic inhibitor agents.

| **ADRENERGIC INHIBITORS** | | | | |
|---|---|---|---|---|
| Vasomotor centre | Neurone | α-Receptor | β-Receptor | α- and β-Receptors |
| Methyl dopa | (Reserpine) | (Phenoxybenzamine) | Acebutalol* | Labetalol |
| (Clonidine) | (Guanethidine) | (Phentolamine) | Atenolol* | Carvedilol |
| | (Bethanidine) | Prazosin | Bisoprolol* | |
| | (Debrisoquine) | Doxasocin | Metoprolol* | |
| | | Terazosin | Esmolol* | |
| | | | Celiprolol* | |
| | | | Nadolol | |
| | | | Pindolol | |
| | | | Timolol | |
| | | | Propranolol | |

* β-blockers with greater selectivity towards cardiac β-receptors.

## CALCIUM ANTAGONISTS

| | Negative chronotropism | Negative inotropism | Flushing/Oedema | Constipation |
|---|---|---|---|---|
| Nifedipine | 0 | 0 | ++ | 0 |
| Verapamil | ++ | ++ | + | ++ |
| Diltiazem | + | + | +− | + |

Table 4.2  Relative effects of calcium antagonists.

given in Table 4.2, but others include nisoldipine, nicardipine, amlodipine and felodipine. The calcium antagonists have little adverse effect on lipids or glucose. The dihydropyridine calcium anatgonists (e.g. nifedipine) are probably the drug of second choice, after diuretics, for elderly hypertensives.

### Renin-angiotensin inhibitors

Adrenergic receptor blockers inhibit renal production of renin from the juxtaglomerular apparatus and it is possible to block the conversion of renin substrate to angiotensin. However, the most widely used of this group of agents in treating hypertension are the ACE inhibitors, such as captopril, enalapril, lisinopril and ramipril, and the more recently developed angiotensin II receptor blockers such as losartan and valsartan. Angiotensin II is a vasoconstrictor and stimulates the production of aldosterone, so blocking its production (ACE inhibitors) or binding to its receptor (A II receptor blockers) will reduce peripheral vascular resistance, with little or no effect on heart rate, cardiac output or body fluid volumes. ACE inhibitors may cause loss of taste, skin rashes and commonly cause an irritating dry cough, probably due to elevation of bradykinin levels. Cough and other side-effects are seen less frequently with the A II receptor blockers. The ACE inhibitors are particularly useful for diabetic nephropathy, where efferent arteriolar dilatation slows the progressive loss of renal function and may reduce proteinuria. They may also improve insulin sensitivity, and have no effect on serum lipids or urate.

### Choice of drug agent

Many hypertensive patients will require drug combinations to achieve adequate BP control. Drug classes generally have additive effects on BP when prescribed together, so submaximal doses of two drugs result in larger BP responses. This approach may be associated with fewer side-effects than maximal doses of a single drug. Rational combinations of drug classes include:

- thiazide diuretic and β-blocker;
- thiazide diuretic and ACE inhibitor;
- β-blocker and calcium antagonist;
- calcium antagonist and ACE inhibitor;
- ACE inhibitor and α-blocker;
- α-blocker and calcium antagonist.

Each hypertensive patient needs to be considered separately when considering the choice of therapy (see Table 4.3), the choice being determined by factors such as age, comorbidity (e.g. diabetes, coronary heart disease, asthma) and the drug's pharmacological profile and side-effects. However, when no other drug is particularly indicated or contraindicated, a thiazide diuretic should be chosen because this group have been shown to be effective, reduce long-term complications of hypertension, to be well tolerated and cost effective.

### Hypertensive crisis

When the BP rises over a few days to levels above around 180/120 mmHg, renal failure and hypertensive encephalopathy may follow. It is important to lower BP but to do so in as controlled and gradual manner as possible because too rapid reduction can result in cerebral and renal underperfusion. Intravenous agents such as labetalol, diazoxide, esmolol, nicardipine and sodium nitroprusside are used, although use of

## DRUGS FOR HYPERTENSION

| Class of drug | Compelling indication | Possible indication | Possible contraindication | Compelling contraindication |
|---|---|---|---|---|
| α-Blockers | Prostatism | Dyslipidaemia | Postural hypotension | Urinary incontinence |
| ACE inhibitors | Heart failure<br>Left ventricular dysfunction<br>Type I diabetic nephropathy | Chronic renal disease*<br>Type II diabetic nephropathy | Renal impairment*<br>Peripheral vascular disease† | Pregnancy<br>Renovascular disease |
| Angiotensin II receptor antagonists | ACE inhibitor induced cough | Heart failure<br>Intolerance of other antihypertensive drugs | Peripheral vascular disease† | Pregnancy<br>Renovascular disease |
| β-Blockers | Myocardial infarction<br>Angina | Heart failure‡ | Heart failure‡<br>Dyslipidaemia<br>Peripheral vascular disease | Asthma/chronic obstructive pulmonary disease<br>Heart block |
| Calcium antagonists (dihydropyridine) | Elderly isolated systolic hypertension | Elderly angina | — | — |
| Calcium antagonists (rate-limiting) | Angina | Myocardial infarction | Combination with β-blockade | Heart failure<br>Heart block |
| Thiazides | Elderly | — | Dyslipidaemia | Gout |

* ACE inhibitors may be beneficial in chronic renal failure but should be used with caution and under specialist supervision.
† Caution with ACE inhibitors and angiotensin II receptor antagonists in peripheral vascular disease because of possible coexistence of renovascular disease.
‡ Blockers may worsen heart failure, but in specialist hands may be used in the long-term treatment of heart failure.

**Table 4.3** The choice of drug class for treating hypertension (adapted from British Hypertension Society Guidelines, 1999).

the last should be limited to a few days because of the risk of thiocyanate accumulation.

## Additional drug therapy

### Aspirin

Aspirin is widely used for the secondary prevention of cardiovascular disease. In the Hypertension Optimal Treatment (HOT) trial of hypertensive patients, 75 mg of aspirin reduced major cardiovascular events, but not fatal events, by 15% but with a significant increase in bleeding events. Overall, the British Hypertension Society recommends that aspirin is not used for routine prophylaxis, but should be used for:

• primary prevention in controlled hypertensive patients <50 years who have evidence of target organ damage, diabetes or a 10-year cardiovascular risk of ≥15%;
• secondary prevention in hypertensive patients where there is evidence of existing cardiovascular disease (e.g. angina, myocardial infarction).

### Statins

This lipid-lowering group of drugs reduces coronary events, all-cause mortality and strokes in patients with coronary heart disease, and although hypertensive patients have not been specifically examined, the evidence supports their use in hypertensives whose 10-year cardiovascular risk is >6%. However, over 50% of all hypertensives fall into this category and if all received statins the cost would be colossal. Taking this into account the British Hypertension Society makes the pragmatic recommendation that statins be used for hypertensive patients in the following circumstances:

• primary prevention in those <70 years with total fasting cholesterol ≥5.0 mmol/L and a 10-year cardiovascular risk of ≥30%;
• secondary prevention in hypertensives <75 years with evidence of existing cardiovascular disease and total fasting cholesterols ≥5.0 mmol/L.

## Further reading

Elliott P, Stamler J, Nichols R et al. Intersalt revisited: further analyses of 24 h sodium excretion and blood pressure within and across populations. BMJ 1996; 312: 1249–53.

Hansson L, Zanchetti A, Carruthers SG et al. Effects of intensive blood pressure lowering and low dose aspirin in patients with hypertension: principal results of the Hypertension Optimal Treatment (HOT) randomised trial. Lancet 1998; 351: 1755–62.

Joint British recommendations on prevention of coronary heart disease in clinical practice. Heart 1998; 80 (Suppl. 2): 1–29.

Ramsay LE, Williams B, Johnston DG et al. Guidelines for the management of hypertension: report of the Third Working Party of the British Hypertension Society. J Human Hypertens 1999; 13: 569–92.

Ramsay LE, Williams B, Johnston DG et al. British Hypertension Society guidelines for hypertension management 1999: a summary. BMJ 1999; 319: 630–5.

# CHAPTER 5

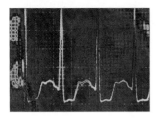

# The Myocardium

## Introduction

### Myocardial structure and function

The myocardium of the left and right ventricles can generate a cardiac output of between 5 and 20 L/min depending on physiological conditions, and contraction is dependent on the highly specialized cardiac cell, the myocyte. Myocytes are connected by intercalated disks, membranes that facilitate electrical and chemical transmission between cells. Each myocyte contains between 100 and 150 thin myofibrils, with each myofibril made up of multiple sarcomeres, the basic unit of contractile myocardial function. Figure 5.1 illustrates the basic composition of the sarcomere unit. The thin, actin filaments are anchored to the Z-line, and are composed of actin molecules with the protein tropomyosin and troponin. The thick myosin filaments interdigitate with the actin filaments and the myosin 'heads' interact with the actin filaments dependent on the concentration of intracellular calcium. The majority of myocardial fibres are orientated circumferentially around the left ventricle (LV) but there are also fibres orientated in a longitudinal direction, many being found in the subendocardial region of the myocardium. During systole, fibre shortening results in left ventricular contraction circumferentially and longitudinally, reducing the short and long axis diameters of the LV, respectively.

### Contraction and relaxation

Electrical stimulation of the myocyte causes influx of calcium through calcium channels in the T-tubules. These are invaginations of the cell membrane related to individual sarcomeres and influx of calcium causes further intracellular calcium release from the sarcoplasmic reticulum. The increase in intracellular calcium causes the myosin heads to move along the actin molecules, causing reduction in sarcomere length and thereby resulting in myocardial contraction, conversion of ATP to ADP providing the energy required. Increasing concentrations of intracellular calcium activate calcium/ATPase pumps, returning calcium to the sarcoplasmic reticulum, and also activate sodium dependent calcium exchange channels which remove calcium into the extracellular space. Reduction in intracellular calcium results in myocardial relaxation. Myocytes are also rich in mitochondria and energy release from metabolic pathways regenerates ATP from ADP and phosphate.

### Preload and the Frank–Starling relationship

Preload is the load on the ventricle before systolic contraction and is a result of ventricular end-diastolic volume, an increase in preload occurring as volume increases. An increase in preload results in augmented ventricular contraction and increased stroke volume. The relationship between preload and augmentation of stroke volume is known as Starling's Law

## THE MYOFIBRIL

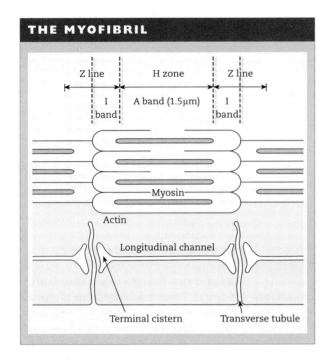

**Fig. 5.1** Schematic diagram of a sarcomere element of the myofibril within a cardiac myocyte.

(Fig. 5.2). Increasing preload stretches the individual sarcomeres and augments contraction by optimizing sarcomere length and increasing sensitivity to calcium. Beyond a certain point, additional stretching causes ventricular stroke volume to fall.

### Afterload

Afterload is the load or wall stress experienced by the ventricle when it contracts during left ventricular ejection, and occurs after the onset of systolic contraction. Major determinants of afterload are the arterial blood pressure and arterial wall compliance. In most clinical circumstances, alteration in blood pressure is a useful indicator of changes in afterload. However, myocardial wall stress, and hence afterload, can also be increased by aortic stenosis (AS), where aortic impedance (or resistance) to ejection is increased but arterial blood pressure may be normal or even low. Wall stress increases with left ventricular dilatation (Law of Laplace) and is reduced by left ventricular hypertrophy.

## LV FILLING AND CONTRACTILITY

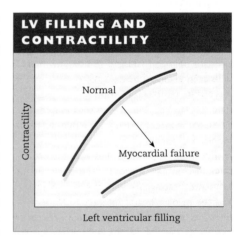

**Fig. 5.2** Frank–Starling curve demonstrating the relationship between left ventricular filling and contractility.

### Contractility

Contractility, or the inotropic state of the myocardium, is the force of myocardial contraction independent of any other haemodynamic factors such as heart rate, preload or afterload. It is well recognized that contractility can be increased with adrenergic stimulation, calcium or other positively inotropic agents such as digoxin or dobutamine, whereas agents such as β-blockers and calcium channel blockers are negatively inotropic agents and reduce contractility. Because measurement of contractility should be independent of other haemodynamic factors, it is almost impossible to measure in the clinical setting but the concept is important, particularly as decreased contractility is often the primary abnormality causing heart failure in primary myocardial disease.

### Myocardial oxygen usage

Determinants of myocardial oxygen consumption ($MVO_2$) are important as they are major factors in the production of myocardial ischaemia, particularly where myocardial oxygen delivery may be reduced as occurs in significant coronary artery disease. The four major determinants of $MVO_2$ are:

1 heart rate;
2 preload;
3 afterload; and
4 contractility.

### Myocardial hypertrophy and dilatation

The left ventricular myocardium responds to pressure overload and volume overload in different ways.

**Pressure overload**: as occurs in conditions such as arterial hypertension or AS. Results in ventricular hypertrophy without any overall change in left ventricular dimension. This so-called concentric hypertrophy results in a reduced cavity size as the ventricular muscle thickens. Myocardial hypertrophy occurs as a result of increasing thickness of individual cardiac myocytes (hyperplasia), due to increasing numbers of myofibrils, rather than an increase in myocyte numbers. This hypertrophy compensates for the increased aortic pressure or impedance and maintains a normal overall wall stress.

**Volume overload**: as occurs in conditions such as aortic or mitral regurgitation. Causes an increase in preload and results in left ventricular dilatation. This is due to myocyte elongation resulting from longitudinal sarcomere proliferation in the myofibrils. The increase in left ventricular internal dimension increases wall stress and there is compensatory myocyte hypertrophy, though this is minimal, sufficient only to normalize wall stress from dilatation.

## Myocarditis

Acute myocarditis is relatively uncommon and the diagnosis is often a presumptive one based on clinical symptoms and signs, though strictly speaking it is a histological diagnosis based on the presence of myocyte necrosis and inflammatory infiltration. The natural history of acute myocarditis is highly variable. In many patients, the condition is mild and self-limiting and the patient may be asymptomatic. However, in some patients, a severe myocarditis may cause severe cardiac failure and death. If the patient survives even a severe acute episode, recovery is highly variable. Some will develop chronic inflammation and heart failure whereas in others the inflammatory process may resolve, leaving many patients with varying degrees of dilated cardiomyopathy. The aetiology of myocarditis is often unknown and labelled as 'idiopathic', though there are many recognized infective and non-infective causes. Almost any infection (bacterial, viral, fungal, protozoal, etc.) can cause acute myocarditis, though viral infections, particularly Coxsackie, are common in Europe and the United States, whereas trypanosomiasis (Chagas' disease) is common in South America. Acute myocarditis can also occur as a manifestation of HIV infection either directly or as a result of opportunistic infection. See Box 5.1 for non-infective causes of myocarditis.

### Clinical features

The presentation of myocarditis is highly variable and may be recognized only because of associated pericarditis, as part of a myopericarditis, although many patients will describe a

## Box 5.1  Non-Infective Causes of Myocarditis

Autoimmune disorders
- Rheumatoid arthritis
- Systemic lupus erythematosus
- Polymyositis
- Systemic sclerosis
- Thyrotoxicosis
- Sarcoidosis
- Diabetes mellitus

Hypersensitivity reactions
- Heavy metals
- Drugs (particularly anthracyclines, cyclophosphamide, fluorouracil)
- Radiation
- Electricity
- Transplant rejection

prodromal flu-like illness. The patient may complain of generalized tiredness and lethargy or occasionally palpitation as a result of ventricular arrhythmias or atrial fibrillation (AF). Dyspnoea is usually an indication of more serious involvement with myocardial dysfunction or a significant pericardial effusion. In severe cases, the presentation may be that of acute pulmonary oedema and severe haemodynamic compromise requiring circulatory support.

### Management
Although the diagnosis is primarily histological, myocardial biopsy is rarely performed in mild cases and may not be performed even in severe myocarditis as there is no evidence that anti-inflammatory agents, in the form of steroids or immunosuppressive therapy, influence the prognosis. Hence, at present, the biopsy result will often not influence patient management although it may allow a firm diagnosis to be made.

Management is largely supportive, with circulatory support and treatment of heart failure in severe cases. If significant pericardial effusion or tamponade is present, pericardial drainage is indicated and may help in determining aetiology. In mild cases, non-steroidal anti-inflammatory agents are often prescribed for pericardial pain.

Steroids and immunosuppresive agents are usually reserved for severe cases, though their value is unproven.

## Dilated cardiomyopathy

Dilated cardiomyopathy is characterized by ventricular dilatation and symptoms and signs of ventricular failure. It is generally regarded as being 'idiopathic' in origin, thereby excluding ventricular dysfunction secondary to ischaemic or valvular heart disease, or hypertension. A similar clinical picture may occur with chronic ischaemia where severe left ventricular dysfunction results with or without symptomatic angina, but this is more usually termed 'ischaemic cardiomyopathy'. The aetiology of 'idiopathic' dilated cardiomyopathy remains unclear. Progression from viral myocarditis to dilated cardiomyopathy has suggested a viral aetiology in some patients. It is recognized that dilated cardiomyopathy may be familial and can occur as a result of alcohol, or in women in the post-partum period. Whether there is an underlying autoimmune or genetic predisposition remains unclear.

### Clinical features
The clinical features are those associated with left and/or right ventricular dysfunction. Tiredness, lethargy and dyspnoea are common and occasionally the patient may present with frank pulmonary oedema. Right heart failure may predominate with a raised jugular venous pressure (JVP), ascites and peripheral oedema, particularly if there is significant tricuspid regurgitation as a result of right ventricular dilatation, though this usually manifests only late in the condition. Palpitation from atrial or ventricular arrhythmias may be present, particularly AF which is a common association. Systemic or pulmonary embolization may occur secondary to atrial or ventricular thrombus formation, particularly if AF is present. Pulsus alternans may be present, the left ventricular apex displaced and a left or right ventricular third heart sound present. There may be clinical evidence of pulmonary

oedema and functional mitral and/or tricuspid regurgitation.

## Investigations

The electrocardiogram (ECG) may be non-specific but may confirm the presence of atrial or ventricular arrhythmias. Poor 'r' wave progression across the anterior chest leads is common as a result of ventricular dilatation. The chest radiograph will often demonstrate pulmonary venous congestion or pulmonary oedema. Echocardiography usually demonstrates dilatation of both left and right ventricles, with globally poor ventricular function and often with associated atrial distension and atrioventricular (AV) valve regurgitation. The global nature of the ventricular dysfunction is important as the presence of regional dysfunction would favour ischaemic heart disease as the likely aetiology. Sluggish blood flow in the dilated, poorly contracting LV may result in the development of thrombus particularly in the apex of the ventricle, often visualized by two-dimensional echocardiography. Exercise testing with assessment of oxygen consumption by respiratory gas analysis can provide an objective assessment of functional capacity, as well as demonstrating underlying ECG abnormalities that may reflect myocardial ischaemia.

Cardiac catheterization allows measurement of pulmonary artery pressure. Pulmonary capillary wedge pressure and left ventricular end-diastolic pressure allow evaluation of the haemodynamic severity of the condition and aids appropriate medical therapy. Left ventricular angiography further characterizes the nature and extent of left ventricular dysfunction, and the severity of functional mitral regurgitation and coronary arteriography excludes ischaemic heart disease as an underlying aetiology. Myocardial biopsy can occasionally be helpful, particularly in myocardial infiltration (see below).

## Management

The management of dilated cardiomyopathy is largely based on the management of heart failure (see Chapter 6).

*Diuretics, digoxin, angiotensin-converting en-zyme (ACE) inhibitors and long-acting nitrates.* All of these have a role, with the ACE inhibitors being of particular importance because of their beneficial effects on mortality.

*β-blockers.* Metoprolol and carvedilol, for example, have also been shown to be effective in some patients though the mechanism remains unclear and may be diverse. Anti-arrhythmic drugs are restricted because many of them have negative inotropic effects and may exacerbate heart failure.

*Amiodarone.* Commonly prescribed for both atrial and ventricular arrhythmias as it is both effective and generally well tolerated, being relatively free from negative inotropy. Aggressive, life-threatening ventricular arrhythmias may occasionally require insertion of an internal defibrillator though currently there is little evidence of their value in these patients.

*Anticoagulation.* Generally recommended in patients with dilated cardiomyopathy especially when associated with atrial arrhythmias or in the presence of ventricular thrombus. However, even in patients without evidence of thrombus and who remain in sinus rhythm, many would still advise anticoagulation if there is severe left ventricular dysfunction and/or atrial dilatation.

*Cardiac transplantation.* Reserved for younger patients with severe functional incapacity or deteriorating heart failure. Difficulty in obtaining sufficient donor organs has led to the development of alternative surgical techniques, such as cardiomyoplasty and ventricular reduction surgery, but these have yet to be shown to provide benefits in morbidity and mortality.

## Hypertrophic cardiomyopathy

Hypertrophic cardiomyopathy (HCM) is characterized by unexplained, usually patchy, hypertrophy of the left ventricular and occasionally right ventricular myocardium. It occurs in the absence of secondary causes of ventricular hypertrophy such as AS or systemic hypertension and is often localized to the upper portion of the interventricular septum (IVS) and anterior free wall of the LV. If the right ventricle is involved, almost always it is in association with left ventricular disease. Histologically, there is hypertrophy associated with myocardial cell disarray as well as disruption of the myofibrillar components within the hypertrophied myocytes. There is usually a variable degree of associated fibrosis.

HCM is inherited as an autosomal dominant disorder and some of the causative genetic mutations have been isolated, including the β-cardiac myosin heavy chain on chromosome 14 and the cardiac troponin T gene on chromosome 1, which account for the majority of the genetic mutations currently isolated. Hence, there may be a family history of the condition, although often there is none, suggesting some cases may be due to spontaneous mutation.

## Clinical features

Symptoms include dyspnoea, chest pain, palpitation, dizziness, or syncope. Occasionally sudden death may be the first presentation. Clinical signs of HCM can be minimal. An ejection systolic murmur at the left sternal edge is most commonly heard. The pulse is usually normal, though a 'jerky' rapidly rising pulse is described. The apex beat may be rather sustained as a function of ventricular hypertrophy.

## Investigations

Transthoracic **echocardiography** (TTE) is the main diagnostic investigation (Fig. 5.3) most commonly demonstrating asymmetric septal hypertrophy of the LV, though isolated apical or posterior wall hypertrophy may also occur. Doppler ultrasound can assess the severity of left ventricular outflow tract obstruction, though the most significant obstruction usually occurs in late systole after most of left ventricular ejection has already occurred. Systolic anterior motion of the mitral valve occurs so that the tips of the mitral leaflets may appose the interventricular septal, and mitral regurgitation of varying degree is commonplace. In families with known HCM, the diagnosis may be made at a screening echocardiographic examination and, in some cases, may be identified incidentally in patients undergoing echocardiography for other reasons. Where the diagnosis is uncertain on conventional TTE, transoesophageal echocardiography (TOE) or magnetic resonance imaging (MRI) provide useful alternatives for diagnostic confirmation.

The **ECG** can show a variety of abnormalities—the QRS complexes may be broad and bizarre, there may be voltage criteria for left ventricular hypertrophy, widespread ST-T changes, interventricular conduction defects and AF—although the ECG is normal in between 5 and 25% of patients. In patients with confirmed HCM, **ambulatory ECG** (Holter) monitoring is important as the presence of sig-

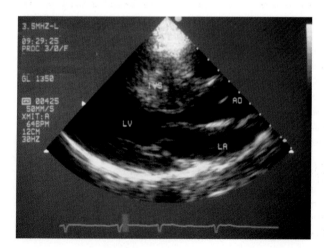

Fig. 5.3 Two-dimensional echocardiogram from a patient with hypertrophic cardiomyopathy. Note the grossly thickened interventricular septum (IVS) in comparison to the normal left ventricular posterior wall.

nificant ventricular arrhythmias can occur in up to 25% of adults and may be asymptomatic. The presence of significant ventricular arrhythmias is associated with increased mortality.

**Cardiac catheterization** may be necessary, particularly in patients with chest pain, in order to determine whether there is coexisting coronary artery disease. Left ventricular angiography often demonstrates left ventricular cavity obliteration during systole. Measurement of the gradient across the left ventricular outflow tract can be performed, confirming the severity of outflow tract obstruction.

## Management

Management is aimed at symptomatic relief and treatment of potentially life-threatening arrhythmias. Symptoms may be due to poor myocardial relaxation, hyperdynamic systolic function with significant left ventricular outflow tract obstruction, arrhythmias, particularly AF or the presence of significant mitral regurgitation. Due to the presence of severe and extensive ventricular hypertrophy, significant ischaemic symptoms can occur in the presence of normal coronaries.

β-blockers and calcium channel blockers, particularly verapamil, have been used to promote myocardial relaxation and reduce ventricular outflow tract obstruction. Where outflow tract obstruction is the predominant feature, surgical myomectomy may be beneficial. Mitral valve replacement may be necessary if MR is severe. Dual chamber cardiac pacing has also been recommended in some patients; alteration in atrial and ventricular electrical activation may augment ventricular filling and reduce outflow tract obstruction. Ventricular arrhythmias are often treated with amiodarone though in some high-risk cases, the role of implantable defibrillators is being assessed.

## Restrictive cardiomyopathy

Restrictive cardiomyopathy is the most uncommon type of cardiomyopathy outside certain geographical regions, such as Africa, where endomyocardial fibrosis is more prevalent. The presentation of restrictive cardiomyopathy is often similar, if not identical, to that of constrictive pericarditis. Differentiation of the two conditions is important as constrictive pericarditis can be successfully treated by surgery whereas the management of restrictive cardiomyopathy is largely supportive. There are a number of other causes of restrictive cardiomyopathy that occasionally occur in adults:

1 amyloid;
2 sarcoid; and
3 haemochromatosis.

## Clinical features

These result from diastolic dysfunction with restricted ventricular relaxation. Systolic contraction is usually well maintained until late in the natural history of the disease when ventricular dilatation and dysfunction develops. Dyspnoea and exercise intolerance predominate and clinical signs are mainly those of right ventricular dysfunction, such as a raised JVP with further increase in inspiration (Kussmaul's sign), peripheral oedema, hepatomegaly and ascites. There may be a third and/or fourth heart sound present. Pulmonary oedema is rarely present until late in the disease process.

## Investigations

ECG and chest radiograph findings are nonspecific although the presence of pericardial calcification strongly favours the diagnosis of constrictive pericarditis rather than restrictive cardiomyopathy. On echocardiography, the myocardium is usually thickened with abnormal left ventricular filling on Doppler ultrasound. In amyloidosis, myocardial deposition produces a characteristic 'ground-glass' textured appearance to the thickened myocardium. The ventricles are not usually dilated until end-stage disease but there is early biatrial dilatation which may become considerable ('giant atria'). Useful information may be obtained on cardiac MRI scanning. Pericardial thickening may be seen in constrictive pericarditis and is best confirmed on computerized tomographic (CT) scanning.

Cardiac catheterization demonstrates raised right atrial pressure with a prominent 'a' wave and rapid 'x' and 'y' descents. Left and right ventricular filling pressures are abnormal with an initial rapid fall in pressure at the onset of diastole, followed by a rapid rise in diastolic pressure in both ventricles to a raised plateau throughout the rest of diastole, the so-called 'dip-and-plateau' or 'square root' appearance. A similar pattern is also seen in constrictive pericarditis, although in constriction ventricular diastolic pressures are closely similar whereas they are often quite different in restriction. In practice, it is often impossible to distinguish the two based on their haemodynamics. Myocardial biopsy is an important diagnostic part of cardiac catheterization. The presence of amyloid, sarcoidosis or haemochromatosis can usually be identified from either right or left ventricular biopsy material.

## Management
This is generally supportive with treatment of fluid retention and arrhythmias. Calcium channel blockers may improve ventricular relaxation. The clinical course is usually that of progressive deterioration, although its onset and rapidity are often quite variable. In haemochromatosis, repeated venesection and the use of chelating agents may be beneficial. If investigations fail to exclude pericardial constriction, then it may be appropriate to consider exploratory thoracotomy, because patients with constriction may respond very well to pericardiectomy and such a treatable condition should not be missed. In restriction, cardiac transplantation should be considered for those most severely affected.

## Miscellaneous

### Acromegaly
The cardiac effects of acromegaly are ill understood. A cardiomyopathy characterized by dilatation of all four chambers occurs late in the disease and appears to be related to elevated levels of growth hormone, which when cor-

rected, results in some improvement in the cardiac dysfunction. Disproportionate cardiac enlargement, compared to other organs, occurs in 75% of affected patients. Histology demonstrates an increase in both collagen and fibrous connective tissue that results in poor contractility. Systemic hypertension is present in 30% of acromegalics and this may result in left ventricular hypertrophy. Other cardiac manifestations of acromegaly include conduction disturbance, arrhythmias, hyperlipidaemia (in the presence of diabetes mellitus which complicates 15–20% of cases), and atherosclerotic coronary disease. Treatment is directed towards suppression of the increased growth hormone secretion by surgical removal or irradiation of the pituitary adenoma, together with conventional treatment for any heart failure.

### Hypothyroidism
Hypothyroidism may be associated with a cardiomyopathy characterized by dilatation of all four cardiac chambers with an increase in interstitial fibrosis and swelling of the myofibrils on histology. The consequent reduction in systolic function causes breathlessness and fluid retention. Pericardial effusions are common, occurring in approximately 30% of patients. There appears to be little correlation between the severity of the biochemical derangement and the severity of any cardiomyopathy or the size of an effusion. Electrocardiographic features include a sinus bradycardia, low voltages, conduction abnormalities and non-specific repolarization changes. Cardiac arrhythmias (including ventricular tachycardia) have also been described. Untreated hypothyroidism is associated with an elevated cholesterol which may predispose to premature coronary artery disease. Treatment involves the cautious administration of thyroid replacement using L-thyroxine (T4), initially at a dose of 25 μg, increasing progressively after a few weeks until the level of TSH returns to normal.

### Connective tissue diseases
A number of connective tissue diseases including rheumatoid arthritis and systemic lupus ery-

thematosus can affect the myocardium, resulting in ventricular dysfunction, though they more commonly cause pericarditis and pericardial effusion. Systemic sclerosis frequently causes myocardial fibrosis as seen at autopsy (80%) but this is not usually sufficient to cause symptomatic ventricular dysfunction. Cardiomyopathy can occur with either a restrictive or dilated pattern.

## Hereditary neuromyopathic conditions

### Erb's limb girdle dystrophy

This is an autosomal recessive condition which is most commonly expressed during the second and third decades of life. Progressive weakness of the limb girdle musculature is the major clinical feature. Cardiac involvement is usually limited to abnormalities of sinus node and AV node function, and the conduction system.

### Facioscapulohumeral dystrophy

This is a rare autosomal dominant condition with marked weakness of the facial, arm and shoulder musculature, and is usually evident at the end of the first decade of life. Atrial standstill is a rare cardiac manifestation.

### Duchenne muscular dystrophy

This is an X-linked recessive disorder. It has an early onset and is rapidly progressive with skeletal muscle weakness and dystrophy. A late onset and less rapidly progressive form (Becker's dystrophy) is also seen. Cardiac muscle may be affected by dystrophic fibrosis and fatty infiltration giving rise to the clinical features associated with a cardiomyopathy. All cardiac structures may be affected, including abnormalities of the specialized conduction system, coronary arteries, and the papillary musculature, in addition to the myocardium. Arrhythmias, valvular disease and systolic and diastolic ventricular dysfunction may all be apparent.

### Dystrophia myotonica

This condition is inherited as an autosomal dominant and is one of the more common neuromuscular disorders. Weakness of the flexor muscles of the neck and sternocleidomastoid muscles are early clinical manifestations. Cardiac abnormalities include disease of the specialized His–Purkinje conduction system, and a dilated cardiomyopathy.

### Friedreich's ataxia

This spinocerebellar degenerative disease is inherited as an autosomal recessive trait and has a spectrum of neurological manifestations, which are classified by their clinical manifestations. Cardiac involvement is common and often the cause of death. Some develop regional ventricular dysfunction, some more global hypokinesia, and others develop a hypertrophic form of cardiomyopathy.

# Heart Failure

## Epidemiology

Heart failure is a condition which has been recognized for centuries but epidemiological studies have been difficult to undertake because of the lack of a single definition of the condition. When few cardiac investigations were available, the definitions of heart failure tended to be pathophysiological, with later definitions placing an increased emphasis on heart failure being a clinical diagnosis (see Box 6.1). Whilst the condition is indeed a clinical syndrome, diagnosis may be difficult in the earlier stages of the condition because of the relative lack of symptoms. Recent definitions have therefore required supportive evidence from cardiac investigations. The most commonly used of these is echocardiography, with left ventricular dysfunction usually defined as ejection fractions of <30–45% in most epidemiological surveys.

Approximately 3–20 per 1000 of the population have heart failure, and its prevalence increases with age (100 per 1000 of those over 65 years), and this is likely to increase further due to an ageing population and improved survival following acute myocardial infarction. In the UK, heart failure accounts for around 100 000 hospital admissions annually, representing 5% of all medical admissions and consuming over 1% of the total healthcare budget.

## Aetiology (see Box 6.2)

Heart failure is a clinical state and not a diagnosis. The cause should always be sought.

Heart failure is most commonly due to failure of myocardial contractility, as may occur with myocardial infarction, longstanding hypertension or the cardiomyopathies. However, under certain conditions, even myocardium with good contractility may be unable to maintain sufficient forward blood flow to meet the body's metabolic needs. Such conditions include mechanical problems such as severe valvular regurgitation and, more rarely, arteriovenous fistulae, thiamine deficiency (beriberi) and severe anaemia. These high cardiac output states may themselves cause heart failure but when less severe may precipitate heart failure in those with underlying cardiac disease.

The prevalence of aetiological factors will depend on the population being studied, coronary heart disease and hypertension being the most common causes in Western societies (>90% of cases), whereas valvular heart disease and nutritional deficiencies may be more important in

## Box 6.1  Definitions of Heart Failure

'A pathophysiological state in which the heart fails to maintain an adequate circulation for the needs of the body despite satisfactory filling pressure.' (Paul Wood, 1958)

'A syndrome in which cardiac dysfunction is associated with reduced exercise tolerance, a high incidence of ventricular arrhythmias and shortened life expectancy.' (Jay Cohn, 1988)

'The presence of heart failure symptoms, reversibility on treatment, and objective evidence of cardiac dysfunction.' (European Society of Cardiology, 1995)

## Box 6.2  Aetological Factors

- Hypertension (10–50%)
- Cardiomyopathy (dilated, hypertrophic, restrictive)
- Valvular heart disease (mitral and aortic)
- Congenital (atrial septal defect (ASD), VSD)
- Arrhythmias (persistent)
- Alcohol
- Drugs
- High cardiac output conditions
- Pericardial (constriction or effusion)
- Right heart failure (pulmonary hypertension)

developing countries. Independent risk factors for the development of heart failure are similar to those for coronary artery disease (raised cholesterol, hypertension and diabetes) but include the presence of left ventricular hypertrophy (LVH) on the resting electrocardiogram (ECG). When present in hypertension, LVH is associated with 14 times the risk of heart failure in those over 65 years. Also, the prevalence of aetiological factors has changed with time. Cohort data from the Framingham Study, which was started in the 1940s, identified a history of hypertension in >75% of patients with heart failure, whereas more recent studies suggest much lower prevalences (10–50%), perhaps due to the better treatment of hypertension. From an overview of clinical trials in hypertension,

effective treatment may reduce the incidence of heart failure by 50%.

Various factors may cause or exacerbate the development of heart failure in patients with underlying cardiac disease.

- **Drugs** such as β-blockers and calcium antagonists may depress myocardial contractility, and chemotherapeutic agents such as doxorubicin may cause myocardial damage.
- **Alcohol** can be cardiotoxic, especially when consumed in large quantities.
- **Arrhythmias** reduce cardiac efficiency, as occurs when atrial contraction is lost (atrial fibrillation, AF) or dissociated from ventricular contraction (heart block). Tachycardias (ventricular or atrial) reduce ventricular filling time, increase myocardial workload and oxygen demand leading to myocardial ischaemia, and, when prolonged, may cause ventricular dilatation and worsening ventricular function. Arrhythmias are common consequences of heart failure itself, whatever the aetiology, with AF reported in up to 20–30% of cases of heart failure at first presentation. Ventricular arrhythmias are a common cause of sudden cardiac death in this condition.

## Pathophysiology

When a primary disturbance of myocardial contractility exists or an excessive haemodynamic burden is placed on a normal ventricle, the heart depends on a number of adaptive mechanisms to maintain cardiac output and blood pressure (see Box 6.3).

### Adaptive mechanisms

Each of these compensatory mechanisms provide immediate haemodynamic benefits but they do so at the expense of longer term adverse consequences, which themselves contribute to the development of chronic heart failure (Fig. 6.1). For instance, **myocardial hypertrophy** increases the mass of contractile elements and improves systolic contraction, but also increases ventricular wall stiffness, impairing ventricular filling and diastolic function.

Reduced renal perfusion causes stimulation of the **renin–angiotensin–aldosterone** (RAA) system, resulting in increased levels of renin, plasma angiotensin II and aldosterone. Angiotensin II is a powerful vasoconstrictor of the renal efferent (and systemic) arterioles, where it stimulates the release of norepinephrine (noradrenaline) from sympathetic nerve endings, inhibits vagal tone and promotes the adrenal release of aldosterone, causing sodium and water retention and renal excretion of potassium. Impaired hepatic function in heart failure may reduce aldosterone metabolism, increasing aldosterone levels still further.

---

**Box 6.3  Adaptive Mechanisms**
- Myocardial hypertrophy
- Neurohormonal
- Activation of renin–angiotensin–aldosterone system
- Activation of sympathetic nervous sytem
- Natriuretic peptides, ADH and endothelin
- Frank–Starling mechanism

---

The **sympathetic nervous sytem** is activated in chronic heart failure via baroreceptors, resulting initially in enhanced myocardial contractility, but later in further activation of the RAA system and other neurohormones, leading to increased venous (cardiac preload) and arterial (cardiac afterload) tone, increased plasma norepinephrine, progressive retention of salt and water, and oedema. Chronic sympathetic stimulation results in the down-regulation of cardiac β-receptors, attenuating the heart's response to stimulation. This, together with baroreceptor impairment, will then lead to further increase in sympathetic stimulation.

**Natriuretic peptides** exert a wide range of effects on the heart, kidney and central nervous system.
- Atrial natriuretic peptide (ANP) is released from the cardiac atria in response to stretch, leading to natriuresis and vasodilatation.
- In humans, brain natriuretic peptide (BNP) is also released from the heart, predominantly from the ventricles, and with actions similar to ANP. The natriuretic peptides act as physio-

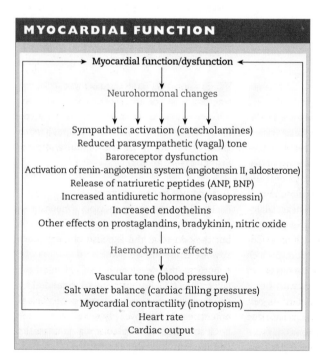

**MYOCARDIAL FUNCTION**

Myocardial function/dysfunction

Neurohormonal changes

Sympathetic activation (catecholamines)
Reduced parasympathetic (vagal) tone
Baroreceptor dysfunction
Activation of renin-angiotensin system (angiotensin II, aldosterone)
Release of natriuretic peptides (ANP, BNP)
Increased antidiuretic hormone (vasopressin)
Increased endothelins
Other effects on prostaglandins, bradykinin, nitric oxide

Haemodynamic effects

Vascular tone (blood pressure)
Salt water balance (cardiac filling pressures)
Myocardial contractility (inotropism)
Heart rate
Cardiac output

Fig 6.1  Diagram showing the relationship between myocardial function, adaptive mechanisms occurring in heart failure and the haemodynamic consequences of these interactions.

logical antagonists to the effects of angiotensin II on vascular tone, aldosterone secretion and renal sodium reabsorption.

**Antidiuretic hormone (vasopressin)** levels are also increased, causing vasoconstriction and contributing to water retention and hyponatraemia.

**Endothelin** is a potent vasoconstrictor peptide secreted by vascular endothelial cells which promotes renal retention of sodium.

Constriction of the systemic veins and sodium and water retention increase atrial pressure and ventricular end-diastolic volume and pressure, sarcomeres lengthen and myofibril contraction is enhanced (**Frank–Starling mechanism**).

With such a complex interplay of influential factors, cardiac output in the resting state is a relatively insensitive index of cardiac function, because these compensatory mechanisms work to maintain it as the myocardium fails but each of these compensatory mechanisms has a price. For instance, catecholamine- and angiotensin-induced vasoconstriction will increase systemic vascular resistance and tend to maintain blood pressure but increase cardiac work and myocardial oxygen consumption.

### Non-cardiac abnormalities

The **vascular endothelium** plays an important role in the regulation of vascular tone, locally releasing constricting and relaxing factors. The increased peripheral vascular tone in patients with chronic heart failure is due to increased sympathetic activity, activation of the RAA system and impaired release of endothelium derived relaxing factor (EDRF or nitric oxide). Some of the beneficial effects of exercise and certain drug treatments (angiotensin-converting enzyme (ACE) inhibitors) may be due to improvements in endothelial function.

### Diastolic myocardial dysfunction

Impaired myocardial relaxation, due to increased ventricular wall stiffness and reduced compliance, results in impaired diastolic ventricular filling. Ischaemic myocardial fibrosis (coronary artery disease) and LVH (hyperten-

sion, hypertrophic cardiomyopathy) are the commonest causes, but may rarely be due to myocardial infiltration, for instance, amyloid. Diastolic dysfunction often coexists with systolic failure but may occur in isolation in 20–40% of patients presenting with heart failure. The diagnosis of diastolic dysfunction is usually made on echocardiographic measurements (Doppler mitral diastolic flow velocity profile). Differentiation between these two components of heart failure makes little difference to management because it remains uncertain how best to treat diastolic dysfunction.

### Myocardial remodelling, hibernation and stunning

After extensive myocardial infarction, regional hypertrophy of the non-infarcted segments, with wall thinning and cavity dilatation of the infarct territory, constitutes the process of remodelling. This is most pronounced when the infarct-related coronary artery remains occluded rather than recanalized. Even after successful reperfusion, myocardial recovery may be delayed (myocardial stunning). This is in contrast to myocardial hibernation, which describes more persistent myocardial dysfunction at rest, secondary to reduced myocardial perfusion, even though cardiac myocytes remain viable and contractility may improve with revascularization. The stunned or hibernating myocardium remains responsive to inotropic stimulation, and can be assessed by stress echocardiography, radionuclide myocardial perfusion scanning or positron emission tomography (PET).

### Clinical presentation

This is determined by the relative contribution of three factors:
1 cardiac damage;
2 haemodynamic overload; and
3 the secondary compensating mechanisms that arise as heart failure develops.

Initially the compensatory mechanisms may be effective at maintaining cardiac output and the symptoms associated with heart failure may only be present on exercise. Symptoms later occur at rest as the condition worsens.

Clinical manifestations are also influenced by the rate of progression of the disease and whether compensatory mechanisms have had time to develop. For instance, the sudden development of mitral regurgitation may be tolerated poorly and cause acute heart failure, whereas the gradual development of the same amount of mitral regurgitation may be tolerated with few symptoms. In the earlier stages of heart failure, symptoms may be non-specific (malaise, lethargy, fatigue, dyspnoea, exercise intolerance) but as the condition progresses the clinical features may become overtly indicative of cardiac disease. AF occurs in 10–50% of patients with established heart failure, and the onset of AF may precipitate an acute deterioration. Ventricular arrhythmias (ectopics, VT) are increasingly common as heart failure progresses.

Heart failure may principally affect the left heart, right heart or both (biventricular), but in practice the left heart is most often affected. Isolated right heart failure may occur due to major pulmonary embolism, pulmonary hypertension or pulmonary stenosis. The ventricles share the interventricular septum, so dysfunction of either ventricle can potentially influence function of the other. Patients often present with a mixture of symptoms and signs related to both ventricles, but it simplifies matters to consider them as if they occur in isolation.

## Left heart failure (see Box 6.4)

An increase in left atrial pressure raises pulmonary venous pressure and results in pulmonary congestion and eventually alveolar oedema, causing breathlessness, coughing and sometimes haemoptysis. Dyspnoea will initially be present on exercise but as LV failure progresses may occur at rest, causing orthopnoea and paroxysmal nocturnal dyspnoea (PND). Examination will often be normal, but as heart failure progresses the following may be observed:
• the **skin** may be cool and pale reflecting peripheral vasoconstriction;

> ### Box 6.4 Clinical Features of Left Heart Failure
>
> Symptoms
> • Reduced exercise capacity
> • Dyspnoea (wheeze, orthopnoea, PND)
> • Cough (haemoptysis)
> • Lethargy and fatigue
> • Reduced appetite and weight loss
>
> Signs
> • Cool skin
> • Blood pressure (high, low or normal)
> • Pulse (normal or low volume (alternans/tachycardia/arrhythmias)
> • Displaced apex
> • Third sound, summation gallop
> • Functional mitral regurgitation
> • Pulmonary crepitations
> • (± Pleural effusion)

• the **blood pressure** may be high in the case of hypertensive heart disease, normal, or low as cardiac dysfunction worsens;
• the **pulse** may be low volume and the rhythm may be normal, or irregular due to ectopics or AF. **Pulsus alternans** may be noted.

Resting sinus **tachycardia** may reflect severe heart failure or be partly reflex due to drug-induced vasodilatation. The venous pressure is normal in isolated left heart failure. On palpation, the **apex** may be displaced laterally (LV dilatation), the beat sustained (LV hypertrophy) or dyskinetic (LV aneurysm). On **auscultation,** there may be a left ventricular third sound (S3), summation gallop and the murmur of mitral regurgitation secondary to dilatation of the mitral valve ring. Other murmurs may suggest intrinsic valvular heart disease. P2 may be accentuated as pulmonary arterial pressure rises secondary to pulmonary venous hypertension. Pulmonary **crepitations** arise due to alveolar oedema and oedema of the bronchial wall may cause wheezing.

## Right heart failure (see Box 6.5)

Symptoms may be minimal, especially if diuretics have already been given, but when present include:
• ankle swelling;

**Box 6.5  Clinical Features of Right Heart Failure**

Symptoms
- Ankle swelling
- Dyspnoea (but not orthopnoea or PND)
- Reduced exercise capacity
- Chest pain

Signs
- Pulse (tachycardia arrhythmias)
- Raised JVP (±TR)
- Oedema
- Hepatomegaly and ascites
- Parasternal heave
- RV S3 or S4
- (Pleural effusion)

---

- dyspnoea (but not orthopnoea or PND);
- reduced exercise capacity.

As right ventricular (RV) pressure rises or the RV becomes more dilated, chest pain is common.

On examination the **pulse** may show similar abnormalities to left heart failure, the **jugular venous pressure** is often elevated, unless reversed by diuretic treatment, and may show large systolic waves of tricuspid regurgitation. Peripheral **oedema**, **hepatomegaly and ascites** may be present. On palpation there may be a left parasternal heave suggesting RV hypertrophy and/or dilatation, and on auscultation a right ventricular S3 or S4. A pleural effusion may be present with right or left heart failure. Most commonly, the right heart fails secondary to left heart disease, but myocarditis and dilated cardiomyopathy may affect each equally. When the right heart fails sufficiently, the symptoms and signs of left heart failure may diminish because of the inability of the right heart to maintain an output sufficient to keep left-sided filling pressures elevated.

The reduction in cardiac output and reduction in perfusion to organs such as the brain, kidneys and skeletal muscle, whether caused by severe left or right heart failure, results in general symptoms such as mental confusion, tiredness and fatiguability and reduced exercise tolerance. The New York Heart Association (NYHA) has classified functional limitation (see Box 6.6).

**Box 6.6  Functional Classification of Heart Failure (NYHA)**

- Class I: no limitation in physical activity
- Class II: slight limitation of exercise (fatigue, dyspnoea)
- Class III: marked limitation of activity (comfortable at rest but slight exertion causes symptoms)
- Class IV: symptoms even at rest

## Prognosis

The 1-year mortality in patients with heart failure is high (20–60%) and correlates with its severity. Framingham data, collected before the widespread use of vasodilator treatment for heart failure, indicated an average 1-year mortality of 30% when all patients with heart failure are grouped together, and over 60% for those in NYHA class IV. The condition therefore carries a worse prognosis than many cancers. Death occurs due to progressive cardiac failure or suddenly (presumed to be due to arrhythmias) with about equal frequencies. A number of factors correlate with the prognosis in heart failure:

1 **clinical:** the worse the patient's symptoms, exercise capacity and clinical appearance, the worse the prognosis;

2 **haemodynamics:** the lower the cardiac index, stroke volume and ejection fraction, the worse the prognosis;

3 **biochemical:** there are strong inverse correlations with plasma norepinephrine, renin, vasopressin and atrial natriuretic peptide. Hyponatraemia is associated with a poorer prognosis; and

4 **arrhythmias:** frequent ventricular ectopics or ventricular tachycardia on ambulatory ECG monitoring indicate a poor prognosis. It is uncertain whether ventricular arrhythmias are just a marker of poor prognosis or whether the arrhythmia is the cause of death.

### Stroke and thromboembolism

The annual overall incidence of stroke or thromboembolism in heart failure is 2%. Predisposing factors include immobility, low cardiac output, ventricular cavity dilatation or aneurysm, and AF. The annual risk of stroke in heart failure trials has been around 1.5% in mild/moderate heart failure and 4% when severe, compared to 0.5% in controls.

## Investigations

• **Chest radiography** will often show cardiomegaly (cardiothoracic ratio (CTR) >50%), especially when heart failure is chronic. A normal heart size does not exclude the diagnosis and may be seen when left ventricular failure is acute, such as occurs with myocardial infarction, acute valvular regurgitation or post-infarct ventricular septal defect (VSD). Cardiomegaly may be due to left or right ventricular dilatation, LVH or occasionally a pericardial effusion. The degree of cardiomegaly correlates poorly with left ventricular function.

Normally, lung perfusion favours the bases but with pulmonary venous congestion (LV failure) upper lobe diversion occurs and, as pulmonary venous pressure rises above 20 mmHg, interstitial oedema develops causing septal (Kerley B) lines especially at the bases. As pressures rise above 25 mmHg, hilar oedema develops in a butterfly or bat's wing distribution, and perivascular oedema produces haziness of the vessels. Engorgement of the superior vena cava (SVC) and azygos veins may be visible. When heart failure causes pleural effusions they are usually bilateral but if unilateral tend more commonly to occur on the right. Unilateral left-sided effusions should make one think of other causes such as malignancy or pulmonary infarction.

• **Electrocardiography** shows some abnormality in most (80–90%) patients, including Q waves, ST/T wave changes, LV hypertrophy, conduction disturbance, arrhythmias.

• **Echocardiography** should be undertaken in all patients in whom there is justifiable clinical suspicion of heart failure. Cardiac cavity dimensions, ventricular function (systolic and diastolic) and wall motion abnormalities can be assessed, and valvular heart disease can be excluded. Mitral regurgitation is often due to left ventricular enlargement causing mitral ring (annular) dilatation.

• **Ambulatory ECG** monitoring should be undertaken if arrhythmias are suspected.

• **Blood tests** are recommended to exclude anaemia and assess renal function before treatment is started. Thyroid dysfunction (both hyper- and hypothyroidism) may cause heart failure so tests of thyroid function should also be requested. In the future, the measurement of biochemical markers (such as the natriuretic peptides) may prove useful in the diagnosis of heart failure and monitoring its progress.

• **Radionuclide imaging** provides another method of assessing ventricular function (ventriculography) and is especially useful when adequate echocardiographic images are difficult to obtain. Myocardial perfusion scanning may be helpful in assessing the functional significance of coronary artery disease.

• **Cardiac catheterization** should be undertaken when coronary artery disease is suspected, in the rare cases of cardiomyopathy or myocarditis where myocardial biopsy is required, or when an assessment of pulmonary vascular resistance is needed prior to consideration of cardiac transplantation. When cardiac catheterization is indicated, contrast ventriculography is usually undertaken and provides another measure of LV function.

• **Exercise testing** is often undertaken, to assess the presence of myocardial ischaemia and in some cases to measure maximum oxygen consumption ($VO_2$ max). This is the level beyond which oxygen consumption does not rise any further despite increasing levels of exertion. It represents the limit of aerobic exercise tolerance and is often considerably reduced in heart failure.

## Management (see Box 6.7)

### General and lifestyle factors

• **Physical activity** should be tailored to the level of symptoms. Judicious exercise training

## Box 6.7 Management of Heart Failure

General and lifestyle factors
- Physical activity
- Oxygen
- Smoking
- Alcohol
- Vaccination
- Nutrition
- Salt and water

Treatment of any underlying cause
- Coronary disease
- Hypertension
- Cardiomyopathy

Correction of any precipitating factors

Drug therapy
- Diuretics
- Digoxin
- Vasodilators
- Sympathomimetics
- β-blockers
- Anticoagulation
- Anti-arrhythmics

Other
- Intra-aortic balloon counterpulsation
- (Ventricular assist devices)
- (Cardiomyoplasty)
- (Left ventricular reduction surgery)

reduces sympathetic tone, encourages weight reduction, and improves symptoms, the sense of well-being and exercise tolerance in stable, compensated heart failure. Exercise has not been shown to improve myocardial contractility or survival. When an acute deterioration in heart failure occurs, a period of rest may be beneficial. Sitting in an upright position will ease the symptoms of pulmonary venous congestion (orthopnoea, PND), and bed rest increases renal blood flow and helps induce a diuresis.

- **Oxygen** is a pulmonary vasorelaxant, decreasing RV afterload and improving pulmonary blood flow.
- **Smoking** tends to reduce cardiac output, increases heart rate, and increases both systemic and pulmonary vascular resistance, and should be strongly discouraged.
- **Alcohol** consumption alters fluid balance, is negatively inotropic, and may worsen hypertension and precipitate arrhythmias (particularly AF). Abstinence has been shown to result in significant symptomatic and haemodynamic improvements. Its consumption should therefore be kept to a minimum or avoided altogether, especially when thought to be the cause of a cardiomyopathy.

Heart failure predisposes towards pulmonary infections, so patients should be considered for **vaccination** against influenza and pneumococcus.

Some patients with chronic heart failure are at increased risk of malnutrition due to poor appetite, malabsorption and an increase in basal metabolic rate (approx. 20%), so adequate **nutrition** is important. Equally, for those who are obese, successful weight reduction can produce significant improvement in symptoms. Before the discovery of diuretics, Kempner described a rice and fruit diet for the treatment of hypertension and heart failure which proved effective in many cases. With the advent of diuretics, and especially with the potent loop diuretics, dietary sodium restriction became less vital. Nevertheless, symptoms may be improved if the normal daily $Na^+$ intake (3–6 g/day) is reduced. Table salt, processed foods (cheese, sausages, chocolate, many tinned foods, smoked fish) and obviously salty foodstuffs (crisps, peanuts, etc.), should be avoided and consumption of fresh fruit, vegetables and fish encouraged. Potassium chloride (KCl) can be used as a substitute in cooking. It is usually advisable to leave fluid intake to the patient's discretion but in advanced heart failure antidiuretic hormone (ADH) is increased and the patient may not be able to excrete a water load, causing dilutional hyponatraemia. Water intake may need to be restricted if serum sodium falls below 125–130 mmol/L. Diuretic treatment also allows modification of this and an improvement in symptoms in heart failure.

### Treatment of underlying causes

The common underlying causes (coronary artery disease, hypertension, cardiomyopathy) should be optimally treated (see Chapters 4, 5 and 8). For patients with coronary artery disease, revascularization (coronary artery bypass graft (CABG) or percutaneous transluminal coronary angioplasty (PTCA)) may improve cardiac function by reducing ischaemia, and prolong survival. Surgery may also be of benefit when significant valve disease (usually aortic or mitral) is present. If diastolic dysfunction is suspected the use of β-blockers, rate-limiting calcium antagonists (verapamil, diltiazem) or ACE inhibitors (reduce LV hypertrophy) have theoretical merit.

### Correction of precipitating factors

Attention should be paid to any factors which may have precipitated or exacerbated heart failure (e.g. infection, alterations in drug therapy, worsening angina, electrolyte disturbance).

Significant bradycardias should be treated by permanent pacing (see Chapter 9) and interest is developing in the place of biventricular pacing in some patients with severe heart failure. Atrial or ventricular arrhythmias should be treated and implantable defibrillators may be used when life threatening arrhythmias are suspected.

## Drug therapy

### Diuretics (see Box 6.8)

• The **loop diuretics** (bumetanide, furosemide (frusemide)) increase renal sodium and water excretion by their effect on the ascending limb of the loop of Henle but their effect when given orally may diminish in chronic severe heart failure due to impaired gut absorption. They cause significant potassium loss and may cause hyperuricaemia.

• The **thiazide diuretics** (bendroflumethiazide (bendrofluazide), chlorothiazide, hydrochlorothiazide, indapamide, xipamide, chlortalidone, mefruside, metolazone) inhibit salt reabsorption in the distal tubule and promote calcium reabsorption. They are less effective at salt and water removal in heart failure than the loop diuretics and are largely ineffective when the glomerular filtration rate falls below around 30% (common in the elderly). The combined use of loop and thiazide diuretics is often synergistic. The thiazides have a direct vasodilatory effect on peripheral arterioles and may cause carbohydrate intolerance, a slight rise in cholesterol and triglycerides, and hyperuricaemia.

• The **potassium-sparing diuretics** fall into two groups: (i) the aldosterone antagonists (spironolactone); and (ii) inhibitors of sodium conductance in the collecting duct (amiloride, triamterene) which diminish renal potassium and hydrogen ion secretion. These agents are generally used to offset the potassium and magnesium-losing effects of the loop diuretics. Magnesium deficiency probably occurs more often than is appreciated because, being principally an intracellular ion, blood levels are maintained at the expense of intracellular depletion.

### Box 6.8 Diuretics and Dosage

| | |
|---|---|
| Bumetanide | 1–5 mg daily |
| Furosemide (frusemide) | 20–120 mg daily |
| Bendroflumethiazide (bendrofluazide) | 2.5–10 mg daily |
| Hydrochlorothiazide | 25–50 mg daily |
| Indapamide | 2.5 mg once daily |
| Xipamide | 20–80 mg daily |
| Chlortalidone | 50–100 mg daily |
| Mefruside | 25–100 mg daily |
| Metolazone | 2.5–10 mg daily |
| Spironolactone | 25–400 mg daily |
| Amiloride | 5–20 mg daily |
| Triamterene | 100–250 mg daily (divided doses) |
| Mannitol | 50–200 g infusion over 24 hours |

Muscle biopsy may provide a guide to intracellular levels but is rarely undertaken because it is invasive and painful. Deficiency may increase the risk of arrhythmias and cause muscle weakness and fatigue. Supplements are best given intravenously because gut absorption is poor. The use of spironolactone may be limited in men by the development of gynaecomastia as a side-effect.

• The **osmotic diuretics** (mannitol) are able to maintain urine flow at low glomerular filtration rate (GFR) and so may be used in acute severe heart failure, as may occur in the early stages following cardiac bypass surgery. They are filtered by the glomerulus but are not re-absorbed or metabolized by the kidney.

Diuretics often improve symptoms but have not been shown to influence survival except for recent supportive evidence for spironolactone.

## Digoxin

In 1785, William Withering of Birmingham described the use of extract of foxglove (*Digitalis purpurea*). Glycosides such as digoxin increase the velocity of myocardial contraction resulting in positive inotropism. The exact mechanism of action is uncertain but digoxin is a potent inhibitor of cellular sodium pump activity, which results in increased Na–Ca exchange and a rise in intracellular calcium. The effect of this is to increase the availability of calcium ions to the myocardial contractile element at the time of excitation-contraction coupling. The main electrophysiological effect of clinical importance is slowing of conduction through the AV node, although in toxic doses various atrial and ventricular arrhythmias may occur.

Digoxin produces no alteration in cardiac output in normal subjects because cardiac output is determined not just by contractility but by loading conditions and heart rate. In heart failure, digoxin may improve contractility and diminish the secondary compensatory mechanisms which can cause symptoms. The RADIANCE and PROVED trials reported symptomatic benefit, and the Digitalis Investigation Group's (DIG) large study confirmed symptomatic benefit and a reduction in hospital admissions, but no significant improvement in mortality. Digoxin is of particular value when AF is present, because of its effect on slowing the ventricular rate. Digoxin should not be used in hypertrophic cardiomyopathy, where increased contractility may increase left ventricular outflow tract obstruction, and in amyloid heart disease where digoxin accumulates in the myocardium. Magnesium or potassium depletion increase the risk of digoxin-induced arrhythmias.

The **serum therapeutic range** for digoxin is narrow (1–2.0 ng/mL), with toxicity increasingly common at levels >2.5 ng/mL. Digoxin toxicity causes anorexia, nausea, headache, fatigue, malaise, confusion and various visual disturbances including changes in colour vision. Treatment involves early recognition, correction of biochemical abnormalities and lidocaine (lignocaine) or phenytoin for arrhythmias. β-blockers are sometimes helpful. Avoid direct current (DC) cardioversion if possible, which may cause ventricular fibrillation. DC cardioversion should be safe if digoxin levels are within the therapeutic range but low energy shocks should be used initially. In severe overdosage, cardiac glycoside-specific antibodies and their Fab fragments have been used successfully.

## Vasodilators

Vasodilatation reduces cardiac afterload and ventricular wall tension, which is the major determinant of myocardial oxygen demand, decreasing myocardial oxygen consumption and increasing cardiac output. Vasodilators may act principally on the venous (nitrates) or arterial (hydralazine) systems or they may have a mixed venodilator and arterial dilator effect (ACE inhibitors, angiotensin receptor antagonists, prazosin and nitroprusside).

**Arterial dilators** tend to increase cardiac output and venodilators tend to decrease pulmonary venous congestion. Because most patients have both problems, the choice is usually an agent with mixed actions or a combination of drugs from both groups. **Venodilators** reduce preload and, in patients who have been on high doses of diuretics, they may reduce cardiac output and cause postural hypotension. However, in chronic heart failure, the beneficial reduction in filling pressure usually outweighs the decrease in cardiac output and blood pressure. In moderate or severe heart failure, the arterial vasodilators may also lower blood pressure.

A **combination** of hydralazine and isosorbide in mild heart failure (VHeFT I trial) was shown to improve survival, and later the ACE inhibitors enalapril (CONSENSUS and SOLVD trials) and captopril (Captopril Multicentre Heart Failure Trial) were shown to improve survival considerably (20–30% reduction), in moderate/severe heart failure. VHeFT II showed enalapril was better than the combination of hydralazine and isosorbide. The effect of these trials has been considerable, with the ACE inhibitors now being considered for all patients with left ventricular dysfunction. Even asymptomatic patients with LV dysfunction have been shown to have an improved survival (SOLVD-P trial) and there is strong evidence for their prognostic benefit after myocardial infarction (GISSI-III, SMILE, ISIS-4, SAVE, AIRE, TRACE). The reduction in mortality appears to be due to a reduction in deaths from progressive heart failure rather than those due to arrhythmias.

• **Sodium nitroprusside** is an extremely short acting venous and arterial vasodilator and may be useful in acute heart failure. Hydrocyanic acid is released which can cause Cn poisoning when used for more than 2–3 days.

• **ACE inhibitors** (see Table 6.1) (e.g. capto-pril, cilazapril, enalapril, lisinopril, perindopril, quinapril, ramipril, trandolapril) are both veno- and arterial dilators but work particularly on the arteriolar bed. They cause a decrease in angiotensin II, a rise in renin and their effects on tissue as well as plasma ACE may also be important. They interfere with the breakdown of the vasodilator bradykinin and decrease circulating catecholamines (angiotensin II promotes the release and inhibits the reuptake of norepinephrine (noradrenaline) in the sympathetic nervous sytem), thus giving additional vasodilator mechanisms. Their effect is to reduce renal and vascular resistance, increase renal blood flow, and lower blood pressure but without a reflex tachycardia, so lowering myocardial oxygen demand. They also increase β-receptor density in the myocardium. They tend to increase serum potassium so caution is required when used with potassium-sparing diuretics. They are relatively contraindicated in patients with renal failure or bilateral renal artery stenosis and where severe hypotension is present (systolic BP <90 mmHg). Adverse effects on renal function are common in patients with hyponatraemia, those on high doses of loop diuretics, and diabetics. The ACE inhibitors should be started at low dose and then gradually increased to the maximum tolerated, because most trials of survival have used high doses, and the ATLAS trial showed improved all-cause mortality with high rather than low doses of lisinopril. Side-effects of the ACE inhibitors include dry cough,

## ACE INHIBITORS

|  | Starting dose (mg) | Maintenance dose (mg) |
| --- | --- | --- |
| Captopril | 6.25 tds | 25–50 tds |
| Enalapril | 2.5 od | 10–20 bd |
| Lisinopril | 2.5 od | 5–20 od |
| Perindopril | 2.0 od | 4.0 od |
| Quinapril | 2.5–5.0 od | 5–10 bd |
| Ramipril | 1.25–2.5 od | 2.5–5.0 bd |
| Trandolapril | 0.5 od | 2.0–4.0 od |

od, once daily; bd, twice daily; tds, three times daily.

Table 6.1 Doses of ACE inhibitors.

dizziness, a deterioration of renal function and rarely angioneurotic oedema.

• **Angiotensin receptor antagonists** (e.g. candesartan, irbesartan, losartan, valsartan) have been recently developed, have similar haemodynamic effects to the ACE inhibitors, and may have fewer side-effects. Their place in the management of heart failure is yet to be clearly defined but they provide a useful alternative to the ACE inhibitors where these cannot be tolerated, due to side-effects such as a cough.

• **Nitrates** (glyceryl trinitrate, isosorbide dinitrate (30–120 mg in divided doses) or mononitrate (20–120 mg in divided doses)) work principally as venodilators in usual therapeutic doses. Nitrate tolerance tends to occur with prolonged use and so intermittent therapy is ideal. Their use is mainly for heart failure patients with angina or those intolerant of the ACE inhibitors and angiotensin receptor antagonists.

• **Hydralazine** (25–50 mg twice daily) acts directly on arteriolar smooth muscle but side-effects (headaches, flushing, nausea, rashes) are common and the drug may cause a lupus-like syndrome. It is rarely used now that the ACE inhibitors and angiotensin receptor antagonists are available.

• **Prazosin** (1.5–15 mg in divided doses) is an α-blocker with action limited to vascular α-1 receptors and little effect on presynaptic α-2 receptors. It acts equally on venous and arterial vessels, but is much less used now that the ACE inhibitors are available.

• **Calcium antagonists** (nifedipine, verapamil, diltiazem, amlodipine (5–10 mg once daily), felodipine) are vasodilator drugs but also tend to be negatively inotropic, may cause peripheral oedema and are not generally used in the treatment of heart failure. Recent trials of amlodipine (PRAISE) and felodipine (VHeFT III) suggest some beneficial effects and that their use is safe, making them potentially useful agents when hypertension or angina coexist with heart failure.

## Sympathomimetic agents

The unwanted effects of naturally occurring sympathomimetic amines have limited their intravenous use. These include an increase in heart rate (epinephrine (adrenaline) and isoprenaline) and vasoconstriction (norepinephrine (noradrenaline)), the development of tolerance and down-regulation of β-receptors in failing myocardium. However, two intravenous agents (dopamine and dobutamine) cause less tachycardia and fewer systemic vascular effects and are now in widespread use in severe heart failure, particularly when acute.

• **Dopamine** is an endogenous catecholamine and immediate precursor of norepinephrine. It acts directly on β-1 receptors in the myocardium and indirectly on the myocardium by releasing norepinephrine from nerve endings. Vasodilatation secondary to specific activation of dopaminergic receptors in the arterial wall is a dose-dependent effect, with higher doses (>5 μg/kg/min) causing vasoconstriction and reduction in renal blood flow due to stimulation of serotonin and α-1 receptors.

• **Dobutamine** (dose 2.5–10 μg/kg/min) is a synthetic sympathomimetic amine which stimulates β-1, β-2 and α-receptors but does not activate dopaminergic receptors and does not release norepinephrine from nerve endings. It reduces systemic vascular resistance and increases cardiac output. It is not a renal vasodilator and the induction of arrhythmias at higher doses can be a problem. It may cause a reduction in serum potassium.

• **Phosphodiesterase inhibitors** (amrinone, milrinone, enoximone) are positive inotropic agents and cause vasodilation through inhibition of phosphodiesterase III which is responsible for breakdown of cAMP, thus raising intracellular levels of cAMP. They are still used intravenously but trials of their oral use have all shown a disappointing increase in mortality due to their arrhythmogenicity.

## β-blockers

β-adrenoreceptor blockers have traditionally been avoided in heart failure because of their negatively inotropic action. However, the long-term sympathetic stimulation that occurs in chronic heart failure results in down regulation of cardiac β-receptors. By blocking at least some sympathetic activity, the β-blockers may increase β-receptor density and result in greater cardiac sensitivity to the inotropic stimulation of circulating catecholamines. They may also reduce arrhythmias and myocardial ischaemia. Recent randomized trials of carvedilol (US Multicentre Carvedilol Study), bisoprolol (CIBIS I and II) and metoprolol (MERIT-HF) have reported that combining β-blockers with conventional treatment (digoxin, diuretics, ACE inhibitors) results in a reduction in hospital admissions, improved symptoms, LV function and survival. Meta-analysis of the effects of β-blockers on mortality and hospital admissions showed an overall 38% risk reduction. In general, a β-blocker should be started at a very low dose (carvedilol 3.125 mg, bisoprolol 1.25 mg, metoprolol 5 mg), under close medical supervision, and titrated upwards over a few months.

### Anticoagulants in heart failure

The risk of both systemic and pulmonary embolism is increased in heart failure but the place of oral anticoagulation (warfarin) is less clear. Patients in AF or with mitral stenosis, and those with evidence of intracardiac thrombus on investigation, should be anticoagulated unless there are contraindications, aiming for an international normalized ratio (INR) of 2.5–3.0. Those with severe left ventricular dysfunction, those who are relatively immobile and those with a past history suggestive of an embolic event should also be considered for anticoagulation. Aspirin has not been shown to have similar benefit.

### Antiarrhythmic agents

Maintenance of sinus rhythm is of symptomatic benefit in heart failure and amiodarone is the most effective agent at helping to prevent AF and of improving the chances of successful cardioversion if AF is sustained. When AF is chronic, digoxin (0.125–0.25 mg daily) is the most appropriate drug for the control of ventricular rate. Ventricular arrhythmias are a common cause of death in severe heart failure

and may be precipitated by hypokalaemia, hypomagnesaemia, digoxin toxicity, myocardial ischaemia and drugs that may affect electrical stability (proarrhythmic effects of anti-arrhythmic and some antidepressant drugs). Most studies have shown no survival benefit of empirical amiodarone in patients with heart failure, except possibly in cases of non-ischaemic cardiomyopathy (GESICA study, CHF-STAT trial). Amiodarone is best reserved for patients with heart failure and symptomatic ventricular arrhythmias, who should also be considered for insertion of an automatic implantable cardioverter defibrillator (AICD).

## Intra-aortic balloon counterpulsation

In severe left ventricular dysfunction, where the natural history of the underlying condition is one of possible improvement (e.g. early following cardiac surgery or myocardial infarction, in acute myocarditis, or occasionally in unstable angina), the use of aortic balloon counterpulsation may help support the circulation for a number of days or even a few weeks. It may also be used as a bridge towards cardiac transplantation while a donor organ is being sought. A long balloon is inserted percutaneously, usually via a femoral artery, and positioned to lie between the upper part of the descending thoracic aorta, just beyond the origin of the left subclavian artery, and the suprarenal section of the abdominal aorta. A predetermined volume of an inert gas is used to fill the balloon, and subsequent inflation by a bedside pump is synchronized with the ECG to occur in diastole, and deflation to occur at the onset of systole. By so doing, coronary perfusion pressure is increased in diastole and left ventricular afterload is reduced in systole. The patient should be anticoagulated with intravenous heparin whilst the balloon is *in situ*. After removal of the balloon, haemostasis is achieved either by local femoral pressure or surgical arterial repair.

## Ventricular assist devices

Various mechanical devices have been designed which support ventricular function as a bridge to more definitive treatment, such as transplantation. These pumps may either be externally placed and connected to the patient's circulation by tubing, or internally implanted. In patients with severe left ventricular dysfunction, in whom intra-aortic balloon pumping is not sufficient to maintain adequate circulatory support, a left ventricular assist device (VAD) may be used. This requires surgical placement with drainage from the left atrium into a pneumatically driven mechanical pump, the output being returned to the ascending aorta. The similarity to cardiopulmonary bypass is obvious, in this case the assistance being purely for the left ventricle rather than providing total circulatory support.

## Cardiac transplantation

In patients with severely limiting symptoms resulting from myocardial dysfunction, cardiac transplantation remains the only method of improving long-term morbidity and mortality. The widespread use of cardiac transplantation is limited by the availability of donor hearts so that the selection of appropriate patients is highly important. Older patients (age >60 years) are less likely to be accepted for transplantation, as are patients with impaired renal function, other comorbidities or a high pulmonary vascular resistance measured at cardiac catheterization. Once the donor heart has been removed and transported to the recipient, the operative procedure itself is relatively straightforward. With the patient on cardiopulmonary bypass, the heart is removed leaving a cuff of the recipient's left and right atria, the former including the pulmonary veins. The aorta and main pulmonary arteries are transected, allowing removal of the heart, and anastomosis of the donor heart can then be performed to the remaining atrial tissue and great vessels.

Survival following heart transplantation is around 85% at 1 year and 60–70% at 5 years in the best centres. Post-operatively, all patients require immunosuppressive therapy to counter rejection and this in turn increases the risk of infection, particularly viral (e.g. cytomegalovirus). Ciclosporin A is the main antirejection agent, though azathioprine and methylprednisolone may also be required particularly during the early post-operative period, or for treatment of an episode of rejection. In order to identify the possibility of developing rejection at an early stage, all patients undergo regular transvenous cardiac biopsy for histological assessment. Other complications of cardiac transplantation include the development of coronary artery disease in the transplanted heart, and the complications of immunosuppressive therapy such as infection, renal failure, insulin-dependent diabetes, malignancy (particularly lymphoma), cataracts and osteoporosis.

## Cardiomyoplasty

Due to the difficulty in obtaining donor hearts for cardiac transplantation, considerable efforts have been made to develop alternative treatment options such as cardiomyoplasty. The concept of this operation is to use skeletal muscle of the latissimus dorsi to provide extra muscle for cardiac contraction. A flap of latissimus dorsi is wrapped around the left ventricle by moving the muscle through the left chest on its arterial pedicle. A pacemaker is used to trigger skeletal muscle contraction and augment myocardial contractility. The difficulty is that skeletal muscle is easily fatigued and is not suited to the sustained repetitive contraction of the myocardium. However, after about 6 weeks, it can be conditioned to behave like cardiac muscle by repetitive electrical stimulation. During this period there is no significant augmentation of myocardial function. Patients considered potentially suitable for cardiomyoplasty must have enough myocardial reserve to undergo cardiac surgery without any expected benefit in the early post-operative period. This procedure is rarely performed and generally restricted to patients with stable but restricting symptoms who are unsuitable for cardiac transplantation.

## Left ventricular reduction surgery

Because wall tension increases as a function of cavity diameter, some have advocated reducing left ventricular cavity size for those with severe dilatation by surgical resection of a large ellipse of left ventricular free wall and subsequent suturing of the borders to close the defect (Battista operation). No long-term data exist concerning the outcome after this procedure and to date it has been undertaken in only a few centres. It has been suggested that this procedure is surgically analogous to the proven prognostic and symptomatic benefit that can be achieved using the vasodilatory ACE inhibitors, but this extrapolation is unproven and probably simplistic.

## Acute left heart failure (see Box 6.9)

The principles of managing acute, sudden-onset left heart failure are similar to those of the more chronic variety. However, when the heart sustains an acute insult the cardiovascular and neurohormonal systems have little time to adapt and initiate compensatory changes. Patients

therefore tolerate acute heart failure much worse than the same degree of cardiac impairment occurring gradually. The chest radiograph may show a normal heart size if the heart had otherwise been normal before the insult because dilatation takes time to develop. Patients present with anxiety, tachycardia, dyspnoea, hypotension, and oliguria. The commonest causes are shown in Box 6.9.

A patient in acute heart failure with pallor, cool skin, hypotension (systolic <90 mmg), oliguria (<30 mL urine per h), pulmonary oedema and a low cardiac output is regarded as having **cardiogenic shock**, which carries a poor prognosis. The Killip classification of heart failure severity, and approximate mortality for each class is shown in Table 6.2.

Acute heart failure should be assessed and treated urgently. The underlying aetiology should be identified and managed and the haemodynamic state of the patient improved using loop diuretics, oxygen, morphine, vasodilators and inotropic support. The use of these agents is outlined above, in the management of chronic heart failure, though in acute circumstances drugs are more often given

### Box 6.9  Causes of Acute Left Heart Failure

- Myocardial infarction
- Myocarditis
- Sustained arrhythmias
- Acute valvular regurgitation (mitral, aortic)
- Post-infarct VSD

### THE KILLIP CLASSIFICATION

| Class | Clinical features | Hospital mortality (%) |
|-------|-------------------|------------------------|
| Class I | No signs of LV dysfunction | 0–6% |
| Class II | S3 gallop with or without pulmonary congestion | 30% |
| Class III | Acute severe pulmonary oedema | 40% |
| Class IV | Cardiogenic shock | >80% |

Table 6.2 The Killip classification of heart failure severity.

intravenously. The patient should ideally be managed in a high dependency or intensive care area and consideration given to inserting a urinary catheter (to monitor hourly urine output), a pulmonary artery flotation (Swan–Ganz) catheter for haemodynamic monitoring, an intra-aortic balloon pump and using mechanical ventilation. Where the problem is valvular or an acute VSD, cardiac surgery should be considered.

## Further reading

Gibbs CR, Davies MK, Lip GYH, eds. *The ABC of Heart Failure*. London: BMJ Publishing Group, 2000.

# CHAPTER 7

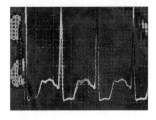

# Thrombosis in Cardiovascular Disease

## Pathophysiology

### Vascular endothelium

Vascular endothelial cells have an important influence on vasomotor tone and local haemostasis. Carrier mechanisms in endothelial cell membranes specifically transport the vasoactive substances serotonin, adenosine and adenine nucleotides, and angiotensin-converting enzyme on the outer cell surface inactivates the vasodilator bradykinin. The cells themselves synthesize vasoactive substances such as prostacyclin, endothelium-derived relaxing factor (nitric oxide) or constricting (endothelin) factors, and platelet activating factors (PAF). In response to vascular injury, smooth muscle in arterioles and venules contracts and prostacyclin production is stimulated by contact with activated platelets or leucocytes. Prostacyclin has strong antiplatelet and vasodilatory properties and is thus the biological antagonist to the platelet-derived vasoconstrictor, thromboxane $A_2$. It has been suggested that a deficiency in endothelial prostacyclin production contributes to the pathogenesis of atherosclerosis.

### Platelets

Vessel injury exposes subendothelial connective tissue to the blood, stimulating platelet adherence. Vascular collagen and fibronectin interact with platelets, particularly with their membrane glycoproteins (Ia/IIa and Ic/IIa), and von Willebrand factor is required for platelet adhesion. Through the action of activators such as collagen, and eventually thrombin and norepinephrine (noradrenaline), the adhered platelets become activated, and in turn express other platelet receptors and release several mediators (calcium, adenosine diphosphate (ADP), serotonin and thromboxane $A_2$) which are potent inducers of further platelet aggregation. Platelet membrane glycoproteins IIb–IIIa interact with plasma fibrinogen and other adhesive proteins such as fibronectin to tighten the platelet aggregate.

### Coagulation

The traditional coagulation cascade is divided into the 'intrinsic' and 'extrinsic' pathways, although interaction between these pathways exists.

• In the **intrinsic pathway**, all participating factors (kininogen, prekallikrein, kallikrein, calcium, factors VIIIa, IX, XI, XII) are present in the circulating blood, and the reaction sequence is initiated by activated platelets.

• In the **extrinsic system**, membrane-bound tissue factor sets off the chain of events which require calcium and factors VII, IX, XI.

Both pathways eventually stimulate factor X which in turn activates prothrombinase (an association of factor Va and factor Xa on a phospholipid), which cleaves prothrombin to produce thrombin.

**Thrombin** represents the culmination of the coagulation cascade and once stimulated, enhances its own production by a positive feedback mechanism. Thrombin acts on the polymer fibrinogen to produce fibrin monomers. A number of proteins circulate in the blood to inhibit the coagulation cascade, particularly antithrombin III (enhanced by heparin) and proteins C and S. However, thrombin, which is bound to fibrin, is protected from antithrombin III, and its release in this protected form during thrombolysis can stimulate rethrombosis.

## Fibrinolysis

This is regulated by controlled activation and inhibition (see Fig. 7.1). Increased levels of PAI-1 activity, resulting in decreased fibrinolytic capacity, have been reported in several thrombotic states including:

- venous thromboembolism;
- sepsis;
- obesity;
- unstable angina;
- acute myocardial infarction.

Both systemically and locally increased PAI-1 concentrations could have a pathogenic role in the development of atherosclerotic disease.

## Antithrombotic drugs

### Heparin

**Unfractionated heparin** refers not to a single structure but rather to a family of mucopolysaccharide chains. It accelerates the action of naturally occurring antithrombin III

and, at high doses, heparin cofactor II. In plasma, approximately 20 times more unfractionated heparin is needed to inactivate fibrin-bound thrombin than to inactivate free thrombin. This explains why more heparin is needed to prevent the extension of venous thrombosis than to prevent formation of the initial thrombus. Heparin is not absorbed through the gastrointestinal mucosa. When in the bloodstream after parenteral administration, heparin binds to endothelial cells, mononuclear macrophages and numerous plasma proteins. Elevated levels of these proteins explain the different individual doses of heparin required to produce the same antithrombotic effect, and the 'heparin resistance' seen in patients with inflammatory and malignant diseases.

The pharmacokinetics of unfractionated heparin are complicated and the dose (usually 24 000–36 000 iu/24 h) needs to be monitored, most commonly by the activated partial thromboplastin time (aPTT). The most common side-effect of heparin is bleeding, which is higher when unfractionated heparin is given by intermittent (14%) rather than continuous infusion (7%), or subcutaneously (4%). Heparin-induced thrombocytopenia occurs in 2.4% of patients receiving therapeutic doses. Some of the limitations of unfractionated heparin can be overcome with **low molecular weight** (LMW) **heparins** (e.g. enoxaparin) which have less protein binding, reduced plasma clearance, less effect on platelets and fewer bleeding complications. Their long half-life, and predictable

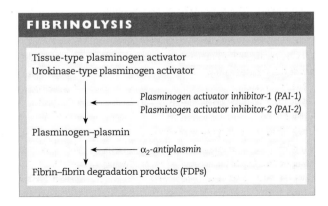

## FIBRINOLYSIS

Tissue-type plasminogen activator
Urokinase-type plasminogen activator

    Plasminogen activator inhibitor-1 (PAI-1)
    Plasminogen activator inhibitor-2 (PAI-2)

Plasminogen–plasmin

    $\alpha_2$-antiplasmin

Fibrin–fibrin degradation products (FDPs)

Fig. 7.1 Fibrinolytic pathway.

anticoagulant response to weight-adjusted doses, allow once- or twice-daily subcutaneous administration without laboratory monitoring. Usual dose of enoxaparin for prophylaxis against deep venous thrombosis (DVT) is 20–40 mg per day, and for more complete anticoagulation (e.g. as treatment for DVT, unstable angina) is 0.75–1.0 mg/kg/12 h.

## Oral anticoagulants

Warfarin and related coumarin agents inhibit the hepatic production of vitamin K-dependent clotting factors (II, VII, IX, X) and of proteins C and S. The intensity of the effect of warfarin differs between patients and varies for the same individual over time. Its action is affected by many drugs, foods and intercurrent illnesses such as hepatic failure, heart failure and hyperthyroidism. The laboratory test used to monitor its effect is the prothrombin time, now standardized into the international normalized ratio (INR). At the start of warfarin treatment the prothrombin time is prolonged but the intrinsic pathway may still be temporarily unaffected. This is the reason why, in switching from heparin to warfarin, heparin should be continued for at least 24 hours after an adequate INR has been achieved. The usual maintenance dose is 1–12 mg once daily. Bleeding is the most common side-effect and is influenced by other factors such as age, hypertension, recent surgery and malignant disease. On average, the overall annual bleeding risk is 6%, with major and fatal episodes being 2% and 0.8%, respectively. A rare complication is coumarin-induced skin necrosis, the aetiology of which is unknown and which occurs on the 3rd to 8th day after starting. Coumarin drugs readily cross the placenta and may be teratogenic, particularly during the first trimester of pregnancy.

## Platelet inhibitors (see Box 7.1)

• The ideal dose of **aspirin** in cardiovascular diseases is unclear but doses between 1 and 2 mg/kg daily produce virtually complete platelet inhibition. Slow release, enteric-coated preparations produce fewer gastrointestinal side-effects.

---

> ### Box 7.1  Reducing Platelet Activity
>
> • Inhibition of prostaglandin synthase (aspirin, sulfinpyrazone, flurbiprofen, indobufen)
> • Inhibition of thromboxane synthase (aspirin)
> • Blockade of endoperoxide-thromboxane receptors
> • Inhibition of the activation pathway or glycoprotein IIb/IIIa (ticlopidine, clopidogrel)

---

• **Ticlopidine** and **clopidogrel** are thenopyridine derivatives that are bioprecursors, requiring production of at least one active metabolite *in vivo*. Clopidogrel is approximately six times as active as ticlopidine in inhibiting human platelet aggregation. The effectiveness of ticlopidine has been demonstrated in a number of clinical scenarios (cerebral ischaemic events, ischaemic heart disease) but may cause bone marrow suppression (leucopenia, thrombocytopenia, pancytopenia) in up to 1% of patients treated, requiring regular blood tests. Clopidogrel (75 mg per day) was developed because it is not toxic to bone marrow, but fewer data are available on its use at present.

Exposure of glycoprotein IIb/IIIa receptors at the platelet surface is the final common endpoint of all pathways leading to platelet aggregation. The **monoclonal antibody** recombinant abciximab, was the first specific IIb/IIIa receptor inhibitor to be developed and was shown to reduce the rate of death and primary cardiovascular endpoints following 'high risk' angioplasty by 35%, but at the expense of bleeding complications. It has to be given intravenously. **Synthetic IIb/IIIa inhibitors** (fradafiban, tirofiban, lamifiban) are reversible receptor antagonists and have the advantages over monoclonal agents of a much shorter duration of action (3 hours as opposed to 3 days) and being active when given orally, although their place in clinical practice when given orally has yet to be established.

## Specific thrombin inhibitors

Recombinant **hirudin** is obtained from *E. coli*

and yeast. Unlike heparin, which requires endogenous cofactors (antithrombin III, heparin cofactor II), does not penetrate thrombus and does not reduce platelet deposition, hirudin is active against thrombin without cofactors, penetrates thrombus, neutralizes thrombin bound to fibrin and reduces platelet deposition and thrombus growth. **Hirulog** is the synthetic analogue of hirudin. Neither has an antidote but the half-life is only around 2 hours. These agents have been used in some trials but only infrequently in routine clinical practice.

## Thrombolytic drugs (see Chapter 8)

• **Streptokinase** is a non-enzyme protein produced by several strains of haemolytic streptococci, and indirectly activates the conversion of plasminogen to plasmin. Most people have circulating antibodies to streptokinase, due to previous streptococcal exposure, so a sufficient dose must be infused to overcome this resistance. Antibody titres rise rapidly a few days after streptokinase administration, so further doses are considerably less effective and produce an allergic response if given within 4–6 months.
• **Anisoylated plasminogen–streptokinase activator complex** (APSAC) was developed to create a more predictable thrombolytic effect. It requires deacylation *in vivo* before being effective in converting plasminogen to plasmin, and antibodies to streptokinase also cross react with APSAC.
• **Urokinase**, a trypsin-like serine protease, can be isolated from human urine or cultured human embryonic kidney cells. It has been used as an alternative to streptokinase in the USA but rarely used in the UK. Recombinant prourokinase was later produced.
• **Recombinant tissue-type plasminogen activator (rt-PA)** is a serine protease which is converted to plasmin by hydrolysis *in vivo*. The presence of fibrin enhances the efficiency of plasminogen activation by rt-PA by two to three times. The high affinity of rt-PA for plasminogen in the presence of fibrin thus allows

activation of the fibrin clot, without plasminogen activation in the plasma.

## Specific cardiovascular conditions

### Risk reduction

Of all the risk factors for cardiovascular events (lipids, smoking, hypertension, family history, etc.), the most important for the prediction of future events is the presence of pre-existing disease. Hence, strategies for risk reduction are much more likely to be effective once the disease is present (secondary prevention) rather than before the disease has declared itself (primary prevention). This is not to say that primary prevention is ineffective, it is merely that the magnitude of the effect is less. For instance, in unstable angina the risk of a recurrent cardiovascular event is 6–10% per year, in stable angina it is around 2–4% per year, and in those not known to have coronary artery disease the risk is approximately 1% per year. If one accepts that aspirin may reduce this risk of a further cardiovascular event by 25–30%, treatment of the highest risk patients with unstable angina will reduce their risk to around <7%, those with stable angina to <3% and those who are asymptomatic to <0.7%. The **relative** risk reduction is the same, but the **absolute** risk reduction is very different. What matters in terms of cost-effective intervention is the absolute risk reduction.

### Unstable angina (see Chapter 8)

Antiplatelet agents have been shown to reduce acute myocardial infarction, and both short- and long-term mortality. Aspirin is the agent most widely used, but ticlopidine has also been shown to be effective. Heparin produces a similar, and possibly slightly greater benefit but its combination with aspirin produces only a small additional effect. However, aspirin reduces the rebound prothrombotic tendency that can occur when heparin is stopped, and in routine practice both heparin and aspirin are usually used together. Hirudin has also been investigated but was found to have a high incidence of bleeding complications. Thrombolytic agents have not been found to be beneficial.

### Acute myocardial infarction (see Chapter 8)

The Fibrinolytic Therapy Trialists' (FTT) Collaborative Group reported an overview of over 58 000 patients enrolled into trials of myocardial infarction and found an overall reduction in mortality of 18%, lowering the absolute risk from 11.5% to 9.6%. The clot specificity of rt-PA compared to streptokinase is an advantage, but rt-PA is considerably more expensive and may be associated with a slightly higher risk of haemorrhagic stroke. In the UK, streptokinase tends to be used as the first-line agent, followed by rt-PA if further thrombolysis is required later on the same admission or within the next 6 months. Achieving early administration of a thrombolytic drug is much more important than the choice of agent. **Aspirin** given as well as a thrombolytic results in even greater benefit, increasing the relative risk reduction in mortality to 42% in the ISIS-2 trial. Most of the data supporting the routine use of heparin preceded the thrombolytic era, but it should be considered in those at high risk who have large infarcts (especially anterior), those in atrial fibrillation (AF) and those who have congestive heart failure. Adjunctive heparin has been shown to enhance the benefit of rt-PA.

### Coronary bypass grafting (see Chapter 8)

The original Mayo Clinic trial on saphenous vein coronary grafts showed aspirin and dipyridamole to reduce the early graft occlusion rate from 10% to 2%. Aspirin (75–300 mg) is usually prescribed indefinitely. Dipyridamole is no longer routinely used. Ticlopidine or clopidogrel can be used as an alternative for those who cannot tolerate aspirin.

### Coronary angioplasty and stenting (see Chapter 8)

Treatment with long-term aspirin (75–300 mg) and periprocedural heparin is usual, but based on extrapolations from data showing benefit in other clinical situations rather than on randomized trials in angioplasty. Glycoprotein IIb/IIIa platelet receptor antagonists have been shown to reduce acute complications following higher risk procedures. Oral anticoagulation used to be used for 3 months following stent insertion but better acute stent thrombosis rates can be achieved with a combination of aspirin (150 mg) and clopidogrel (150 mg preprocedure and 75 mg once daily for 2–4 weeks postprocedure), and with a significantly lower bleeding complication rate.

### Stable coronary disease (see Chapter 8)

• **Aspirin** (75–300 mg) reduces mortality by 13%, reinfarction rate by 31% and non-fatal stroke by 42% following acute myocardial infarction.
• **Warfarin** also reduces the frequency of the same complications, but is not used routinely as its benefit is no greater than aspirin's, and it is more inconvenient to administer and more expensive.

### Primary prevention

Because of its proven benefit in secondary prevention, aspirin has been investigated in two large trials of primary prevention involving male medical practitioners in the USA and UK. No benefit was demonstrated in the UK trial, but a reduction in myocardial infarction from 0.4% to 0.2% was seen in the trial from the USA, although this benefit was confined to those over 50 years of age. As can be seen, the absolute risk reduction was small. No data are yet available for women.

### Atrial thrombosis in valvular disease

This occurs mainly in patients with mitral valve disease, and especially in those with mitral stenosis (MS) in AF. Transoesophageal echocardiography (TOE) provides useful data because it gives excellent images of the left atrium (LA) and atrial appendage, and may show evidence of sluggish atrial blood flow (see Chapter 3). On the basis of autopsy studies in non-anticoagulated patients with rheumatic heart disease, about 50% of patients with AF have atrial thrombus compared to 15% of those in sinus rhythm. Up to 75% of clinically significant embolic episodes from LA thrombus involve the cerebral circulation. The risk of emboli increases with age and previous episodes of embolization. In the absence of AF, pure mitral regurgitation (MR) has a low incidence of embolic episodes. Mitral valve prolapse and aortic valve disease have a very low incidence.

No prospective trial has investigated the benefit of oral anticoagulation in MS, probably because this treatment has been accepted clinically to be beneficial for so many years that it would be unethical to randomize patients to no anticoagulation. Patients in AF with MS are at highest risk and should be anticoagulated to an INR of 2.5–3.5. Patients with mixed MS and MR or severe pure MR should be maintained at an INR of 2.0–3.0. Those with mitral valve prolapse and a history of a transient cerebral event (transient ischaemic attack (TIA)) should be treated with aspirin, but those who have had a stroke, in the absence of an alternative cause, should be considered for anticoagulation (INR 2.0–3.0). Anticoagulation is not required for aortic valve disease or infective endocarditis, unless AF is present.

## Non-valvular AF

AF carries a substantially increased risk of embolic stroke even in the absence of valvular disease — as high as 5% per year in the elderly (six times the normal risk). However, the absolute risk of emboli in idiopathic AF depends crucially on the presence of other risk factors, being positively correlated with:

- increasing age;
- presence of systemic hypertension;
- diabetes;
- recent heart failure;
- previous stroke;
- cerebral TIA.

Echocardiographic predictors of increased risk include an enlarged LA and impaired left ventricular function. TOE is a particularly useful investigation to stratify patients at risk.

Those without additional risk factors should be advised to take daily aspirin (300 mg) and those with additional risk factors should be anticoagulated (INR 2.0–3.0). Data is lacking for anticoagulation in those >75 years, who may actually be at high risk, because the benefit of anticoagulation is significantly offset by a higher incidence of bleeding complications.

## Cardioversion

Systemic embolization is a complication of electrical and pharmacological cardioversion, when the ineffective atrial contraction of AF is converted to the mechanically more efficient sinus rhythm. No randomized trials have been undertaken but, in the absence of a contraindication, it is generally accepted that all patients who have been in AF for longer than 48 hours should be anticoagulated (INR 2.5–3.0) for 3 weeks before, and at least 3 weeks after, successful cardioversion. Little data are available for patients with AF of <48 hours, but most would anticoagulate with heparin. Increasingly, TOE is undertaken in this situation to help determine whether intracardiac thrombus is present.

## Ventricular thrombus

Left ventricular thrombus occurs in approximately 30% of anterior myocardial infarcts, compared to only 5% of those with inferior ones. Other factors that predict the development of thrombus include poor ejection fraction (<35%), size of infarct and the presence of AF. Combining the data from several large trials, the risk of stroke (from any cause) after MI averages 2.9%, although this has probably now fallen with more widespread use of thrombolytic agents. When ventricular thrombus does occur, it generally does so in the first 7 days after infarction. About 75–90% will be detectable on transthoracic echocardiography (TTE). Meta-analysis of a number of trials suggest that anticoagulation reduces the risk of emboli. During hospitalization, many advocate the use of subcutaneous heparin (12 500 IU twice daily) for all patients with anterior infarcts, and oral anticoagulation (INR 2.0–3.0) after discharge for those with large anterior infarcts.

In the first 3 months after infarction, left ventricular aneurysms have a 10% risk of embolization and oral anticoagulation is advisable for this period. Chronic left ventricular aneurysms carry a surprisingly low risk of embolization in the long term and do not routinely require anticoagulation. Patients with aneurysms and global severe left ventricular dysfunction, mobile thrombus in the left ventricle (LV) or those with previous emboli, should be anticoagulated long term (INR 2.0–3.0).

## Dilated cardiomyopathy

In dilated (idiopathic) cardiomyopathy autopsy studies show a high risk of mural thrombi (50% in LV, 25% in right ventricle, 20% in right atrium (RA), 8% in LA). Patients not receiving anticoagulants have an overall risk of around 18% of an embolic episode (14% if in sinus rhythm and 33% if in AF). The risk increases with the severity of LV dysfunction. Anticoagulation (INR 2.0–3.0) is advisable in the absence of contraindications for all patients who are significantly affected by this condition. For some reason, the risk of emboli is much lower in ischaemic cardiomyopathy and anticoagulation is indicated only for those in AF, those with previous embolism and those with poor ejection fraction together with LV thrombus visible on echocardiography.

## Prosthetic heart valves

The risk of thromboembolism varies depending on the type of valve (bioprosthetic or mechanical), the particular design (e.g. Starr Edwards, St Jude, Carbomedics, etc.), the position (mitral or aortic) into which it is inserted and the presence of other factors (AF, LV dysfunction, previous emboli, etc.). Overall, there has been a decreasing risk of thrombus formation on prosthetic valves as their design has improved, and hence the degree of anticoagulation required has tended to decline. A balance has always to be struck between optimum protection from thrombus development and minimizing the risk of bleeding complications. Perhaps the most important thing to stress to patients requiring anticoagulation is the need to maintain adequate and as consistent anticoagulation as possible.

General agreement exists that all mechanical prostheses should be anticoagulated, with the risk of emboli being higher for valves in the mitral than the aortic position. An INR of 2.5–3.5 is sufficient for those with no other embolic risk factors, but an INR of 3.0–4.5 should be achieved for those at higher risk. Several trials have suggested an even lower rate of embolism and death when antiplatelet agents (usually aspirin) are combined with warfarin, but this additional benefit may mostly have been due to a reduction in the rate of myocardial infarction in these patients. In the absence of other risk factors, bioprostheses do not require long-term anticoagulation, although some advocate 3 months anticoagulation (INR 2.0–3.0) after surgery, a time when the risk of thrombus forming on the bioprosthesis is higher.

Patients with prosthetic valves requiring anticoagulation should not have their anticoagulants stopped unless absolutely necessary. When patients undergo non-cardiac surgery, and anticoagulation is felt to be hazardous, warfarin can be stopped 3–4 days before the proposed surgery and heparin substituted to maintain an aPTT ratio of 2.0–2.5 times normal. The heparin can then be stopped 4–6 hours preoperatively, allowing near normal coagulation for the operative period, and restarted as soon as haemostasis is felt to be satisfactory.

Patients with a prosthetic valve who are anticoagulated and have a stroke should have a computerized tomographic (CT) or magnetic resonance imaging (MRI) scan of the head. If the stroke is embolic and only of moderate size, anticoagulation should be continued unless temporarily contraindicated by severe systemic hypertension, and the later addition of an antiplatelet agent should be considered. If the stroke is haemorrhagic or due to a large embolic infarct, anticoagulation should be omitted for 5–7 days.

## Further reading

Fuster V, Verstraete M. Haemostasis, thrombosis, fibrinolysis and cardiovascular disease. In: Braunwald E, ed. *Heart Disease*. London: WB Saunders Co, 1997: 1809–43.

# CHAPTER 8

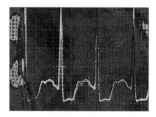

# Coronary Heart Disease

## Epidemiology

In the UK, cardiovascular disease kills one in two of the population, and accounted for nearly 250000 deaths in 1998. One in four men and one in five women die annually from CHD, which represents approximately half of the deaths from cardiovascular disease. There is a misconception that CHD occurs rarely in women: in fact, there is little difference in the incidence of the disease taking into account the longer life expectancy of women compared with men.

Although CHD remains the main cause of premature mortality in the UK, death rates have been falling progressively over the last 20 years. This is particularly true for the younger age groups, where, for example, there has been a 33% fall for men aged 35–74 years and a 20% fall for women in a similar age range over the last 10 years. Many other countries including Australia, Sweden, France and the US, have exceeded the UK's fall in mortality.

Death rates for CHD in the UK remain some of the highest in the Western world, exceeded by only Ireland within Europe. In the UK, there are marked regional, socio-economic and ethnic differences in the prevalence of CHD, rates being higher in the north of England and Scotland, in manual workers and in the Asian population.

A reduction in death rate from CHD was one of the ambitious targets in *The Health of the Nation* paper (Department of Health, 1996). *The Health Survey for England* (Department of Health, 1996) suggests that 3% of adults suffer from angina and that 0.5% of adults have had a myocardial infarct within the last 12 months, equating to 1.4 million and 246000 people, respectively. CHD accounts for approximately 3% of all hospital admissions—that is 284292 admissions with a mean length of stay of 6.6 days.

CHD costs the National Health Service in the UK £1630 million per year. Of these costs, inpatient care accounts for 54%, and primary prevention only 1% (£12 million). Sixty five million working days are lost each year due to CHD, representing 9% of all working days lost. Thus, the total economic burden of CHD in the UK is approximately £10000 million per year. The provision for the investigation and treatment of patients with CHD in the UK falls far behind Europe, with a significant minority of the population not having immediate access to a specialist cardiologist in their local hospital. The recently published *National Service Framework for Coronary Heart Disease* (Department of Health, 2000) sets a series of targets for the investigation and treatment of the patient with CHD, from primary through to tertiary care; the document also attempts to standardize access to facilities across the United Kingdom.

## Box 8.1  Selected Risk Factors for CHD

- Elevated cholesterol
- Smoking
- Obesity
- Diabetes mellitus
- Systemic hypertension
- Male gender
- Family history (CHD)
- Personality
- Physical activity
- Clotting disorders

## Risk factors (see Box 8.1)

### Lipids and diet

The percentage of food energy derived from fat in the British diet has fallen gradually over the last 20 years from 42% to 39%. More impressive has been the shift away from saturated fat intake, from 20% to 16%. The significant regional differences in fat intake are matched by the increase in fresh fruit and vegetable consumption in the south, particularly amongst the professional classes.

There is a direct relationship between the risk of CHD and levels of blood cholesterol. In the UK, cholesterol levels are high.
- In men the mean blood cholesterol is 5.8 mmol/L.
- In women it is 6.0 mmol/L.
- Approximately one-third of the UK population have levels in excess of 6.5 mmol/L which would be regarded as high.

Cholesterol is transported in the blood in the form of lipoproteins, 75% as low density lipoprotein (LDL) and 20% as high density lipoprotein (HDL). Low levels of LDL cholesterol are implicated in CHD and there is an inverse relationship between HDL levels and the incidence of CHD.

The role of triglycerides as a risk factor for CHD is controversial. Grossly elevated triglyceride levels are associated with pancreatitis and should be treated. Similarly combined hyperlipidaemia (e.g. in diabetics) warrants intervention, but the power of triglyceride as a risk factor once cholesterol has been normalized is weak.

Increased levels of lipoprotein (a) are an independent risk factor for CHD. The function of this protein is unclear, but it has been implicated in familial CHD risk and can be found in atherosclerotic plaque in association with fibrinogen.

### Smoking

Approximately 24% of deaths from CHD in men and 11% in women are due to smoking. Although there has been a progressive decline in the proportion of the population who smoke since the 1970s, in 1996 29% of men and 28% of women still smoked. Of particular concern is the prevalence of smoking in teenagers, which is increasing, especially in young girls. Non-smokers who live with smokers (i.e. passive smokers) have a 20–30% increase in risk compared with those living with other non-smokers. The risk of developing CHD from smoking is dose related with those smoking 20 or more cigarettes daily having a risk of two to three times that of the general population of developing a major coronary event.

The role of smoking in the pathogenesis of CHD is complex and includes:
- promotion of atherosclerosis;
- increase in thrombogenesis and vasoconstriction (including coronary artery spasm);
- increase in blood pressure (BP) and heart rate;
- provocation of cardiac arrhythmias;
- increase in myocardial oxygen demand;
- reduction in oxygen-carrying capacity.

The risk of developing CHD from smoking falls to 50% 1 year after smoking cessation, and to normal within 4 years of quitting the habit.

Smoking is also a major risk factor in the development of:
- lung cancer;
- chronic airflow obstruction (chronic bronchitis and emphysema);
- cerebral and peripheral vascular disease;
- abdominal aortic aneurysm;
- recurrent angina following coronary revascularization procedures (coronary artery bypass grafting (CABG) and coronary angioplasty).

## Obesity

There is an interrelationship between weight, an elevated BP, raised blood cholesterol, non-insulin dependent diabetes mellitus and low levels of physical activity. The proportion of the population who are classified as obese (body mass index (BMI) >30 kg/m$^2$) in the UK has increased progressively in the last 20 years. Approximately 17% of men and 20% of women are obese, and an additional 45% of men and 33% of women are judged to be overweight (BMI 25–30 kgs/m$^2$).

## Diabetes mellitus

Diabetics have more severe, more aggressive, more complex and more diffuse CHD than do age-matched controls. In general, coronary disease develops at a younger age than in the non-diabetic patient. In insulin dependent diabetes, premature coronary disease is detectable in population studies from the 4th decade, and by the age of 55 years up to one-third of patients have died from the complications of CHD: the presence of microalbuminaemia or diabetic nephropathy increases the risk of CHD significantly.

The risk of developing CHD in the patient with NIDDM is two to four times higher than the general population and does not appear to relate to either the severity or the duration of the diabetes, possibly because the presence of insulin resistance may predate the onset of clinical symptoms by 15–25 years.

Diabetes, although an independent risk factor for CHD, is also associated with the presence of abnormalities of lipid metabolism, obesity, systemic hypertension and an increase in thrombogenesis (increased platelet adhesiveness and elevated levels of fibrinogen). Late results of CABG are less favourable in diabetics, and diabetics have both an increased early mortality and a higher risk of restenosis following coronary angioplasty.

## Systemic hypertension (see Chapter 4)

The risk of CHD is directly related to BP: for each 5 mmHg reduction in diastolic BP the risk of CHD is reduced by approximately 16%. BP values for the UK population are generally high:
approximately 10% of men and 8% of women are hypertensive, defined as a systolic BP of more than 160 mmHg and a diastolic pressure of more than 95 mmHg.

## Gender and sex hormones

Morbidity from CHD in males is twice that in females and the condition occurs approximately 10 years earlier in men compared with women. Endogenous oestrogen is protective in women, but after the menopause the incidence of CHD rises steeply and parallels that seen in men. Smokers have an earlier menopause than non-smokers. Symptoms from CHD in women may be atypical: this, coupled with gender bias, difficulties with interpretation of standard investigations (e.g. treadmill exercise test) leads to the under-investigation of females compared with males. Furthermore, the results of revascularization procedures are more beneficial in men and are associated with a higher perioperative complication rate in women.

The use of oral contraceptives increases the risk of CHD approximately threefold with some evidence that the risk with the newer third generation preparations may be less. There is a synergistic relationship between oral contraceptive use and smoking, with a relative risk for myocardial infarction of more than 20 : 1.

## Family history

A family history of CHD in a first-degree relative aged less than 70 years is an independent risk factor for the presence of CHD, with an odds ratio of two to four times that of a control population. Family aggregation of CHD suggests a genetic predisposition to the condition. There is some evidence that a positive family history may influence the age of onset of CHD in near relatives.

## Race

Asians living in the UK have a higher incidence of premature death from CHD than the indigenous population, which is matched by a lower rate for Afro-Caribbeans.

## Geography

Death rates from CHD are higher in Northern

Ireland, Scotland and the north of England, and may reflect in part differences in diet, water hardness, smoking, the socio-economic structure and urban living.

## Social class

Socio-economic gradients in CHD mortality are widening, such that premature death rates from CHD are three times higher for male unskilled workers compared with members of the professions (e.g. doctors, lawyers). Furthermore, the wives of manual workers are at least twice as likely to die prematurely from CHD as the wives of non-manual workers. Other risk factors are interrelated, including diet, cigarette consumption, obesity and exercise etc.

## Personality

Stress, either physical or mental, is a risk factor for CHD. In the present era, the work environment has become a major cause of stress, and there is an interrelationship between stress and abnormalities of lipid metabolism.

Coronary prone behavior (Type A personality) includes aggression, competitiveness, hostility, cynicism, desire for recognition and achievement, sleep disturbance, road rage etc. Both anxiety and depression are important predictors of CHD.

## Physical activity

Regular aerobic activity reduces the risk of CHD, although only 11% of men and 4% of women meet government targets for exercise. It is estimated that one-third of men and two-thirds of women cannot sustain a normal walking pace up a gradual slope (3 mph up a 5% gradient). Regular exercise may be associated with a 20–40% reduction in the incidence of CHD.

## Clotting

A number of thrombogenic elements may influence the incidence of CHD, including levels of fibrinogen, endogenous fibrinolytic activity, blood viscosity and the levels of Factors VII and VIII. Inhibitors of plasminogen activators (e.g. plasminogen activator inhibitor PAI-1) appear to be increased in some patients with CHD. The increased incidence of CHD in patients with the rare autosomal recessive disorder of homocystinuria may be manifest through altered clotting.

## Infection

Infection with *Chlamydia pneumoniae*, an intracellular Gram-negative organism and a common cause of respiratory disease, does appear to be linked to the presence of atherosclerotic coronary disease.

## Alcohol

Although there is a theoretical basis for the protective effect of low-to-moderate doses of alcohol, this is controversial. Alcohol in low dose increases endogenous thrombolysis, reduces platelet adhesion and increases circulating levels of HDL, but the literature is not uniformly supportive of the concept. Increasing doses of alcohol are associated with an increase in cardiovascular mortality due to arrhythmias, systemic hypertension and dilated cardiomyopathy.

## Pathophysiology

Angina pectoris occurs as a consequence of myocardial ischaemia. Oxygen supply fails to meet oxygen demand, due invariably to a reduction in supply as a consequence of impaired coronary artery flow. Major determinants of myocardial oxygen consumption ($MVO_2$) include systolic wall tension, contractile state and heart rate. The subendocardium is particularly sensitive to ischaemia, and the redistribution of myocardial perfusion in the presence of coronary stenoses may account for susceptibility for subendocardial infarction. The presence of ventricular hypertrophy is an additional factor affecting the likelihood of subendocardial ischaemia.

## Fixed obstruction

The effect of an atherosclerotic stenosis on coronary flow dynamics is complex, and may be affected by numerous variables including lesion severity, complexity, length, coronary vascular tone, pressure drop across the lesion, branch points, turbulence etc. At rest, luminal diameter must be reduced by >75% to affect flow, but maximal flow (e.g. during exercise) may be reduced when the lumen is impaired by as little as 30%. In clinical practice, a lesion of $\geq$50% on a coronary arteriogram is judged 'significant'.

## Coronary artery spasm

Alterations in coronary vascular tone via endogenous nitric oxide production may account for much of the variation in 'angina threshold' between one patient and another, and one day and the next. Many factors modulate coronary artery tone including hypoxia, endogenous catecholamines, and vasoactive substances, which may be derived from platelets (e.g. serotonin, adenosine diphosphate) or endothelium (e.g. endothelium-derived relaxing factor).

## Collaterals

The presence of collateral vessels may offer alternative routes of myocardial perfusion when a major epicardial coronary artery is either stenosed or occluded. These channels are dormant in normal circumstances but within a few hours existing collaterals dilate and go on to develop the characteristics of a mature vessel. Numerous factors determine the collateral response to myocardial ischaemia, but it is clear that collateral blood flow can develop very rapidly, for example during balloon occlusion of a vessel during coronary angioplasty.

## Plaque-fissure

A sudden change in the pattern of angina from stable to unstable or the occurrence of an acute myocardial infarct is usually related to the presence of a plaque-fissure. At points of high shear stress (e.g. on the acute margin of the right coronary artery (RCA)), and often in association with a minor atherosclerotic plaque, the wall of the artery (the internal elastic lamina) is breached and the thrombogenic constituents of the arterial wall are exposed to the lumen (Fig. 8.1). This results in platelet deposition, thrombus formation, and a rapid reduction in coronary blood flow: thus, a minor lesion may over a period of a few minutes progress to coronary dissection (Fig. 8.2a & b) and acute occlusion.

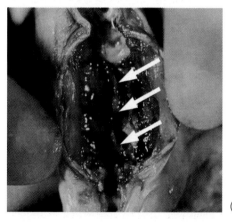

(a)

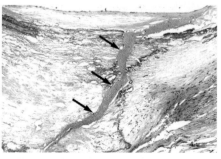

(b)

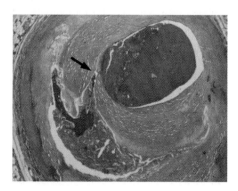

Fig. 8.1  Plaque-fissure.

Fig. 8.2  (a) Coronary artery dissection. (b) Histology of the early stages of a coronary dissection with blood tracking deep into the arterial wall.

## Angina: clinical syndromes (see Box 8.2)

### Stable angina

Having a clinical diagnosis of chest pain with other symptoms provoked by a number of stimuli (see below), stable angina is relieved by rest or removal of the stimulus. Symptoms are provoked by myocardial ischaemia, usually occurring as a result of impaired myocardial blood supply as a consequence of a significant ($\geq$50%) stenosis (either fixed or dynamic) of an epicardial coronary artery. In stable angina, symptoms are reversible and not progressive.

### Unstable angina

The term 'unstable angina' should be restricted to describing a small subgroup of patients who exhibit angina of increasing frequency and severity, with attacks that are often prolonged and only partially relieved by sublingual nitrates. The history is usually short (weeks) and the prognosis poor, with a significant likelihood of progressing to acute myocardial infarction or sudden death. Symptoms stop short of acute myocardial infarction, although the distinction has recently become blurred with the appreciation of intermediate high-risk acute coronary syndromes (e.g. minimal myocardial damage, (MMD)).

### Silent ischaemia

Ambulatory (Holter) monitoring in patients with CHD frequently demonstrates episodes of prolonged and significant (>1 mm) S–T segment depression. These episodes may occur with or without associated symptoms, and there is evidence that reversible abnormalities of myocardial metabolism (confirmed on positron emission tomography (PET) scanning), and

function (both diastolic and systolic) may occur, even in the absence of symptoms. It has been suggested that asymptomatic episodes of S–T segment depression ('silent ischaemia') may be the harbinger of symptomatic episodes that occur later in the natural history of the disease. Silent ischaemia appears to show a diurnal variation, with higher frequencies in the early hours, and may occur in the setting of autonomic dysfunction (e.g. in diabetics) or following myocardial infarction.

### Syndrome X

This syndrome should be reserved to describe the patient with symptoms of typical angina, often not exercise related, but provoked by emotion, anxiety or being diurnal in character, in the setting of normal epicardial coronary arteries on coronary arteriography. The condition is probably heterogeneous in aetiology, but should not be used to include the patient with atypical symptoms. In the absence of large vessel coronary artery disease, the microvasculature is likely to be abnormal, either in terms of structure or functional integrity. There would appear to be an association with ventricular hypertrophy, systemic hypertension, glucose intolerance and insulin resistance. Myocardial scintigraphy may be abnormal in the patient with Syndrome X.

### Prinzmetal's variant angina

Described by Prinzmetal in 1959, variant angina describes symptoms of angina at rest in association with S–T segment elevation on the electrocardiogram (ECG) indicating transmural ischaemia. This uncommon condition appears to relate to the presence of augmented coronary artery tone, which is rapidly relieved by nitroglycerine and may be provoked by acetylcholine. Variant angina may occur in structurally normal coronary arteries, in the presence of mild 'fixed' coronary disease or in the setting of severe occlusive coronary stenoses.

### Clinical history

Eliciting a good clinical history in the patient suffering from angina pectoris is fundamental to making an accurate diagnosis of possible CHD.

---

### Box 8.2  Classification of Angina

- Stable angina
- Unstable angina
- Syndrome X
- Prinzmetal angina

This is especially true as physical examination is frequently non-contributory due to the paucity of physical signs. The hallmark is the presence of chest pain.

## Chest pain

Many patients favour a description of their symptoms that does not include the word 'pain': 'tightness', 'heaviness', 'pressure' and 'ache' are all descriptors of the sensation which is frequently localized to the midline, in the retrosternal region. The use of non-verbal clues, for example a clenched fist or the flat of the hand applied firmly to the chest, is helpful as an additional pointer to the diagnosis. Very well localized pain, superficial pain and chest wall discomfort that is tender to the touch are not typical of myocardial ischaemia. Symptoms may be localized to the arm (most commonly on the left side), the jaw or neck, and less commonly to the epigastrium. Angina tends to radiate from the axilla down the inside of the arm rather than down the lateral aspect of the arm, which is more typical of musculoskeletal pain originating in the cervical spine. Sensory symptoms in the arms (numbness, heaviness, and loss of use) are common.

Anginal pain is short lived, lasting less than 5 min and is usually provoked by exertion, emotion, food, anxiety, change in ambient temperature or smoking a cigarette. Exercise with the arms (e.g. shaving, brushing teeth) appears to be particularly potent in provoking angina. Exercise tolerance may be abbreviated when walking after a meal (post-prandial pain) because of the necessary increase in cardiac output required for digestion. Typically, attacks are relieved by rest, removal of the emotional stimulus or by the administration of sublingual nitrates. More prolonged attacks suggest the presence of unstable angina or impending myocardial infarction. In women, attacks may be more atypical, occurring at rest or at night, with, at other times, a normal exercise tolerance. Angina on lying down (decubitus angina) occurs as a result of an increase in venous return and cardiac output, and pain at night is more common during REM sleep or in association with dreaming. Some patients can 'walk through' their pain

(second wind phenomenon) due to the recruitment of collaterals.

## Breathlessness

Apprehension, sweating and breathlessness may occur in association with chest pain. Occasionally, breathlessness without chest pain may occur in the patient with severe coronary disease or associated left ventricular dysfunction, as a result of a raised left ventricular end-diastolic pressure (LVEDP) and a transient reduction in pulmonary compliance.

## Altered consciousness

Syncope is rare in angina and should alert the clinician to an alternative diagnosis. Dizziness or presyncope in association with palpitation may indicate the presence of an arrhythmia.

## Physical signs

Whereas the clinical history in the patient with angina is the key to diagnosis, physical examination is often unrewarding unless symptoms are occurring as a result of a condition other than CHD (Box 8.3). It can be helpful to examine the patient during an episode of chest pain which may reveal the presence of transient added heart sounds (third sound (S3) or fourth sound (S4)) or murmurs (e.g. secondary to mitral regurgitation (MR)).

## Stigmata of hyperlipidaemia

A corneal arcus senilis may be significant in younger patients, but can be a normal finding in patients over the age of 40 years and not neces-

---

**Box 8.3 Disease Associated with Angina Pectoris**

- Atherosclerotic coronary artery disease
- Coronary artery spasm
- Coronary arteritis (e.g. SLE, Kawasaki)
- Coronary artery ectasia
- Aortic stenosis
- Aortic regurgitation
- Hypertrophic cardiomyopathy
- Primary pulmonary hypertension
- Pulmonary stenosis (rare)
- Mitral stenosis (rare)

sarily be indicative of hyperlipidaemia. Xanthelasma (intracellular lipid deposits, usually around the eye) are correlated with levels of triglyceride but are often seen in patients with normal lipid levels. Tuberous, tendinous and eruptive xanthomas should be sought on the elbows, knees, Achilles tendon, dorsum of the hand and elsewhere as they are indicative of hyperlipidaemia.

## Systemic blood pressure
An elevated BP is an important risk factor for CHD.

## Pulse
Pulse is frequently normal in the patient with stable angina. During an acute attack, a tachycardia or a transient arrhythmia (e.g. atrial fibrillation (AF), ventricular tachycardia) may be evident. A resting tachycardia or pulsus alternans may indicate severe ischaemic myocardial dysfunction as a consequence of previous infarction.

## Venous pressure
Normal in uncomplicated angina but venous pressure may be elevated as a result of previous myocardial infarction.

## Precordial palpation
A dyskinetic or displaced apex may be indicative of previous myocardial infarction with ventricular dilatation or the presence of a left ventricular aneurysm, otherwise examination of the precordium is normal.

## Auscultation
During attacks of angina, a reduction in ventricular compliance causes an increase in left atrial pressure with an audible S4. Prolonged ventricular ejection may result in paradoxical (reversed) splitting of second sound (S2). An S3 is unusual in patients with angina unless there is pre-existing myocardial damage. Papillary muscle ischaemia or abnormalities of papillary muscle alignment (which may be transient) may result in the late systolic murmur of mild MR. Of rare interest is the mid diastolic murmur audible at the left sternal edge and apex from a proximal coronary artery stenosis.

## Evidence of other vascular disease
Physical examination of the patient with coronary disease should include an examination of the peripheral and extracranial vasculature for the presence of bruits or absent pulses. Abnormal abdominal pulsation from an aortic aneurysm formation may also be present.

## Differential diagnosis (see Box 8.4)

Having elicited an accurate clinical history, there is frequently little doubt that the patient is suffering from angina. The characteristic pain and radiation, the temporal relationship to exercise or other provocative factors, and the relief by rest or sublingual nitrates is typical. Chest wall pain is usually well localized, sharp, fleeting, rarely in the midline and may be postural. This type of pain may also be associated with anxiety, dizziness, lassitude, sighing and hyperventilation (neurocirculatory asthenia or Da Costa's syndrome). Pain and swelling of the costal cartilages (Tietze's syndrome) is rare. Left-sided chest pain is more common probably because most patients are aware that their heart is on the left side. Disease of the cervical spine may cause pain over the anterior chest, axilla and arm, but is usually associated with limitation of movement, clinical findings of reduced movement, muscle weakness and absent or attenuated reflexes in the upper limb.

Gastrointestinal pain may cause real difficulty as there are features shared with angina,

---

**Box 8.4 Differential Diagnosis of Angina**

- Chest wall pain
    Da Costa's syndrome
    Tietze syndrome
- Pleurisy
- Pulmonary embolism
- Diseases of the cervical spine
- Gastrointestinal pathology

and sublingual nitrates may relieve oesophageal spasm. The association of gastrointestinal pathology (e.g. hiatus hernia, gastritis, peptic ulceration, gall bladder disease and biliary colic) with eating certain foodstuffs, the presence of dyspepsia or acid reflux and the relief by antacids, all help point to the gastrointestinal tract. Widespread availability of endoscopy and oesophageal motility testing can confirm the diagnosis.

## Investigations (see Box 8.5)

### Resting electrocardiogram

A normal resting ECG does not exclude a diagnosis of angina, although there may be evidence of pre-existing myocardial infarction (Q waves, T wave inversion, LBBB). Conversely, the presence of minor ST–T segment (repolarization) abnormalities are common in the population at large and are not necessarily indicative of underlying coronary disease. The sensitivity of the resting ECG (when compared with coronary arteriography) is approximately 50% and the specificity approximately 70%. Reversible changes in the baseline ECG occurring with episodes of chest pain (S–T segment shift, T wave inversion) are indicative of occlusive coronary disease. Widespread ECG changes are associated with a poor prognosis as they are commonly associated with severe and diffuse coronary disease.

### Chest radiograph

Chest radiography is usually normal in the patient with angina. Cardiac enlargement and/or an elevation in venous pressure may indicate previous myocardial infarction or left ventricular dysfunction. Occasionally, the presence of a left ventricular aneurysm results in the characteristic bulge or calcification within the cardiac silhouette (Fig. 8.18) but these radiographic findings may be unreliable.

### Exercise testing

The treadmill exercise test is pivotal in the investigation of the patient with chest pain. It should be viewed as a natural extension to the clinical examination, allowing firm decisions to be made regarding the need for further invasive investigation (coronary arteriography). A well supervised, maximum, symptom-limited exercise test using one of the standard protocols allows the patient to be stratified for future risk of subsequent cardiac events.

A number of parameters are evaluated during the test, and although there is emphasis on ECG changes, the appearance of the patient, the occurrence of symptoms, BP and heart rate response, and the amount of work achieved are all important determinants of prognosis.

Indications and contraindications to exercise testing are listed in Boxes 8.6 and 8.7. Exercise tests should be supervised by a physician or technical personnel trained in advanced life support in an area equipped with full resuscitation

### Box 8.5 Investigations in Stable Angina

- Resting ECG
- Chest radiograph
- Exercise ECG
- ± Echocardiogram
- ± Radionuclide scan
- ± Coronary arteriography

### Box 8.6 Indications for Exercise Testing

- Assessment of objective exercise tolerance
- Nature of symptoms limiting exercise (chest pain, fatigue, breathlessness etc.)
- Evaluation of haemodynamic response to exercise
- Document S–T segment changes occurring with exercise or during the recovery period
- Evaluation of exercise induced arrhythmias
- Document beneficial effects of surgical procedures, PCI or medical therapy
- Risk stratification following acute myocardial infarction
- Guide to rehabilitation following acute myocardial infarction
- Risk stratification in patients with hypertrophic cardiomyopathy

facilities. An exercise protocol should be applicable to a wide variety of patient groups, including children and the elderly, and allow the aerobic threshold to be reached in the majority of patients within a few minutes. A number of protocols are available, but in practice the modified or full Bruce protocol is in use in the majority of centres (Table 8.1). In most exercise laboratories, a treadmill rather than bicycle ergometry is used as the stimulus to exercise. The treadmill has the advantage that it is under the control of the supervisor resulting in a higher level of achieved exercise.

Physical exercise results in an increase in myocardial oxygen requirement ($MVO_2$), which will provoke angina in the patient with significant CHD. During dynamic exercise, increasing $MVO_2$ is linearly related to increasing cardiac output that is mainly brought about by an increase in heart rate. BP increases during exercise, and an increase in systolic BP is particularly marked. The 'double product' (peak heart rate × peak systolic BP) correlates well with peak $MVO_2$. A full 12-lead ECG should be recorded during exercise and following completion of the test at intervals until the heart rate and BP have fallen to pretest levels. ECG changes occurring during the recovery period (coinciding with the time of oxygen debt) are a sensitive indicator of the presence of CHD, as is the time taken for normalization.

In patients with CHD, myocardial ischaemia is reflected as S–T segment depression, which is seen most frequently in the lead with the tallest R wave (usually $V_5$). Criteria for 'significant' S–T segment depression represent a compromise between sensitivity and specificity (Fig. 8.3). Most series define positivity as >1mm planar (horizontal) or downsloping S–T segment depression measured 80msec after

## Box 8.7 Contraindications to Exercise Testing

- Unstable angina
- Acute pericarditis
- Acute myocarditis
- Uncontrolled blood pressure
- Heart failure
- Critical aortic stenosis
- Sustained ventricular arrhythmia
- High grade atrioventricular block
- Acute systemic illness

## EXERCISE STRESS TEST PROTOCOLS

**Full (standard) Bruce protocol**

| Stage | Speed (mph) | Gradient (%) | Duration (min) |
|-------|-------------|--------------|----------------|
| I | 1.7 | 10 | 3 |
| II | 2.5 | 12 | 3 |
| III | 3.4 | 14 | 3 |
| IV | 4.2 | 16 | 3 |
| V | 5.0 | 18 | 3 |
| VI | 5.5 | 20 | 3 |
| VII | 6.0 | 22 | 3 |

**Modified Bruce protocol**

| Stage | Speed (mph) | Gradient (%) | Duration (min) |
|-------|-------------|--------------|----------------|
| I | 1.7 | 0 | 3 |
| II | 1.7 | 5 | 3 |
| III | 1.7 | 10 | 3 |
| IV | 2.5 | 12 | 3 |
| V | 3.4 | 14 | 3 |
| VI | 4.2 | 16 | 3 |
| VII | 5.0 | 18 | 3 |

Table 8.1 Exercise stress test protocols.

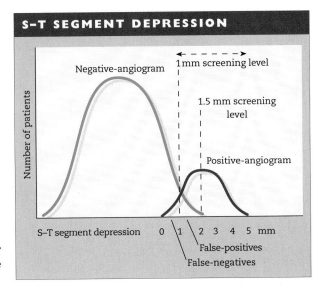

**Fig. 8.3** Relationship between sensitivity and specificity of S–T segment depression on exercise testing.

the J point (Fig. 8.4). Changes in T wave morphology may be provoked by respiration or changes in posture and do not reliably indicate myocardial ischaemia. Similarly, J point depression accompanies a tachycardia due to shortening of the pulmonary regurgitation (PR) interval and repolarization of the atria. Rate dependent aberrancy is an unreliable indicator of ischaemia. Some patients exhibit S–T segment elevation, 'pseudonormalization' of inverted T waves or an increase in R wave amplitude, all of which may be provoked by ischaemia.

Reasons for terminating an exercise test are listed in Box 8.8. A number of other conditions may give rise to repolarization changes on exercise (Box 8.9).

### Radionuclide scintigraphy

Radionuclide imaging is not usually necessary in the routine investigation of patients with angina, but it may be useful in certain subgroups (Box 8.10). The patient is exercised using a standard protocol and the radionuclide (e.g. $^{201}$Tl or $^{99m}$Tc-sestamibi) is injected into a peripheral vein, which is then taken up by perfused myocardium. The patient is then scanned using a gamma camera and a series of tomographic (single photon emission computed tomography (SPECT)) images recorded in a variety of planes.

**Box 8.8 Reasons for Terminating an Exercise Test**

- Symptomatic (chest pain, breathlessness, exhaustion)
- Fall in systemic blood pressure
- Peripheral circulatory insufficiency (claudication)
- Sustained arrhythmia (eg ventricular tachycardia)
- Symptomatic heart block
- Failure of treadmill or ECG apparatus
- Diagnostic ST segment shift
- Target heart rate or grade of exercise achieved
- Extreme elevation of blood pressure (>250 mmHg systolic)

These images are then compared with a second series of resting images recorded from similar angles (Fig. 8.5). Thus, areas of reversible ischaemia and/or infarction can be demonstrated and localized. Attention to technical detail and careful interpretation of the images, taking care not to over report are important if 'false-positives' are to be avoided. Pharmacological stress using a variety of agents may be helpful in the patient who is unable to exercise (e.g. adenosine, arbutamine, dobutamine and dipyridamole).

## INFEROLATERAL S-T SEGMENT DEPRESSION

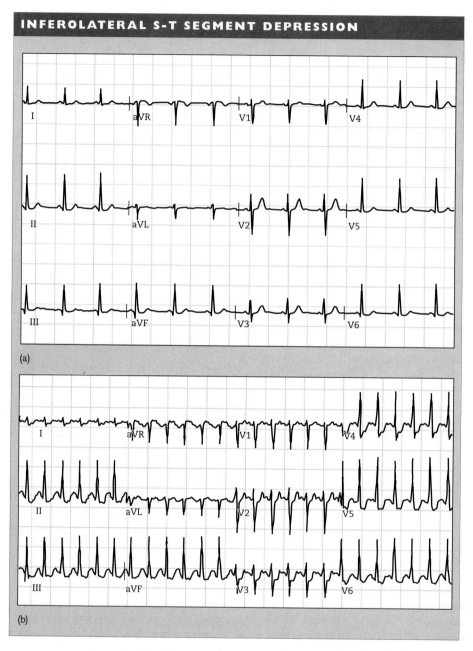

(a)

(b)

Fig. 8.4 (a) 12-lead ECG (rest). (b) 12-lead ECG (exercise) showing inferolateral S–T segment depression.

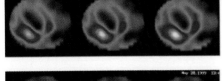

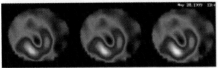

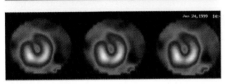

(a)

(b)

(c)

**Fig. 8.5** Radionuclide scintigraphy using thallium with adenosine as a stress agent: (a) rest; (b) redistribution; and (c) reinjection traces.

**Box 8.10 Indications for Radionuclide Stress Imaging**

- Patients who are unable to exercise
- Patients with abnormal conduction on the resting ECG (eg LBBB)
- Assessment of regional myocardial ischaemia in a patient with a moderate coronary artery lesion
- Accurate risk stratification of patients with documented coronary artery disease or following acute myocardial infarction
- Assessment of myocardial viability in the presence of left ventricular dysfunction

**Box 8.9 Causes of a 'False Positive' Exercise Test Result**

- Systemic hypertension
- Aortic stenosis
- Cardiomyopathy
- Mitral valve prolapse
- Pre-excitation
- Hyperventilation
- Hypoglycaemia
- Hypokalaemia
- Digoxin
- Anaemia
- Mitral regurgitation
- Aortic regurgitation

### Stress echocardiography

See Chapter 3.

### Coronary arteriography

Coronary arteriography is currently the only method of accurately delineating the coronary anatomy. The majority of clinical trials depend on a demonstration of the coronary anatomy to determine prognosis, and arteriography is a necessary prerequisite to CABG or coronary angioplasty.

In the UK, the relatively low numbers of cardiologists and catheter laboratories available limits the number of coronary arteriograms performed annually.

- In 1998, it was estimated that 1429 procedures/million population were undertaken in the UK, compared with 3584 procedures/million in France and 6441 procedures/million in Germany.
- In the US, there are now more than 1.5 million angiograms performed annually, whereas in Europe the rate of investigation and treatment of CHD appears to be static (Fig. 8.6).

Coronary arteriography, although an invasive investigation, is a low-risk procedure with a morbidity of 0.8% and a mortality of 0.12% in elective patients. Complications are higher in unstable patients, those with additional aortic valve disease and in the setting of acute myocardial infarction or cardiogenic shock. Coronary arteriography is most commonly performed using a percutaneous femoral approach, the Judkins technique, in which preformed catheters are advanced retrogradely into the left ventricle, and each of the two coronary arteries in turn. An alternative approach is by means of the brachial artery, accessed by either a cut-down (modified Sones technique) or using the percutanous route.

Coronary anatomy varies from patient to patient. There are two coronary arteries, the left and right (Fig. 8.7). The first segment of the left coronary artery, the left main stem, is the common trunk that divides into: the anterior branch, the left anterior descending (LAD) and

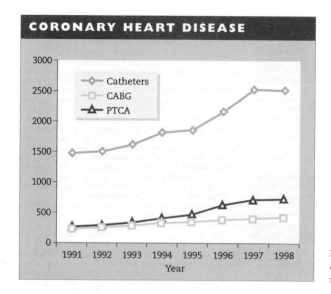

## CORONARY HEART DISEASE

Fig. 8.6 Coronary artery disease: investigations and treatment in Europe.

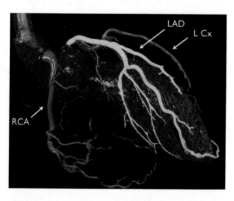

Fig. 8.7 Coronary anatomy (RCA, right coronary artery; LAD, left anterior descending; L Cx, left circumflex).

the posterior branch (the left circumflex). The RCA does not usually have major branches, but supplies the AV nodal artery and the posterior descending artery in about 90% of cases (right dominant anatomy). In the remaining 10% of patients, the posterior descending arises from the left circumflex (left dominant anatomy). The term 'three vessel disease' refers to involvement of all three major branches (i.e. the LAD, the left circumflex and the RCA). Coronary arteriography is usually combined with left ventriculography to assess ventricular

systolic function and abnormalities of wall motion.

Indications for invasive assessment will differ from one centre to another, but there is a general consensus that coronary arteriography is indicated in some groups of patients (Box 8.11).

### The 'open access' chest pain clinic

In the last few years, many centres have offered open access clinics for the assessment of the patient with chest pain. The patient is seen by a dedicated team (who may include a cardiologist or physician, a technician and a nurse practitioner), who will take a clinical history, provide a treadmill exercise test, screen for risk factors and advise regarding risk factor modification. The general practitioner is then notified of suggested treatment options and the need for further investigation. These very successful clinics are likely to dramatically increase the requirement for increased facilities and personnel to undertake cardiac catheterization and coronary revascularization.

## Box 8.11 Indications for Coronary Arteriography

- Symptoms of coronary artery disease despite adequate medical therapy
- Determination of prognosis in a patient with known coronary artery disease
- Stable chest pain with marked ischaemic changes on an exercise test
- Widespread reversible ischaemia on a myocardial perfusion scan
- Patients with chest pain in whom the aetiology is unclear
- Unstable coronary syndromes (particularly with elevated troponin T or I)
- Following non-Q wave myocardial infarction
- Following Q wave myocardial infarction in high risk patients (determined by exercise testing or myocardial perfusion scanning)
- Survivors of near miss sudden death
- Patients with sustained or recurrent ventricular arrhythmias (e.g. ventricular tachycardia)
- Recurrent symptoms following coronary intervention (PCI or CABG)
- In patients undergoing surgery for valvular heart disease
- Prior to surgical correction of infarct related ventricular septal defect or papillary muscle rupture
- In patients with heart failure where the aetiology is unclear
- To determine the cause of chest pain in hypertrophic cardiomyopathy

## Medical management

### General measures
#### Smoking
Epidemiological evidence suggests that the risk of subsequent myocardial infarction in patients suffering from angina is reduced by stopping smoking (see page 96).

#### Diet and weight reduction
The evidence that weight reduction *per se* favourably affects coronary risk is lacking, but there is a clear interrelationship between obesity, systemic hypertension and abnormalities of lipids. Given that many patients who quit smoking put on weight, they should be advised

that the cardiac risk of being an ex-smoker and overweight are significantly less than being a thin smoker.

### Exercise and lifestyle
Regular physical exercise reduces the risk of CHD, and is likely to be associated with a more healthy lifestyle. Exercise may have a cardioprotective effect as well as being of therapeutic use following acute myocardial infarction.

### Specific therapy (see Box 8.12)
#### Aspirin
All patients with angina should receive aspirin unless there is a specific contraindication. A variety of doses have been used in the available trials, but a small dose of 75 mg daily has been shown to be adequate and is only rarely associated with gastrointestinal side-effects. Aspirin reduces platelet adhesiveness and prolongs the bleeding time. Clopidogrel, although expensive, is a more potent platelet agent which is suitable for patients intolerant or allergic to aspirin. This drug is widely used in percutaneous coronary intervention (see page 119).

#### Nitrates
The actions of nitrates are complex and include a reduction in preload due to pooling of blood in venous capacitance vessels, reduced afterload and a fall in systemic BP, direct epicardial coronary dilatation, increased coronary perfusion pressure, and redistribution of myocardial blood flow. Nitrates may also enhance coronary collateral flow.

A number of nitrate preparations are available including sublingual, buccal, oral, transcutaneous and intravenous formulations (Table 8.2).

## Box 8.12 Medical Treatment in Stable Angina

- Aspirin
- β-blockade
- Calcium antagonist
- Nicorandil
- ± Lipid lowering therapy

**NITRATE PREPARATIONS**

| Drug name | Trade name | Route | Dose | Cost* |
|---|---|---|---|---|
| Glyceryl trinitrate | Cor-nitro, Glytrin, Nitrolingual, Nitromin, Generic | Sublingual | 0.3–0.6 mg (prn) | £3.13 (0.4 mg × 200) |
| | Sustac | Oral | 2.6–30 mg daily (bd or tds) | £5.12 (2.6 mg × 90) |
| | Susard | Buccal SR | 2–6 mg daily (tds) | £9.38 (1 mg × 100) |
| | Deponit, Minitran, Nitro-Dur, Transiderm-Nitro | Patch | 5–20 mg daily (om) | £12.49 (5 mg × 30) |
| | Percutol | Ointment | ¹/₂–2 inches (tds or qds) | £10.98 (60 g) |
| | Nitrocine, Nitronal | IV | Infusion | £16.85 (50 mL × 1) |
| Isosorbide dinitrate | Cedocard, Isoket, Sorbid SA | Oral | 40–160 mg daily (bd) | £3.47 (20 mg × 56) |
| | Isordil | Oral, sublingual | 40–120 mg daily (bd or tds) | £0.72 (10 mg × 112) |
| | Isocard | Dermal spray | 30–120 mg daily (om or bd) | £17.50 (30 mg × 65) |
| | Isoket | IV | Infusion | £17.96 (50 mL × 1) |
| Isosorbide mononitrate | Elantan, Imdur, Isib, Ismo, Isodur XL, MCR-50, Monit, Mono-Cedocard, Monomax | Oral | 20–120 mg (bd or tds) | £6.05 (25 mg × 28) |

* Cost for cheapest preparation.

om, every morning; bd, twice daily; tds, three times daily; qds, four times daily; prn, as required.

Table 8.2  Nitrate preparations.

Sublingual nitrates remain one of the most effective and convenient forms of drug treatment for an acute attack of angina. The metered aerosol spray has the advantage of a 3-year shelf life, whereas GTN tablets have a shelf life of only 2 months which can be prolonged to 6 months by refrigeration. An advantage of the tablet preparation is that the partially dissolved tablet can be removed from the mouth once the attack has been relieved, thereby reducing the side-effects of headache, flushing and postural dizziness. Side-effects can be minimized by taking the drug whilst sitting. Many patients are given inadequate instruction on nitrate use, which can and should be administered both prophylactically and for the relief of an angina attack once it occurs; used in this way the beneficial effects may last up to 1 hour. Administration of sublingual nitrates may be a useful diagnostic test for the differentiation between angina and other causes of chest pain. Peak levels of the drug occur within 2 min with a plasma half-life of 7 min: 75% of patients obtain symptomatic relief within 3 min and a further 15% within 15 min.

Long-acting mononitrates have largely replaced dinitrates because of the virtually complete bioavailability without the disadvantage of extensive first-pass hepatic metabolism. Tolerance to long-acting nitrates, which is an ill-understood phenomenon, is common if there is not a nitrate free period of at least 8 hours in every 24 hours.

## β-blockade

β-blocking drugs remain the mainstay of drug treatment for angina, although in the last few years calcium antagonists have made a significant impact and are now used as monotherapy in a number of patients. β-blocking drugs are competitive inhibitors of catecholamine binding at β-receptor sites. They reduce $MVO_2$ by two routes: (i) a direct myocardial action reduces LV systolic pressure, and the rate of pressure rise ($\delta p/\delta t$) (i.e. contractility), and (ii) the 'double product' (heart rate × systolic BP) is reduced in response to exercise. β-blocking drugs are effective in reducing frequency and severity of attacks of angina and also improve prognosis by reducing the incidence of major cardiac events.

Choosing the appropriate β-blocking preparation depends on a number of factors, including the dosing regimen, cardioselectivity, and the side-effect profile. Side-effects sufficient to cause withdrawal of the drug occurs in 5–10% of patients. β-blockers are contraindicated in patients with severe airflow obstruction, high-grade atrioventricular block or severe peripheral vascular disease.

Many of the secondary characteristics of β-blocking drugs (e.g. partial agonist activity, membrane stabilizing activity and local anaesthetic action) have little practical clinical importance. Low lipid solubility may be beneficial, as a failure to cross the blood brain barrier reduces the likelihood of CNS side-effects.

Commonly used preparations are listed in Table 8.3.

## Calcium antagonists

These are a heterogeneous group of drugs that inhibit the slow current channel, by which calcium ions enter the cell to initiate smooth muscle contraction and intracardiac conduction. Thus, the administration of calcium channel blockers relaxes smooth muscle, reduces afterload, and has a direct effect on coronary vasomotor tone, thereby reducing coronary artery spasm. Calcium antagonists have little effect on venous capacitance vessels. All calcium antagonists are negatively inotropic, which may in clinical practice be masked by the vasodilator effect. There has been concern raised over the possible excess in cardiac mortality when hypertensive patients or those with CHD are treated with nifedipine. As a result of a number of studies, it is clear that nifedipine should be avoided as monotherapy without concomitant β-blockade. Diltiazem is well tolerated and probably the best first-generation calcium antagonist used in the treatment of angina. The properties of the calcium antagonists are very different (Table 8.4).

## Lipid-lowering therapy

An elevation in blood cholesterol is an impor-

## β-BLOCKING DRUGS

| Drug name | Trade name | Selectivity | Secondary properties | Lipid solubility | Dose | Cost* |
|---|---|---|---|---|---|---|
| Acebutolol | Sectral | + | ISA, MSA | Low | 400–1200 mg daily (om or bd) | £2.57 (50 mg × 56) |
| Atenolol | Tenormin | + | – | Low | 25–100 mg daily (om or bd) | £4.41 (25 mg × 28) |
| Bisoprolol | Emcor, Monocor | + | – | Moderate | 10–20 mg (om) | £9.61 (10 mg × 28) |
| Labetalol | Trandate | – | – | Low | 200–2400 mg daily (bd, tds, or qds) | £5.05 (50 mg × 56) |
| Metoprolol | Betaloc, Lopresor | + | – | Moderate | 50–300 mg daily (bd or tds) | £3.30 (50 mg × 100) |
| Nadolol | Corguard | – | – | Low | 40–160 mg daily (om) | £3.76 (40 mg × 28) |
| Oxprenolol | Trasicor | – | ISA | Moderate | 80–320 mg daily (bd or tds) | £1.29 (20 mg × 56) |
| Pindolol | Visken | – | ISA, MSA | Moderate | 2.5–15 mg daily (om, bd, or tds) | £4.07 (5 mg × 56) |
| Propranolol | Beta-Prograne, Inderal | – | MSA | High | 80–240 mg daily (bd or tds) | £5.40 (80 mg × 28) |
| Timolol | Betim | – | – | Low | 20–60 mg daily (bd) | £2.45 (10 mg × 30) |

* Cost for cheapest preparation.

om, every morning; bd, twice daily; tds, three times daily; qds, four times daily; ISA, intrinsic sympathomimetic activity; MSA, membrane stabilizing activity.

Table 8.3  β-Blocking drugs.

## CALCIUM ANTAGONISTS

| Drug name | Trade name | Dose | Cost* |
|---|---|---|---|
| Amlodipine | Istin | 5–10 mg (om) | £11.85 (5 mg × 28) |
| Diltiazem | Adizem, Angitil, Dilzem, Slozem, Tildiem, Viazem XL | 60–120 mg (tds) | £7.50 (60 mg × 100) |
| Felodipine | Plendil | 5–10 mg (om) | £8.12 (5 mg × 28) |
| Nicardipine | Cardene | 20–40 mg (tds) | £8.38 (20 mg × 56) |
| Nifedipine | Adalat, Adipine, Angiopine, Cardilate, Coracten, Fortipine LA, Tensipine | 5–20 mg (bd or tds) | £7.74 (10 mg × 90) |
| Nisoldipine | Syscor | 10–40 mg (om) | £9.36 (10 mg × 28) |
| Verapamil | Cordilox, Securon, Univer | 80–120 mg (tds) | £0.33 (40 mg × 20) |

* Cost for cheapest preparation.

om, every morning; bd, twice daily; tds, three times daily.

Table 8.4 Calcium antagonists.

tant risk factor for CHD, but should be considered in the context of other risk factors such as smoking, raised BP and a lack of exercise. A significant number of patients will respond to a low-fat diet and weight reduction alone, but up to 40% will require additional lipid lowering therapy; this is particularly true of patients with a family history of CHD. Patients who have undergone revascularization procedures should be treated aggressively as there is clear evidence that long-term graft function following CABG and the rate of restenosis following percutaneous transluminal coronary angioplasty (PTCA) can be improved with lipid lowering therapy.

The Standing Medical Advisory Committee in the UK has suggested that statins which are the most effective group of lipid lowering drugs should be reserved for patients suffering from angina with a total cholesterol of 5.5 mmol/L or more. For people without symptomatic CHD, who are found to have a high cholesterol on screening, treatment with statins should be reserved for those with a risk of a major coronary event (myocardial infarction or sudden death)

of 3% per year or more, as a high cholesterol in isolation is a weak predictor of coronary risk. The Sheffield Table for primary prevention of CHD shows the serum cholesterol in relation to other recognized risk factors that confers a 3% risk of CHD per year and should be treated with statins (Fig. 8.8). Classification of hyperlipidaemia and a simple treatment algorithm is shown in Table 8.5, and the expected changes in lipids and lipoproteins in Table 8.6.

### Other drugs

Nicorandil offers a useful alternative in the treatment of angina, usually in combination with other drugs. This potassium channel blocker relaxes smooth muscle as well as providing direct vasodilatation of the coronary arteries. Side-effects are similar to those seen with oral nitrates.

In the absence of impaired ventricular function, angiotensin-converting enzyme (ACE) inhibitors have no role in the treatment of angina. Interestingly, ACE inhibitors have been shown to reduce the long-term risk of developing unstable angina or sudden death in patients with left ventricular dysfunction.

Hormone replacement therapy reduces the

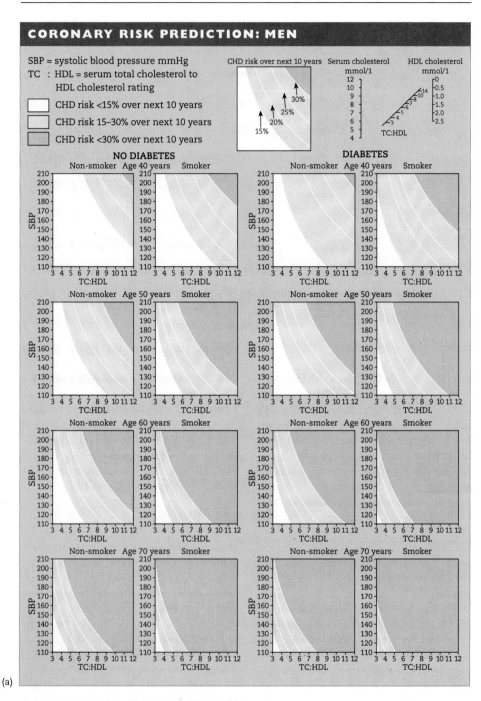

(a)

**Fig. 8.8** Coronary risk prediction chart: (a) men; (b) women.

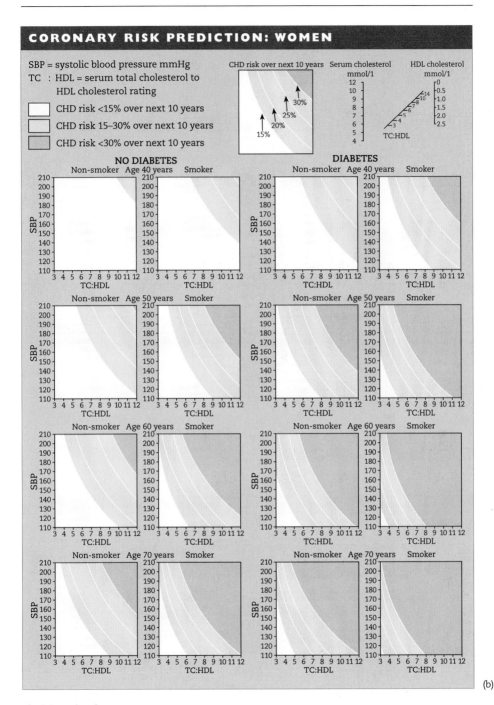

**CORONARY RISK PREDICTION: WOMEN**

SBP = systolic blood pressure mmHg
TC  : HDL = serum total cholesterol to
HDL cholesterol rating

CHD risk <15% over next 10 years

CHD risk 15–30% over next 10 years

CHD risk <30% over next 10 years

(b)

Fig. 8.8 *continued.*

## PRIMARY LIPID DISORDERS

| Lipoprotein (Frederickson) type | Molecular disorder | Genetic transmission | Estimated incidence | Cholesterol | Triglycerides | Clinical features |
|---|---|---|---|---|---|---|
| I | LPL, ApoC-II | Autosomal recessive | Rare | +++ | +++ | Eruptive xanthomas, hepatosplenomegaly, pancreatitis |
| IIa | LDL, ApoB-100 | Autosomal dominant | 1:500 | ++ | Normal | Tendon xanthomas, premature atherosclerosis |
| IIb | Unknown | Autosomal dominant | 1:200 | + | + | Premature atherosclerosis |
| III | Apo-E | Autosomal recessive | Rare | ++ | + | Palmar and tuberoeruptive xanthomas, premature atherosclerosis |
| IV | Unknown | Autosomal dominant | 1:500 | + | ++ | Usually none or premature atherosclerosis |
| V | Unknown | Autosomal dominant | 1:500 | +++ | +++ | Eruptive xanthomas, premature atherosclerosis |

**Table 8.5** Classification of primary lipid disorders.

## BLOOD LIPIDS AND DRUGS

| Drug | Lipids (% change) | | Lipoproteins (% change) | |
|---|---|---|---|---|
| | Cholesterol | Triglyceride | LDL | HDL |
| Statins | ↓20–33% | ↓10–30% | ↓25–45% | ↑2–15% |
| Fibrates | ↓10–20% | ↓30–50% | ↓20–25% | ↑10–25% |
| Nicotinic acid | ↓15–30% | ↓20–60% | ↓15–40% | ↑10–20% |
| Probucol | ↓5–15% | ↓0–5% | ↓8–15% | ↓10–25% |
| Fish oils | ↓↑ | ↓10–60% | ↓↑ | ↑5–10% |

Table 8.6 Expected changes in blood lipids with drug treatment.

risk of acute myocardial infarction and sudden cardiac death in post-menopausal women. All women with a coronary history, or who are known to have other risk factors for CHD, should be commenced on hormone replacement therapy HRT unless there is a specific contraindication.

### 'Stepped' drug therapy in the management of stable angina

All patients should be treated with aspirin 75 mg daily. For very occasional episodes of angina, sublingual nitrates may be adequate. Most patients require treatment with a cardioselective β-blocker, or alternatively a calcium antagonist. In 10–20% of patients, additional drugs will be needed in the form of long-acting oral nitrates, or alternatively a calcium antagonist can be added to the β-blocker. Resistant patients may require 'triple therapy' (β-blocker + calcium antagonist + nitrate) or 'quadruple therapy' ('triple therapy' + Nicorandil) which necessitates investigation with a view to revascularization in the majority.

### Medical management of unstable angina
(see Box 8.13)

In view of the early risk of acute myocardial infarction or sudden death, patients with true unstable angina should be admitted to hospital, commenced on aspirin, heparin (either unfractionated or low molecular weight (LMW)) and

### Box 8.13 Medical Treatment in Unstable Angina

- Aspirin
- Heparin (LMW)
- Intravenous nitrates
- Calcium antagonist
- ± β-blockade
- ± Nicorandil
- IIb/IIIa antagonist

intravenous nitrates as well as additional oral anti-anginal medication, with a view to early invasive investigation and revascularization. Early data suggests that the powerful antiplatelet II/IIIa antagonists (e.g. Abciximab, Eptifibatide, Tirofiban) have a major role in treating patients with unstable angina and non-Q wave myocardial infarction, reducing the risk of subsequent percutaneous coronary intervention. If the patient is stabilized in hospital and sent home there is a high chance of recurrent symptoms or a major cardiac event.

## Coronary revascularization

### Coronary artery bypass grafting

Surgical revascularization using CABG was first performed in the early 1960s and is now one of the most common surgical procedures undertaken. In the UK, more than 25 000 CABG procedures were performed in 1998. Reversed saphenous vein has been the graft conduit of choice for many years but the superior patency rates of arterial conduits (e.g. internal mammary artery) has resulted in most patients nowadays receiving at least one artery graft. Early perioperative mortality for elective CABG is 1–3%. Risk factors for death include:

- poor myocardial function;
- recent myocardial infarction;
- haemodynamic instability;
- older age;
- female gender;
- diabetes mellitus;
- diffuse small vessel disease;
- environmental and institutional factors, including the choice of surgeon.

Early complications include perioperative myocardial infarction, bleeding, stroke, wound infection and atrial arrhythmias. Following successful surgery, 75–90% of patients are free from angina. Vein grafts occlude at the rate of 2–5% per annum, whereas the patency of a left internal mammary artery graft to the LAD is >95% at 10 years (Fig. 8.9).

In groups of patients with high-risk coronary anatomy, CABG has been shown to improve prognosis as well: these include patients with a left main stem stenosis, triple-vessel disease, two-vessel disease including a proximal stenosis of the LAD, two-vessel disease and impaired ventricular function.

## Coronary angioplasty/stenting

PTCA was first performed by Andreas Gruentzig in 1977, and by 1990 the number of PTCA procedures worldwide exceeded the number of CABG operations. Recent data show that in 1997 the number of PTCA procedures worldwide had increased to 1 210 000, with 50% undertaken in the US, 31% in Europe, 9% in Japan and 10% in other countries. In experienced centres, early mortality is approximately 1% depending on case mix, and the rate of major complications (death, myocardial infarction and emergency CABG) is usually between 3 and 5%. Initially, PTCA was used to treat single, proximal, short, discrete, non-calcified lesions in large (≥3 mm diameter) arteries. PTCA was carried out in centres with

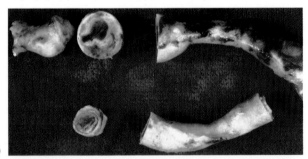

(a)

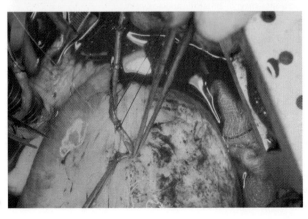

(b)

Fig. 8.9 (a) Diffuse graft atherosclerosis in an old vein graft. (b) Left internal mammary artery graft.

on-site surgical facilities (still the preferred option) because of the risk of abrupt vessel closure which followed successful dilatation in approximately 5% of patients. Abrupt vessel closure occurring as a result of arterial dissection and/or thrombus formation may result in the need for emergency CABG, acute myocardial infarction, or sudden death. The major late problem of PTCA is restenosis, which may be apparent clinically in 15–20% of patients who develop recurrent angina, or angiographically defined as ≥50% diameter restenosis in the target vessel. Restenosis occurs as a result of the migration of fibroblasts and connective tissue into the area of barotrauma resulting from balloon dilatation and intimal disruption. Restenosis appears to be more common in certain subsets of patients, including those with:

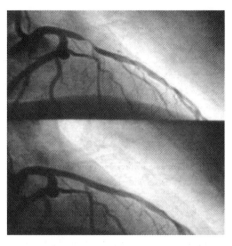

Fig. 8.10 Severe proximal stenosis (left anterior descending), before and after stent insertion.

- proximal LAD lesions;
- vein graft disease;
- long lesions;
- unstable angina;
- diabetes;
- restenotic lesions; and
- patients who continue to smoke or who have untreated hypercholesterolaemia.

No drug therapy has been shown to reduce the incidence of restenosis following PTCA.

The first human implants of intracoronary stents were undertaken in 1986. The development of the stent was a landmark in interventional cardiology because the advent of intracoronary 'scaffolding' reduced the incidence of abrupt vessel closure, acute myocardial infarction, sudden death and the need for emergency CABG (Fig. 8.10). It subsequently became clear from the BENESTENT and STRESS trials that stenting compared with simple balloon angioplasty reduced the incidence of late restenosis. In 1997, 600 000 stents were implanted worldwide, 57% in the US, 30% in Europe, 5% in Japan and 8% in other countries. The advent of stents has increased the applicability of percutanous intervention to other patient subsets including multivessel disease, long lesions and vein grafts. Antiplatelet therapy in stented patients includes pretreatment with aspirin and Clopidogrel, periprocedural heparin,

and post-procedural Clopidogrel for 1 month and low-dose aspirin continued indefinitely. With current antiplatelet regimens, early stent thrombosis occurs in approximately 0.5% of patients. High-risk subgroups (e.g. diabetics, patients with small vessels (<3.0 mm diameter), those undergoing multivessel intervention) are often treated with a IIb/IIIa antagonist (e.g. Abciximab), which has been shown to reduce risk of subsequent cardiac events.

PTCA is effective in reducing or abolishing attacks of angina in selected patients with lesions amenable to balloon dilatation. At present, there is little evidence that PTCA improves life expectancy when compared with medical therapy, and it is probably similar to CABG in terms of morbidity and mortality when similar patient groups are compared. Early trials comparing PTCA and CABG prior to the advent of stents demonstrated a high redo rate in the PTCA group, with significant numbers of patients with recurrent symptoms crossing to the surgical arm. Currently, there are a number of trials comparing the use of stents vs. CABG in multivessel disease. Until the results of these trials are available, PTCA/stenting tends to be reserved for patients at the 'simple' end of the spectrum with one or two lesions, and patients with three-vessel disease are treated with

CABG. In many ways, the two revascularization techniques should be viewed as complementary rather than in competition. A comparison of the two techniques is shown in Table 8.7.

## PMR/TMR

The utility of percutanous and transmyocardial revascularization using laser energy as a method of increasing direct myocardial perfusion from the left ventricular cavity is being investigated. Small 1–2 mm diameter channels are created using a carbon dioxide laser, either from the epicardium through to the ventricular cavity using an open chest left thoracotomy approach, or more recently from the left ventricular cavity into the myocardium using a percutanous retrograde arterial approach. At present, studies are limited to patients in whom conventional revascularization (CABG or PTCA) is not technically feasible. Symptomatic improvement following the procedure is seen in the majority of patients, confirmed objectively on exercise testing. Favourable prognostic data are lacking, and the results of the recently published DIRECT trial suggests that laser revascularization is no better than placebo in the majority of patients.

## Natural history

It is clear from the literature that the prognosis of the patient with stable angina has improved with the passage of time. Patients can now be more easily divided into high- and low-risk subsets on clinical history, treadmill exercise testing and coronary arteriography. Furthermore, aggressive risk factor modification coupled with effective drug therapy and successful methods of revascularization has reduced risk and improved prognosis. Prognosis in individual patients is difficult to estimate but varies from an annual mortality of 1–2% for single vessel disease, 3.5–7.5% for three vessel disease, to 10–13% for left main stem disease.

Table 8.7 Comparison between percutaneous coronary intervention and coronary artery bypass grafting.

## PCI AND CABG COMPARISON

| Percutaneous coronary intervention (PCI) | Coronary artery bypass grafting (CABG) |
| --- | --- |
| *Indications* | |
| Discrete single vessel disease | Diffuse multivessel disease |
| Multivessel disease | Small calibre vessels |
| Complex disease (e.g. bifurcations) | Long lesions |
| Chronic total occlusions | Left main stem disease (±) |
| Left main stem disease (±) | Additional valve surgery |
| Primary PCI (AMI) | |
| Rescue PCI (AMI) | |
| Salvage PCI (cardiogenic shock) | |
| *Advantages* | |
| Short hospital stay | More complete revascularization |
| Major surgery avoided | Good symptomatic relief |
| Fewer cerebral events | ? Improved prognosis |
| Less periprocedural infarcts | |
| *Disadvantages* | |
| Less complete revascularization | Longer hospital stay |
| Symptom recurrence | Increased initial costs |
| More subsequent procedures | Periprocedural complications |

## Acute myocardial infarction

### Epidemiology

The true incidence of acute myocardial infarction is unknown but approximately 150 000 deaths from CHD occurred in the UK in 1995. The incidence and mortality of acute myocardial infarction is improving with time as a result of efforts targeted at primary prevention and risk-factor reduction, patient awareness, paramedic ambulance personnel, coronary care units, drug therapy (e.g. aspirin, β-blockade, ACE inhibitors), thrombolysis, rehabilitation, post-infarct risk stratification and revascularization (PTCA, CABG).

### Pathophysiology

An acute myocardial infarct occurs when myocardial ischaemia, usually occurring as a result of atherosclerotic coronary artery disease, is sufficient to result in irreversible necrosis of cardiac muscle.

#### Coronary thrombosis

Angiographic and post-mortem studies of patients very early after the onset of symptoms demonstrate a high (>85%) incidence of occlusive thrombus in the culprit artery (Fig. 8.11). The thrombus is a mixture of white (platelet rich) and red (fibrin/erythrocyte rich) clot. Even without treatment, the incidence of thrombosis falls to 65% by 24 hours, suggesting that spontaneous thrombolysis occurs if the patient survives the acute event.

#### Plaque fissure

Coronary thrombosis commonly occurs in association with a plaque fissure (see page 99).

#### Coronary artery spasm

In a small minority (<5%) of patients, acute myocardial infarction occurs in the setting of normal coronary arteries. It is assumed that coronary artery spasm plays a role in some of these cases. Spasm may also be superimposed on 'fixed' atherosclerotic disease that can lead to a critical occlusion, often with added thrombus sufficient to cause infarction.

#### Collateral vessels

One of the major determinants of the extent of myocardial necrosis is the presence of a collateral blood supply to the area undergoing infarction. In patients suffering acute myocardial infarction, following a long history of chronic stable angina, collateral vessels may be well developed such that the size of the infarct is small. In the young patient with a sudden occlusion of the LAD, the consequence is usually an extensive anterior infarct because of the paucity of collateral vessels.

### Clinical history (see Box 8.14)
#### Chest pain
The majority (>80%) of patients present with chest pain. The symptoms are typical and can be compared with a prolonged attack of severe

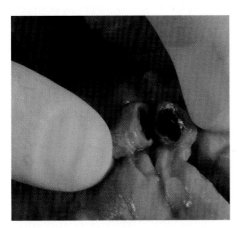

Fig. 8.11 Coronary thrombosis.

> ### Box 8.14 Symptoms in Acute Myocardial Infarction
>
> - Prolonged chest pain
> - Anxiety, apprehension
> - Sweating
> - Breathlessness
> - Nausea

angina. Whereas a typical attack of angina lasts 5–10 min, the chest pain of myocardial infarction usually lasts at least 30 min. The pain or tightness is oppressive and may be associated with sweating or fear.

Although the pain may radiate to the arm(s) or jaw, occasionally the symptoms may be mainly arising from the epigastrium, which may cause diagnostic difficulty. In the elderly and diabetics, pain may be slight or absent.

An acute infarct often occurs after extremes of exertion or emotion, rarely at the peak of exercise. Up to 50% of patients are awoken from sleep by chest pain and approximately one-third of patients continue with their activities despite the presence of chest pain. On direct questioning, many patients admit to vague symptoms in the days or weeks before the event including malaise, fatigue or non-specific chest pain.

### Breathlessness

Breathlessness may be due to a sudden rise in left ventricular end diastolic pressure, indicative of incipient ventricular failure, and may occasionally occur as the sole manifestation of myocardial infarction.

Anxiety may result in hyperventilation. In silent infarction, late breathlessness is indicative of significant left ventricular dysfunction.

### Gastrointestinal symptoms

An increase in vagal activity results in nausea and vomiting and is said to be more common in inferior infarction.

Diaphragmatic stimulation in inferior infarction may also cause hiccoughs.

### Other symptoms

These include palpitation, dizziness or syncope from ventricular arrhythmias, and symptoms from arterial embolism (e.g. stroke, limb ischaemia).

### Physical examination

#### General appearance

The patient appears pale, sweaty and apprehensive due to sympathetic overactivity.

There may be obvious respiratory distress with tachypnoea and breathlessness.

A moderate fever of usually less than 38°C occurs 12–24 hours after the infarct and may be useful in diagnosis if cardiac enzyme estimations are not yet available.

### Pulse and BP

A sinus tachycardia (100–120/min) occurs in one-third of patients; with adequate analgesia, the pulse usually slows unless there is impending cardiogenic shock.

A slow heart rate may indicate a sinus bradycardia or heart block complicating the infarct. A moderate increase in BP is attributable to catecholamine release.

Hypotension occurs as a result of vagal overactivity, dehydration, right ventricular infarction, or may be indicative of cardiogenic shock.

### Examination of the heart

Palpation of the precordium may reveal an area of dyskinesia, particularly in patients who have sustained an extensive anterior infarct.

An S4 is common, but may be transient. More severe left ventricular dysfunction is accompanied by an S3, and/or reversed splitting of the S2.

Late systolic murmurs of mild MR come and go depending on ventricular loading conditions.

Pericardial friction rubs are rarely heard until the second or third day, or much later (up to 6 weeks) as a feature of Dressler's syndrome (see page 203).

### Examination of the lungs

End inspiratory crackles may be evident, even in the absence of radiographic pulmonary oedema.

Frank pulmonary oedema is seen as a complication of extensive, usually anterior, infarction.

### Other features

Clinical evidence of hyperlipidaemia, peripheral vascular disease, diabetes, and hypertensive retinopathy may all be present.

## Investigations (see Box 8.15)
### Cardiac enzymes

Following death of myocardial tissue, the cytoplasmic constituents of myocardial cells are liberated into the circulation. Creatine phosphokinase (CPK) is detectable 6–8 hours after acute infarction peaking at 24 hours and returning to normal after another 24 hours. An isoenzyme (CPK-MB) is specific for heart muscle, but can also be released in myocarditis, cardiac trauma and following direct current (DC) countershock. Aspartate amino transferase (AAT), a non-specific enzyme commonly run as part of a biochemical screen, can be detected as early as 12 hours, peaks at 36 hours and returns to normal by 4 days. Hepatic congestion, primary liver disease and pulmonary embolism may all be associated with an elevation in AAT. Like CPK, AAT is also found in skeletal muscle.

---

**Box 8.15  Investigations in Acute Myocardial Infarcton**

- FBC, ESR, CRP
- Resting ECG
- Cardiac enzymes
- Troponin I or T
- Echocardiography
- Exercise testing
- ± Coronary arteriography

---

An increase in the non-specific enzyme lactate dehydrogenase (LDH) occurs late in myocardial infarction: elevated levels are detectable at 24 hours, peaking at 3–6 days with an increase which may remain detectable for 2 weeks. Its isoenzyme $LDH_1$ is more specific but its clinical use has been superseded by measurement of the troponins (see below).

Serial estimates of a panel of cardiac enzymes are measured daily for the first 3 days: a significant elevation is defined as twice the upper limit of the laboratory normal. Time-activity curves of the various enzymes are shown in Fig. 8.12.

### Troponins

The troponins (T&I) are regulatory proteins located within the myocyte contractile apparatus. Both are sensitive markers of myocardial cell injury and can be measured by a bedside test kit. Troponins appear to be raised both in acute myocardial infarction and in some high-risk patients with unstable angina when CPK levels remain normal. The diagnostic criteria for acute myocardial infarction have recently been redefined based on troponin estimations (see *Eur Heart J* 2000; **21**: 1502–1513).

### Other blood tests

Non-specific changes in routine blood tests

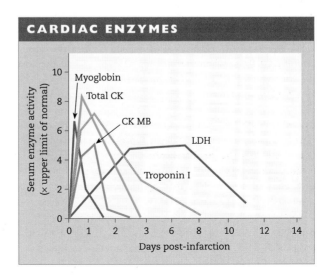

**Fig. 8.12** Time-activity curves for a panel of cardiac enzymes.

include an elevated white cell count after 48 hours, typically 10–15 000, predominately polymorphs, and an elevated erythrocyte sedimentation rate (ESR) and C-reactive protein (CRP) peaking at day 4 with a second peak as a feature of Dressler's syndrome. Mild hyperglycaemia as a result of carbohydrate intolerance may persist for some weeks. Catecholamine release, recumbency and a change in diet alter estimates of lipid levels, which should therefore be deferred for 4–6 weeks.

## Electrocardiography

The combination of a typical history in association with elevated cardiac enzymes is more reliable than the ECG in the diagnosis of acute myocardial infarction. The ECG has a positive predictive accuracy of approximately 80%; thus a normal ECG does not exclude infarction. Serial ECGs are valuable in documenting the evolution of electrical disturbances. ECG changes evolve in a well-defined order (Fig. 8.13). Incomplete repolarization of damaged myocardium causes S–T segment elevation ('current of injury') overlaying the affected region. In patients seen very early after infarction, tall, symmetrical T waves may be apparent which invert as the S–T segments rise. Reciprocal S–T segment depression is seen in the leads opposite the infarct. The S–T segments return to the isoelectric line within a few days depending on the magnitude of the infarct, followed by T wave inversion which may remain indefinitely. Subsequently, pathological Q waves, defined as a duration >30 msecs and an amplitude >25% of the ensuing R wave, develop in the area of infarction. Q waves are not specific as they may be seen in cardiomyopathy and ventricular hypertrophy. In one-third of patients, Q waves resolve within 18 months of the acute event. A proportion of the 20% of patients who have a documented infarct by clinical and enzyme criteria have the infarct in an area that is electrically silent to the surface 12-lead ECG.

The relationship between the ECG and the pathological severity of infarction is unreliable, thus, a patient with Q waves may have sustained a transmural or a subendocardial infarct. The same is true for the patient with S–T segment depression or fixed T wave inversion (non-Q wave infarction), which is not specific for subendocardial infarction. Although subendocardial infarction is less likely to result in cardiogenic shock or myocardial rupture, minor degrees of infarction may result in sudden death from ventricular arrhythmias or be the harbinger of a later transmural infarct (the so-called 'stuttering' infarct). The prognosis of a non-Q wave infarct is less favourable than Q-wave infarction.

## Echocardiography

Following myocardial infarction, regional wall motion abnormalities, reduced fractional shortening and ejection fraction, mural thrombus, pericardial fluid and abnormalities of valve function can all be detected by cross-sectional echocardiography (see Chapter 3).

## Radionuclide scintigraphy

Infarct avid myocardial scintigraphy with a radionuclide with a short half-life ($^{99m}$Tc-pyrophosphate) can be used to make a semiquantitative assessment of infarct size but this is not used as routine investigation (see Chapter 3).

## Coronary arteriography

Urgent coronary arteriography may occasionally be required if there remains doubt over the diagnosis in a patient with atypical symptoms in the absence of the characteristic ECG changes. Coronary arteriography is usually reserved for patients undergoing primary PTCA or stenting.

## Differential diagnosis

### Aortic dissection

Retrosternal pain radiates through to the back, with clinical evidence of reduced or absent pulses and/or aortic regurgitation.

Diagnosis is confirmed by computerized tomographic (CT)/magnetic resonance scanning or transoesophageal echocardiography (see Chapter 3).

## SERIAL ECG CHANGES

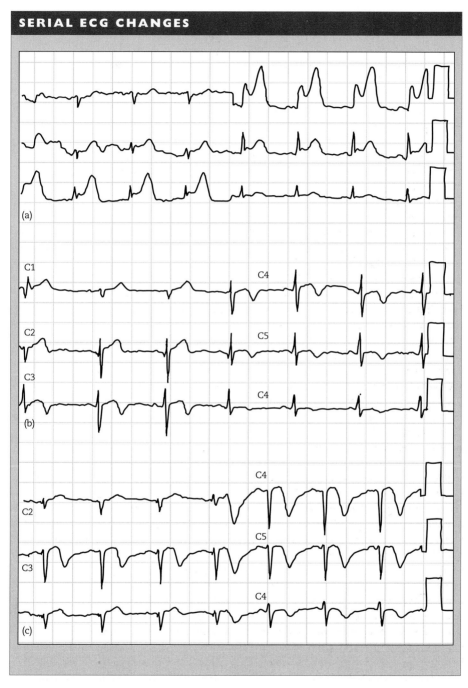

**Fig. 8.13** Serial ECG changes in an evolving anterior infarct (a–c).

## Acute pericarditis

• Chest pain is relieved by sitting forward.
• Previous viral infection, fever, systemic upset, friction rub and typical ECG (see Chapter 13).

## Acute pulmonary embolism

• Marked breathlessness with little or no chest pain.
• Pleuritic pain and haemoptysis may accompany peripheral emboli.
• Elevated venous pressure, right-sided S3, pleural rub.
• Arterial hypoxaemia, typical ECG, oligaemic chest radiograph.
• Confirm with V/Q scan, spiral CT, pulmonary arteriography (see Chapter 16).

## Chest wall pain

• Differentiated on the clinical history.
• Superficial, localized pain, often transient, may be provoked by activity or changes in posture. Responds to minor analgesics or NSAIDs. Similar symptoms from costo-chondritis (Tietze's syndrome) localized to costo-chondral junction (often the second).

## Gastrointestinal disorders

Disorders of the upper GI tract (oesophageal reflux, spasm, hiatus hernia, peptic ulceration or acute pancreatitis) may all cause diagnostic difficulty in occasional patients.
• ST/T wave changes and a response to nitrates may occur with oesophageal spasm, pancreatitis and cholecystitis.
• A careful clinical history and investigation of the GI tract will help clarify the diagnosis.

## **Treatment** (see Box 8.16)
### General measures

Once admitted to hospital, the patient should be transferred rapidly to the coronary care unit. In some hospitals, thrombolysis is administered in the Accident and Emergency Department; in others, the patient is admitted to the cardiac care unit (CCU) first. Either way, there should be the shortest possible delay before the patient is monitored for disturbances of heart rhythm, and a venous cannula inserted for vascular ac-

---

> ### Box 8.16  Treatment in Acute Myocardial Infarction
>
> • Analgesia (opiate)
> • Aspirin
> • Heparin (LMW)
> • Thrombolysis
> • β-blockade
> • ± Diuretics
> • ± ACE inhibitor
> • Oxygen

---

cess. Rather than undergo a formal admission procedure, it is preferable for the patient to be admitted to the CCU inappropriately and then moved to another ward if it transpires that the diagnosis was incorrect. Central venous cannulation and arterial access is not required in uncomplicated patients (Killip I).

Routine blood tests should include haematology and a biochemical screen including a panel of cardiac enzymes. A portable (AP) chest radiograph is taken together with daily ECGs. Depending on bed availability, uncomplicated patients usually remain in CCU for 24–48 hours and are discharged from hospital after 5–7 days.

### Analgesia

Adequate analgesia and if necessary light sedation is important, as a comfortable, relaxed patient is less likely to suffer from arrhythmias, and a reduction in endogenous catecholamines will reduce the chance of subendocardial ischaemia. Small doses of intravenous opiates (diamorphine 2.5–5.0 mg or morphine sulphate 5–10 mg) are effective analgesics with additional vasodilating properties, which may be particularly useful in the patient suffering from pulmonary oedema. Because of the side-effects of nausea and vomiting, prophylactic anti-emetics (prochlorperazine 10 mg, metoclopramide 10 mg or cyclizine 50 mg) should also be administered. The initial pain usually settles within 24 hours in Killip I patients. Recurrent pain after a few days may be indicative of pericarditis, or later still, Dressler's syndrome, both of which are best treated with NSAIDs.

Anxious patients may benefit from a short acting benzodiazepine (e.g. lorazepam 0.5–1.0 mg). Bedrest is only necessary as long as the patient is in pain, or there is evidence of arrhythmia or haemodynamic disturbance.

There is little evidence that oxygen supplements are necessary in the uncomplicated infarct, although many patients will experience psychological benefit from oxygen which is widely prescribed. Nasal cannulae delivering 2–4 L/min of humidified oxygen are convenient, although oxygen delivery is variable. In patients with pulmonary oedema, transcutaneous oxygen monitoring is helpful, and arterial blood gas estimates usually unnecessary.

### Antiplatelet therapy

The benefit of the early administration of aspirin 300 mg has been documented in a number of clinical trials (e.g. ISIS-2). Long-term treatment with aspirin following myocardial infarction also reduces all-cause mortality, including reinfarction and non-fatal stroke. The beneficial effect of aspirin is especially marked in non-Q wave myocardial infarction. The minimum effective and best tolerated dose is 75 mg daily which should be continued indefinitely. Data from the CURE trial suggest that a combination of aspirin 75 mg and clopidogrel 75 mg is superior to aspirin alone in non-Q wave infarction.

### Anticoagulation

Heparin reduces the risk of systemic and pulmonary embolism and has also been shown to facilitate the resolution of apical thrombus demonstrated on echocardiography. Most of the data favourable to the routine use of heparin preceded the thrombolytic era. Heparin can either be administered by the subcutaneous or intravenous route; LMW heparin is convenient to administer as it does not require routine monitoring. Formal anticoagulation with heparin followed by warfarin should be reserved for patients with extensive myocardial infarction, cardiogenic shock, left ventricular aneurysm or sustained atrial arrhythmias. In the GUSTO-I trial, clinical outcome in patients treated with heparin following myocardial infarction was clearly related to the level of anticoagulation: the optimal range for the activated partial thromboplastin time (aPTT) was 50–70 s, more aggressive anticoagulation was associated with an increased risk of bleeding.

### Thrombolytic therapy

Early mortality and long-term outcome following acute myocardial infarction relates to early and complete reperfusion as judged by normal (TIMI-3) flow in the target artery.

The rapid intravenous administration of a thrombolytic agent has been shown to improve prognosis in a number of clinical trials (e.g. ISIS-3, GISSI-2, GUSTO-I). Arterial patency at 90 min following infusion appears to be the main determinant of long-term outcome: a patent vessel favourably improves survival, ventricular function and the incidence of late sudden death. A number of thrombolytic agents are effective (Table 8.8), and although accelerated t-PA is superior to streptokinase, the routine use of t-PA is prohibitive.

All patients should be considered for thrombolytic therapy following myocardial infarction with relatively few contraindications (Box 8.17). It is important to emphasize that the clinical (bedside) assessment of reperfusion is unreliable. Normalization of the S–T segment is not a surrogate for arterial patency, although this combined with the resolution of chest pain and a 'reperfusion' arrhythmia (e.g. accelerated idioventricular rhythm) is highly suggestive of a restoration of arterial patency.

### β-blockade

β-blocking drugs reduce heart rate, systemic BP and cardiac output. Cardiac work and peak $\delta p/\delta t$ are lowered, thus there is a significant reduction in $MVO_2$. In numerous clinical trials, β-blockers have been shown to reduce all-cause mortality, including sudden death and non-fatal reinfarction. The absolute benefit is most marked in the elderly, those with a previous myocardial infarct, diabetes mellitus, left ventricular dysfunction and electrical instability. β-blockade is well tolerated in the majority of patients. Despite the widespread use of other

## FIBRINOLYTIC AGENTS

| Drug name | Trade name | Dose | Cost* |
|---|---|---|---|
| Alteplase | Actilyse | 100 mg IV over 90 min (symptoms < 6 h) or over 3 h (symptoms 6–12 h) | £135.00 (1 pack, 10 mg) |
| Anistreplase | Eminase | 30 units IV over 4–5 min (symptoms < 6 h) | £495.00 (1 pack, 30 units) |
| Reteplase | Rapilysin | 2 × 10 units IV over < 2 min, 30 min apart (symptoms < 12 h) | £716.25 (1 pack, 20 units) |
| Streptokinase | Kabikinase | 1.5 million units IV over 1 h | £81.18 (1.5 million units) |
| Streptokinase | Streptase | 1.5 million units IV over 1 h | £89.72 (1.5 million units) |

*Cost for cheapest preparation.

Table 8.8 Fibrinolytic agents for use in acute myocardial infarction.

### Box 8.17 Contraindications to Thrombolysis

Absolute
• Previous haemorrhagic stroke (at any time)
• Other strokes or cerebrovascular events (within 1 year)
• Intracranial neoplasm
• Active internal bleeding
• Suspected aortic dissection

Relative
• Severe or uncontrolled systemic hypertension (BP >180/110 mmHg)
• History of previous cerebrovascular event
• Current use of anticoagulants
• Known bleeding diathesis
• Recent major trauma, including head injury (within 4 weeks)
• Recent major surgery (within 4 weeks)
• Prolonged cardiopulmonary resuscitation
• Non-compressible vascular punctures (especially arterial)
• Recent internal bleeding (within 4 weeks)
• Prior administration (within 2 years) or allergic reaction to streptokinase or anistreplase
• Active peptic ulceration
• Pregnancy

drugs post-infarction (e.g. aspirin, ACE inhibitors), there is evidence that β-blockers offer an additional benefit over the other drugs. The majority of benefit is seen in the first year following infarction, but late sudden death is reduced by β-blockade suggesting that the drug should be continued in the long term. A once daily selective β-blocking agent (e.g. atenolol 25–50 mg daily) is commonly prescribed.

### Nitrates
Most of the data relating to the beneficial effects of nitrates are derived from the prethrombolysis era. Nitrates are commonly used for the relief of chest pain and are particularly effective when combined with heparin in the management of the patient with unstable or post-infarction angina. They are effective venous and arteriolar dilators and may therefore be used to control systemic hypertension, or to offload the myocardium in the patient with cardiogenic shock. If nitrates are used in the post-infarct patient, the intravenous route is preferable in doses sufficient to reduce systolic BP to 100 mmHg.

### ACE inhibitors
A variety of ACE inhibitors have been studied following acute myocardial infarction using a variety of dosing regimens, either in unselected

patients (e.g. CONSENSUS II, GISSI-3, ISIS-4) or selected high-risk patients (e.g. SAVE, AIRE). In general, the trials show a significant reduction in all-cause mortality, including late sudden death and reinfarction. Secondary endpoints also show a significant reduction in the incidence of heart failure and the need for early revascularization.

ACE inhibitors should be started early (within 24 hours) and are most beneficial in the elderly, and in patients with clinical evidence of heart failure or left ventricular dysfunction on echocardiography. ACE inhibitors are well tolerated with side-effects (e.g. systemic hypotension, cardiogenic shock, renal dysfunction) occurring in only a small minority of patients. The benefit of ACE inhibitors appears to occur in addition to the benefit seen with the concomitant use of β-blockers.

## Calcium channel blockade

The calcium antagonists are a heterogeneous group of drugs with differing clinical properties. The short-acting dihydropyridines (e.g. nifedipine) have no role in treating the post-infarction patient, except possibly in combination with β-blockade. Used alone, a number of trials have shown that nifedipine and similar agents may actually increase mortality compared with placebo. Diltiazem may have a role in patients with non-Q wave myocardial infarction, and verapamil in patients in whom β-blockers may be contraindicated. Both drugs are usually well tolerated although side-effects of heart failure, hypotension or symptomatic heart block may occasionally be seen.

## Diuretics
See Chapter 6.

## Other vasodilators
See Chapter 6.

## Inotropic support
See Chapter 6.

## Anti-arrhythmic agents
See Chapter 9.

## Magnesium
See Chapter 9.

## Mechanical support
See Chapter 6.

## DC cardioversion
See Chapter 9.

## Endocardial pacing
See Chapter 9.

## Primary angioplasty/stenting

A number of small clinical trials have demonstrated superior TIMI-3 (i.e. normal) flow in patients undergoing primary angioplasty, with or without stenting, following myocardial infarction when compared with a variety of thrombolytic agents. Vessel patency, myocardial salvage, reinfarction and the incidence of cerebral haemorrhage are all superior following balloon angioplasty. There is no doubt that a strategy of primary intervention requires a huge resource, including a dedicated and experienced team, 24-hour catheter laboratory availability and a mechanism for rapid access to allow the shortest possible elapse from the onset of chest pain to restoration of arterial patency. This approach will only ever be applicable to a minority of patients in the UK, and it remains to be determined which will benefit most in a health care system with limited resources.

## Complications

## Arrhythmias
See Chapter 9.

## Cardiogenic shock
See Chapter 6.

## Acute mitral regurgitation

Mild MR following myocardial infarction is heard in up to 50% of patients and occurs as a result of abnormal papillary muscle geometry, malaligned mitral cusps or annular dilatation. Typically, a late systolic murmur comes and goes depending on loading conditions.

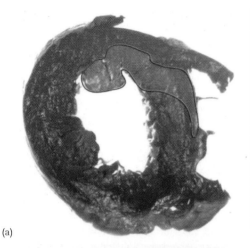

(a)

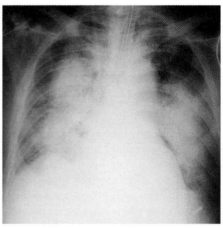

Fig. 8.15 Chest radiograph demonstrating acute pulmonary oedema in a patient with papillary muscle rupture (note small heart).

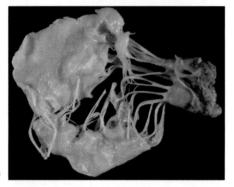

(b)

Fig. 8.14 (a) Transmural infarction involving a papillary muscle. (b) Papillary muscle rupture.

Severe MR as a result of papillary muscle rupture is rare (Fig. 8.14), occurring in <1% of all infarcts. It is seen more frequently complicating inferior infarcts because the posteromedial papillary muscle has only a single blood supply and is therefore more susceptible to ischaemic insult. Typically, the patient appears in acute pulmonary oedema (Fig. 8.15) or cardiogenic shock within the first 10 days after an infarct; sudden death may also occur. A pansystolic murmur, which may be inconspicuous and cannot be differentiated on clinical grounds from an infarct-related ventricular septal defect (VSD) may be present. Cross-sectional echocardiography is diagnostic with a flail leaflet prolapsing into the left atrium in association with detachment of all or part of the subvalve apparatus.

Without surgical intervention (mitral repair or replacement), more than 75% of patients are dead within 24 hours. Surgical mortality should be in the order of 10% depending on the condition of the patient.

## Ventricular septal defect

Acquired VSD occurs in 1–3% of cases of acute myocardial infarction (Fig. 8.16). VSD complicating anterior infarction is more common than those involving inferior infarcts, although the latter have a worse surgical mortality. Necrotic muscle results in a 1–2 cm defect in the muscular septum, often in association with a left ventricular aneurysm. Most patients with an acute VSD have had a sizeable infarct, whereas patients with acute MR have often sustained only a small infarct involving the papillary muscle. Diagnosis is confirmed on cross-sectional imaging, with Doppler flow clearly visible from left to right ventricle. Cardiac catheterization is usually required to document the coronary anatomy and/or to insert an intra-aortic balloon. Operative mortality is in the region of 20–30% in experienced centres, and right ventricular function appears to be a major determinant of late survival. Immediate resuscitation and surgical referral reduce the chance of multi-

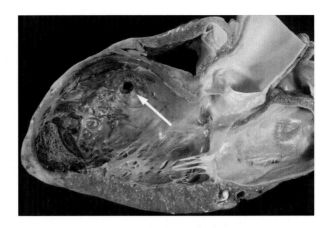

**Fig. 8.16** Anterior myocardial infarct complicated by an acute VSD.

system failure occurring as a consequence of low cardiac output.

### Free-wall rupture

Up to 15% of patients dying suddenly following myocardial infarction die from free-wall rupture (Fig. 8.17). This complication appears to have reduced in frequency since the routine use of β-blockade. Cardiac rupture is more common in the elderly, in females and following extensive transmural infarction. A small minority of patients survives the acute event as a result of a sealed off tamponade or pseudoaneursym formation. Diagnosis is usually evident on echocardiography and the treatment is surgical.

### Systemic thromboembolism

Even in the presence of mural thrombus on echocardiography, systemic thromboembolism is rare, occurring in less than 5% of patients overall. Systemic emboli usually pass to the cerebral circulation. Formal anticoagulation (heparin followed by warfarin) should be reserved for patients with poor ventricular function (ejection fraction <40%), left ventricular aneurysm or atrial arrhythmias (especially AF).

### Pulmonary embolism

As a result of the liberal use of heparin and thrombolytics, coupled with rapid mobilization, the incidence of pulmonary embolism has fallen.

Pulmonary embolism if it occurs should be treated in the routine manner (see Chapter 16).

### Pericarditis and the post-myocardial infarction syndrome

Early pericarditis (within 1 week of infarction) is characterized by typical pericardial pain (see Chapter 13) and an audible friction rub in association with ST/T wave changes. It is more common following extensive transmural infarction, but seems to be occurring less frequently since the advent of thrombolytic therapy, now reported in 6–7% of patients. Symptoms respond rapidly to NSAIDs in the majority of patients.

Post-myocardial infarction (Dressler's) syndrome consists of pleuropericarditis occurring 2–6 weeks after myocardial infarction, in association with a fever elevated ESR, CRP and white count. The condition appears to have an immune basis, and may occur without preceding (early) pericarditis. A minority of patients has a pericardial effusion, and occasional cases of pericardial tamponade or constriction have been reported. The syndrome is indistinguishable from post-cardiotomy syndrome following cardiopulmonary bypass procedures. Symptoms usually respond rapidly to NSAIDs, but some patients require a short course of oral steroids.

### Left ventricular aneurysm

Transmural apical infarction is particularly prone to aneurysm formation. Early infarct ex-

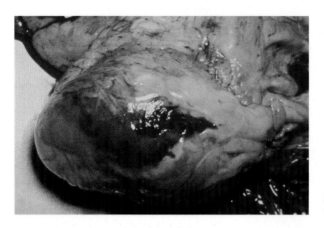

**Fig. 8.17** Left ventricular free wall rupture.

pansion may be associated with myocardial thinning, dilatation and fibrosis such that a discrete bulge occurs, within which there is paradoxical movement (i.e. systolic expansion), thereby detracting from overall ventricular function. Symptoms of recurrent chest pain, breathlessness, intractable arrhythmias and systemic thromboembolism are typical. Clinical features include a dilated heart, dyskinetic or paradoxical apex, an S3 and possible MR. Chronic cases have a typical appearance on the chest radiograph, often with calcification within the wall of the aneurysm (Fig. 8.18). The diagnosis can be confirmed on cross-sectional echocardiography (which often demonstrates thrombus within the aneurysm), magnetic resonance scanning or cine-angiography.

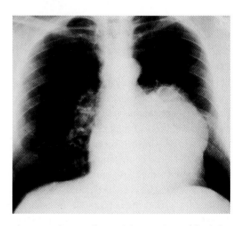

**Fig. 8.18** Chest radiograph in a patient with a left ventricular aneurysm.

The early use of ACE inhibitors and thrombolytics has reduced the incidence of aneurysm formation. Left ventricular aneurysm formation ± CABG has an early mortality of less than 5% in experienced centres.

### Rehabilitation and risk factor modification

Prior to leaving hospital, patients should be counselled by a cardiac rehabilitation nurse. During their inpatient stay, the patient will be receptive to reassurance and encouragement, and the opportunity should not be missed to address the correction of risk factors. Explanations are important and lead to realistic expec-

tations in the post-infarct recovery period. Specific advice should be given regarding diet, smoking, physical activity, sex, and plans for return to work. If facilities are available, a formal rehabilitation programme and group activity should be encouraged with emphasis on a progressive increase in dynamic (isotonic) exercise (e.g. walking, swimming, cycling).

### Post-infarct investigations
*Lipids*

Estimation of blood lipids may be unrepresentative early after a myocardial infarct. It is therefore recommended that a fasting lipid profile be checked 4–6 weeks after the acute event. This is conveniently arranged at the first post-infarct clinic visit. Approximately 75% of patients who have sustained a myocardial infarct will have an abnormal lipid profile. Aggressive reduction of total cholesterol with a statin following myocardial infarction significantly reduces all-cause mortality, reinfarction, ventricular dysfunction (heart failure), hospital readmission, stroke and the need for subsequent revascularization. Reduction in cholesterol using statins is at least as effective as aspirin and β-blockade in reducing mortality following myocardial infarction. A fasting total cholesterol greater than 5.2 mmol/L should be treated with a statin. In patients with combined hyperlipidaemia, fibrates may be an alternative approach, which are effective in reducing triglycerides although they may be less effective than statins at lowering cholesterol.

## Functional testing and risk stratification

Post-infarct exercise testing is a simple non-invasive test that will identify the presence of inducible ischaemia and thus be able to stratify patients for risk and the need for subsequent coronary arteriography. Most of the studies of post-infarct exercise testing relate to the pre-thrombolytic era. As most of the studies show a very low (1–2% at one year) mortality in patients receiving thrombolysis, the value of routine exercise testing has recently been questioned, particularly in relation to 'false-positive' responders. Nevertheless, a predischarge or 6-week post-infarct exercise test does provide useful information, and can determine the need for further investigation (Box 8.18).

## Coronary arteriography and revascularization

The routine use of coronary arteriography and revascularization following myocardial infarction does not improve prognosis in unselected groups of patients. The primary indication for invasive investigation is symptomatic recurrent ischaemia, intractable arrhythmias or poor performance on the treadmill.

## Natural history and prognosis

Early 30-day and late mortality following myocardial infarction is related to the territory and extent of the ECG changes. Limited inferior infarcts have a 30-day and 12-month mortality of 4.5% and 6.7%, respectively, whereas anterior infarcts with widespread S–T segment elevation and bundle branch block have mortalities of 19.6% and 25.6% respectively. Additional information can be gained from classification according to the haemodynamic (Killip) class:

---

**Box 8.18 Exercise Testing Following Myocardial Infarction**

Poor prognostic features:
- Exercise induced chest pain (angina)
- S–T segment depression
- Abnormal blood pressure response
- Flat heart rate response (chronotropic incompetence)
- Exercise induced ventricular arrhythmias

---

**Box 8.19 Factors Associated with a Poor Prognosis Following Myocardial Infarction**

- Increasing age
- Female gender
- Extensive infarction (determined by cardiac enzymes or widespread ECG changes)
- Mechanical complications of myocardial infarction (e.g. VSD, free wall rupture, acute mitral regurgitation)
- Anterior infarction
- Inferior infarction with right ventricular involvement
- Diabetes mellitus
- Previous angina or myocardial infarction
- Impaired ventricular function (S3, pulmonary oedema)
- Failure to perfuse with thrombolysis
- Anterior infarction associated with atrioventricular block
- Recurrent infarction/ischaemia whilst still an inpatient
- Electrical instability (e.g. secondary VT/VF)
- Depressed heart rate variability
- Abnormal late potentials

- the majority of patients (85%) have no evidence of heart failure (Killip I);
- an S3 and bibasal crackles define Killip II (10%);
- Frank pulmonary oedema (Killip III) and cardiogenic shock (Killip IV) together account for only 5% of patients.

The major determinants of prognosis after myocardial infarction are age, systolic BP, heart rate, infarct location and Killip class. Factors associated with a poor prognosis are listed in Box 8.19.

# CHAPTER 9

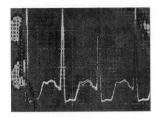

# Pacing and Electrophysiology

## Introduction

Cardiac myocyte contraction generates the mechanical force of atrial and ventricular systole.
• Individual myocyte contraction is the end result of a complex of ionic fluxes that cause cell membrane depolarization and repolarization.
• The transmembrane voltage changes (the consequence of ionic flux across the cell membrane) which occur during this process can be recorded using specialized techniques and are depicted as the action potential (Fig. 9.1).

Cell membrane depolarization and repolarization trigger activation and subsequent relaxation of the actin/myosin complex. Co-ordination of myocyte mechanical activity through the heart is achieved by the cardiac conduction system, itself a complex arrangement of cells that depolarize and repolarize.

Potential gradients, created by myocardial depolarization, can be detected by body surface electrodes. These may be translated into an electronic or pen and ink inscription showing potential gradient variation with time in any given recording electrode. Recording electrodes may be bipolar or unipolar, and potential differences recorded in a standardized way, in either frontal or coronal planes.

Thus, summation of the electrical activity of the heart is used to generate the surface electrocardiogram (ECG).

### The conduction system (Fig. 9.2)
Heart rate and co-ordination of atrioventricular (AV) contraction are determined by an electrical control system comprising:
• **sinus node** (SN);
• **atrial conduction channels**;
• **atrioventricular node** (AVN);
• **His–Purkinje system**.

Disease in any of these or atrial or ventricular myocardium can cause abnormality of heart rate or incoordination of cardiac contraction.

The **SN** is located in the superior aspect of the right atrium (RA), close to the SVC. It is composed of specialized pacemaker tissues which spontaneously depolarize. The rate of spontaneous depolarization is governed by intrinsic cellular properties, exogenous catecholamines and autonomic nervous tone. A wave of excitation spreads from the area of the SN through the atria along **specialized conduction channels**. The **AVN** is then activated but conduction through it is slow due to its characteristic decremental conduction features (the greater the frequency of depolarization the slower the conduction through AV nodal tissues). This protects the ventricles from an

## THE ACTION POTENTIAL

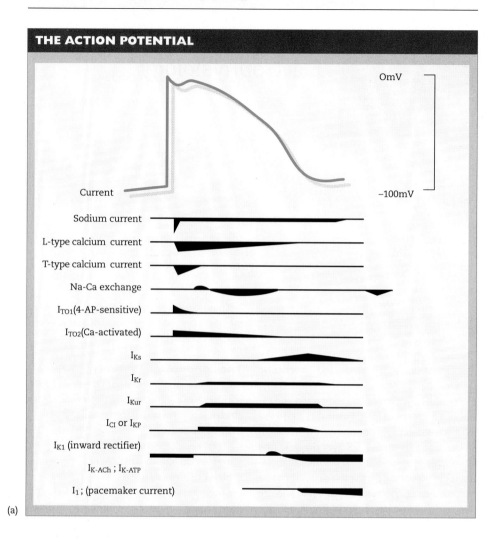

(a)

Fig. 9.1 (a) The relationship between transmembrane voltage gradient and time inscribes the action potential, the component currents of which are shown. Outward currents are grey, inward currents, black. (b) A schematic of the phases of the action potential.

after it arises from the main bundle, the left bundle divides into anterior and posterior fascicles. Repolarization of atria and ventricles is organized such that those areas depolarizing first repolarize last, an arrangement which may help to protect against reactivation of myocardium by myocardial depolarization at adjacent sites.

excessively fast rate response to atrial tachy-arrhythmias (in particular atrial fibrillation (AF)). The excitation wavefront then exits through the **His–Purkinje system**, passing into left and right conduction bundles before disseminating distally down the conduction system and into ventricular myocardium. Soon

## Arrhythmia

### Abnormalities of cardiac rhythm
• **Tachycardia**: abnormally fast rate (defined as more than 100 b.p.m.).

## THE ACTION POTENTIAL

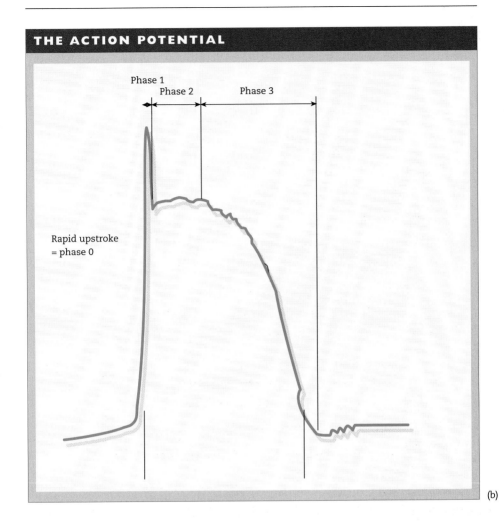

Phase 1

Phase 2          Phase 3

Rapid upstroke
= phase 0

(b)

Fig. 9.1 *continued.*

- **Bradycardia**: abnormally slow rate (defined as less than 60 cardiac b.p.m.).
- **Irregularity of rhythm**.

### Symptoms

- **Palpitation:** awareness of the heart beating, often due to an abnormality of rhythm, but sometimes an exaggerated awareness of sinus rhythm, or an increase in stroke volume (e.g. aortic or mitral regurgitation) or a sinus tachycardia (e.g. anxiety, fever, hyperthyroidism). Not all patients associate tachycardia with palpitation and may use the term to describe the irregularity of heart beat which comes, for example, with ventricular ectopic activity.

- **Dizziness, presyncope** or **syncope** can occur with systemic arterial hypotension causing hypoperfusion of the brain. Although an assessment of these symptoms requires exclusion of non-cardiac causes, systemic arterial hypotension may be the consequence of tachycardia, bradycardia, intravascular volume depletion, arterial vasodilatation or low cardiac output.

- **Non-specific symptoms** such as malaise, poor exercise tolerance and dyspnoea may occur with persistent bradycardia. Dyspnoea

## THE CARDIAC CONDUCTION SYSTEM

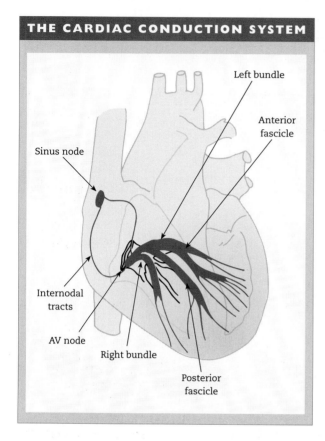

Left bundle

Anterior
fascicle

Sinus node

Internodal
tracts

AV node

Right bundle

Posterior
fascicle

**Fig. 9.2** The cardiac conduction
system.

and chest pain, often anginal in character, may
occur in tachycardia.

### Electrophysiological investigations (Box 9.1)

#### Surface ECG (Fig. 9.3)
The atrial chambers are thin walled. They possess a less specialized conduction system than
the ventricles, with their greater muscle mass,
which are served by the His Purkinje system
emanating from the AVN. The electrocardiographic deflections are arbitrarily termed:
- **P wave** (atrial mass depolarization);
- **QRS** (ventricular mass depolarization);
- **T** wave (ventricular mass repolarization); and
- **U** wave (genesis disputed).

The ventricles can be considered as three

> ### Box 9.1 Electrophysiological Investigations
>
> - ECG
> - Signal-averaged ECG
> - 24-hour tape and patient-activated recorders
> - Implantable loop recorder
> - Tiltable test
> - Carotid sinus massage
> - EP study

muscle masses: (i) interventricular septum; (ii)
right ventricle (RV); and (iii) left ventricle (LV).
The first portion of the ventricular mass to
depolarize is on the left side of the interventricular septum with subsequent spread of activation from left to right across the septum.
Simultaneous depolarization then occurs from
endocardial surface to epicardial surface in both

## ECG COMPONENTS

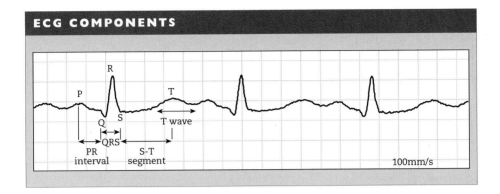

Fig. 9.3 The components of the ECG: P wave, atrial depolarization; QRS, ventricular depolarization; T wave, ventricular repolarization.

right and left ventricular muscle masses. The larger left ventricular mass generates greater voltages and so predominates in the QRS deflection. The precise features of the normal QRS deflection are determined by the recording lead's orientation. Each ECG recording lead has positive and negative poles.

- Standard leads I, II and III are bipolar and orientated in the coronal plane.
- Leads AVR, AVL and AVF ('A' for augmented as instrumental augmentation is necessary because of the low potential at the extremities) are unipolar leads orientated in the coronal plane.
- Leads VI to V6 are unipolar leads orientated in the horizontal plane.

The vectorial orientation of these leads is illustrated in Fig. 9.4. Box 9.2 defines the six chest leads. Abnormalities of the ECG which are caused by structural cardiac disease are discussed in the relevant chapters dealing with specific cardiac disorders.

### Signal-averaged ECG

This employs computer analysis of ECG recordings to identify late potentials in electrical activity related to myocardial depolarization in regions of myocardial abnormality, which may be the substrate for re-entry ventricular arrhythmia.

### Box 9.2 Einthoven's Triangle and the Chest Leads

The six chest leads are defined by international convention:
1 fourth interspace at right bottom of sternum
2 same interspace left sternal border
3 midway between 2 and 4
4 fourth interspace mid-clavicular line
5 same level as 4 in anterior axillary line
6 same level as 4 and 5 in mid-axillary line

### Ambulatory ECG monitoring

These devices (Holter monitors) are mini-ECG recorders, about the size of a small personal stereo. They continuously record two ECG leads via electrodes attached to the anterior chest wall over a 24-hour period, during which time the patient continues with their usual activities. They keep a diary of any symptoms which can be correlated with the ECG.

### Patient-activated recorders

Patient-activated devices will record a single ECG lead which can be analysed later or transmitted by telephone to a central recording station. Their particular value is in the assessment of patients whose symptoms are infrequent, but the ECG recordings are often of poor quality.

### Implantable recording devices

Small subcutaneous recording devices can be implanted as a minor procedure. ECG is stored

## EINTHOVEN'S TRIANGLE

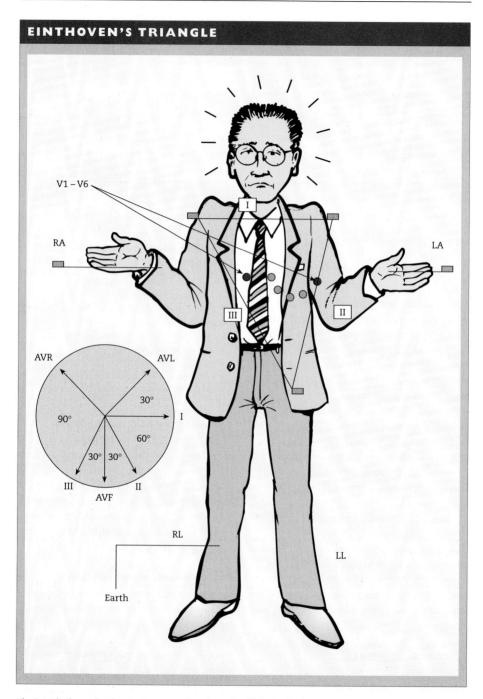

**Fig. 9.4** Einthoven's triangle: there are three 'standard' bipolar limb leads (I–III) and three augmented unipolar limb leads (AVR, AVF and AVL).

in the device prior to patient activation so that events which give rise to immediate loss of consciousness can be recorded after the event. This feature and long device life facilitate capture of infrequent events.

## Tilt table testing and carotid sinus massage

Patients lie on a couch which can be tilted (head up) to 60°. Continuous monitoring of blood pressure, heart rate and ECG is performed. Tilting usually continues for 45 min but is stopped if bradycardia (cardioinhibition) or hypotension (vasodepression) occurs. In some centres there may be additional use of sublingual nitrates or intravenous isoprenaline to stress vagotonic reflexes.

Patients with carotid sinus hypersensitivity syndrome may also have vagal cardioinhibition on inadvertent stimulation of the carotid sinus. Carotid sinus massage under controlled conditions and after assessment of carotid artery disease may unmask this.

## Exercise stress testing

Exercise stress testing will demonstrate inability of the SN to mount a tachycardia in response to physiological demand (chronotropic incompetence).

## Electrophysiology study

Catheters mounted with recording electrodes are introduced through the femoral or subclavian veins using a standard Seldinger technique under local anaesthetic. These are passed to the heart using standard cardiac catheterization techniques and positioned in the atria, at the AVN, and in the RV. Electrical activity from the endomyocardium apposed to the electrodes is filtered, amplified and recorded in unipolar or bipolar configurations as electrograms. The timing of electrical activity recorded from the endocardial surface (electrograms) at these sites and the response of electrical activity to cardiac pacing and extrastimulation (addition of premature paced beats during steady rate pacing), allows assessment of sinus and atrioventricular nodal activity and the integrity of the con-

duction system. Extrastimulation techniques are also used to assess inducibility and mechanism of tachycardias.

## Bradycardia

Bradycardia can be a secondary feature in a number of non-cardiac disorders:

- hypothyroidism;
- raised intracranial pressure;
- jaundice.

Cardiac causes of bradycardia include:

- **SN disease** with a slow atrial rate;
- **atrioventricular nodal disease** with a reduced frequency of nodal and therefore ventricular depolarization in response to a normal atrial rate;
- **abnormality of autonomic function** (vasovagal syndrome).

## Causes of bradycardia

### Sinus node disease

This may be due to degenerative disease of the SN, which is commoner with increasing age, or result from ischaemic heart disease or viral infection or autoimmune disease such as lupus. The SN may depolarize slowly or there may be a delay in electrical activity leaving the SN ('exit block').

### Atrioventricular node disease and conduction disease

AVN disease causes **heart block**. This may be caused by or follow:

- ischaemic heart disease;
- autoimmune disease (for example lupus or related to aortopathy in Reiter's or ankylosing spondylitis);
- sarcoidosis;
- destruction by infection (aortic root abscess);
- prosthetic aortic or mitral valve insertion.

Interruption of AVN conduction may be incomplete and produce degrees of block. Conduction disease distal to the AVN may either give rise to impairment of AV conduction or an altered pattern of ventricular depolarization with altered left or right bundle branch conduction. Right bundle branch block may occur in the normal heart. Left bundle branch block is regarded as usually indicating underlying cardiac disease, although it may be difficult to determine the cause. Isolated bundle branch block has no effect on cardiac rate and requires no treatment as a lone finding. Disease of the right bundle and left anterior fascicle with first degree heart block (so-called 'tri-fascicular block') carries a high risk of development of complete heart block and is usually considered an indication for prophylactic ventricular pacemaker implantation.

*First degree heart block*
Prolongation of the P to QRS (PR) interval >200 msec on the surface ECG. It is indicative of AVN disease. In isolation it requires no treatment but may be the only manifestation of conduction disease in a patient with intermittent complete heart block.

*Second degree heart block*
• **Type 1:** there is prolongation of successive PR intervals with failure of conduction of the ultimate P wave of a series (P wave not succeeded by a QRS complex). Again, as an isolated finding it requires no treatment but may be the only manifestation of conduction disease in patients with symptomatic intermittent higher degree heart block.
• **Type 2:** there is intermittent but regular failure of P waves to conduct through the AVN (fixed P wave to QRS relationship 1 : 2/1 : 3/1 : 4, etc.) with consequent bradycardia, the ventricular rate being 1/2, 1/3 or 1/4, etc. of the atrial rate. Prophylactic pacemaker implantation is indicated regardless of symptomatic status, as progression to complete heart block with the risk of a slow ventricular escape rhythm or even asystole is common.

*Complete heart block (third degree heart block)*
There is failure of atrioventricular nodal conduction so that there is complete AV dissociation. The ventricular rate is always slower than the atrial rate (note that AV dissociation is not complete heart block when the atrial rate is

slower than the ventricular rate as can occur during periods of increased vagal tone).

## Vasovagal syndrome
There is a complex interrelationship between cardiac rate and vasomotor tone to maintain systemic arterial pressure. Autonomic tone is a determinant of both cardiac rate and vasomotor tone. Enhancement of vagal tone may slow cardiac rate or cause vasodilatation or both and by either mechanism can lead to a fall in systemic arterial pressure. A sudden **increase in vagal tone** can cause a precipitous fall in arterial pressure whether **bradycardia** (due to **cardioinhibition**) or **vasodilation** (due to **depression of vasomotor tone**) is the principal cause. Increased vagal tone may follow external stimuli as, for instance, may occur in individuals susceptible to needles or the sight of blood, or can occur spontaneously, when it is termed vasovagal syndrome.

**Carotid sinus syndrome** is a similar entity. Sensitivity of the carotid sinus to mechanical pressure is the cause of a surge in vagal tone, in turn causing cardioinhibition and vasodepression which cause profound systemic arterial hypotension. Sinus bradycardia may be a normal finding in individuals with a high level of physical fitness and increased vagal tone. Excessive training can lead to exaggerated vagal tone and a condition colloquially called 'athlete's heart' in which the patient is susceptible to aspects of vasovagal syndrome.

## Investigations for bradycardia
### Electrophysiology study
Invasive electrophysiology study can assess the performance of the SN, AVN and conduction systems. A combination of electrogram recordings and extrastimulation techniques enables assessment of the functional integrity of the sinus and atrioventricular nodes and specialized electrical systems.

### Ambulatory monitoring or patient-activated recorders
Spontaneous episodes of bradycardia due either to SN disease or AV conduction failure

may be identified and should be correlated with patient symptoms using a patient diary.

## Implantable recorder

Implantable devices are available which continuously record an ECG. Activation of the device using a hand-held, patient-activated control unit holds up to 42 min of the ECG.

## Pacemaker implantation and drug therapy for bradycardia

### Drug therapy

Drug treatment is inadequate for long-term symptomatic relief of symptomatic SN disease or conduction disease, but isoprenaline administered parenterally or sublingually may be useful for emergency treatment. Where treatment is considered necessary, pacemaker implantation is usually the treatment of choice. Vasovagal syndrome may have a partial response to treatment with β-blockers which, by reducing sympathetic tone, helps to counter the decreased vasomotor tone that can be a feature of increased vagotonia. Recently there has been interest in agents which act in the central nervous system and address the underlying neurological disorder.

### Cardiac pacemakers (Fig. 9.5)

Permanent pacemaker implantation was first performed in a human in 1958. Since that time it has become the mainstay in the treatment of bradycardia with 20000 devices implanted annually in the UK. Pacemakers may be implanted to correct symptomatic bradycardia or to act as prophylaxis against asystolic sudden death (AV block without a ventricular escape rhythm). Pacemakers are classified according to:

1 their **sensing** capabilities;
2 their **pacing** capabilities;
3 their **programmability features** (which determine the pacemaker response to sensed events); and
4 their ability to increase spontaneously heart rate in **response to physical activity** (rate responsive pacemaker).

Depolarization of ventricular myocardium is achieved by delivery of electrical charge via

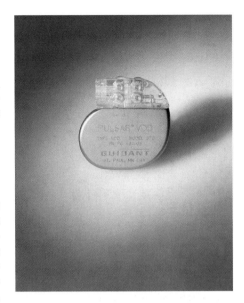

Fig. 9.5 Cardiac implantable pacemaker.

unipolar or bipolar pacing electrodes. A potential difference as small as 0.1 mV is often sufficient to achieve a propagating activation wavefront.

The British Pacing and Electrophysiology Group (BPEG)/North American Society of Pacing and Electrophysiology (NASPE) pacemaker classification (Table 9.1) was devised as a shorthand means of communicating pacemaker capability and has since been further refined in response to the need for a means of categorizing the capabilities of increasingly sophisticated pacemakers.

### Single chamber pacemakers

These sense and pace a single cardiac chamber (either RA or RV). Hysteresis may be used by which the generator is set to pace at a level higher than the heart rate (sensed rate) at which the pacemaker is set to be triggered.

### Dual chamber pacemakers

These pacemakers maintain AV synchrony. Thus, both atrium and ventricle can be either sensed, paced or both, depending on pacemaker programming and spontaneous cardiac

## BPEG/NASPE GENERIC PACEMAKER CODE

| Position | I | II | III | IV | V |
|---|---|---|---|---|---|
| Category | Chamber paced | Chamber sensed | Response to sensing | Programmability | Anti-arrhythmic function |
| | 0, none | 0, none | 0, none | 0, none | 0, none |
| | A, atrium | A, atrium | T, triggered | P, simple programmability | P, pacing (antitachycardia) |
| | V, ventricle | V, ventricle | I, inhibited | M, multiprogrammable | S, shock |
| | D, dual (A+V) | D, dual (A+V) | D, dual (T+I) | C, communicating | D, dual (P+S) |
| | S, single | S, single | | R, rate modulation | |

Table 9.1 The BPEG/NASPE generic pacemaker code.

activity. The interval between atrial and ventricular pacing (AV delay) can be set to optimize cardiac function as there is evidence that the duration of the AV delay can influence the dynamics of ventricular filling and may favourably affect ventricular function.

### Rate responsive pacemakers
These increase their pacing rate in response to physical activity. This is achieved by use of either a device that generates current in response to vibration (e.g. piezoelectric crystal) or by the action of an accelerometer which increases pacing rate in response to a sensed physiological event, such as a shortening of the QT interval which occurs with increased sympathetic tone or changes in respiratory rate. Programmability of the relationship between an increase in heart rate and the 'sensed' physiological parameter activity, allows the pacing rate to be adjusted to suit the physiological demands of the individual.

### Mode-switching pacemakers
Patients who undergo AV node ablation (see p. 150) for paroxysmal atrial fibrillation/flutter may benefit from implantation of 'mode switching' pacemakers. AV synchronous pacing occurs when the patient is in sinus rhythm but auto- matically mode switches to single chamber ventricular pacing at the onset of atrial arrhythmia.

### Temporary pacemakers
Complete heart block complicating myocardial infarction may be temporary with return of AV conduction up to 1–2 weeks later. If a patient is in heart block and haemodynamically compromised, temporary cardiac pacing of the RV ($\pm$ RA) can be performed via temporary pacing lead(s) to the right heart, connected to an external pacing generator which the patient carries until permanent pacemaker implantation or AV conduction recovery.

## Pacing for vasovagal syndrome
When bradycardia due to cardioinhibition is a major component of vasovagal syndrome, implantation of a pacemaker may cure or ameliorate symptoms. Single chamber pacemakers can exacerbate vasovagal syndrome by a mechanism similar to pacemaker syndrome. Thus AV synchrony should always be maintained in the treatment of vasovagal syndrome. The value of specific rate increasing pacemakers when vasodilatation is the principal component is under evaluation.

Similarly, increased vagal tone may follow stimulation of a hypersensitive carotid sinus. This phenomenon appears to be common in some elderly patients and carotid sinus massage is an important investigation in elderly syncopal or presyncopal patients or patients with a history of unexplained falls.

## Non-bradycardia indications for cardiac pacing (Box 9.3)

### Antitachycardia pacing

The pacing system delivers pacing pulses to the heart at a rate greater than that of a re-entry tachycardia mechanism. This may allow 'capture' of the re-entry circuit such that on cessation of pacing the tachycardia is terminated. However, this is not always successful and the patient must be able to tolerate the paced rate. The technique is employed in antitachycardia pacing devices for supraventricular tachycardia infrequently because of the availability of curative ablation techniques, but has an important role in implantable cardioverter defibrillator therapy. Temporary pacing may also be used to pace-terminate arrhythmias, particularly ventricular tachycardia (VT), when drug therapy is ineffective, not established or other interventional therapies are awaited.

### Multi-site atrial pacing

This is a possible therapy for paroxysmal AF. Pacing both in RA and in or near coronary sinus (effectively left atrium (LA)) alters atrial susceptibility to AF.

### Heart failure

Biventricular cardiac pacing, with appropriate modulation of timing of chamber contraction by pacing settings, can offset some of the adverse haemodynamic consequences of ventricular dysfunction. Left ventricular pacing is achieved by access of the coronary venous system via the coronary sinus. Pervenous epicardial pacing is then used to stimulate the LV. It is probably most beneficial in patients with left bundle branch block (LBBB).

### Hypertrophic cardiomyopathy

Dual chamber pacing with variation in the paced AV interval, together with pacing from specific locations in the RV, may alter features of ventricular systole and diastole so as to optimize haemodynamics. The impact both on patient well-being and prognosis, however, is uncertain.

## Choice of pacemaker generator

This is determined by the mechanism giving rise to bradycardia and individual patient requirements. Pacemaker choice requires careful consideration. One approach would be to give every patient the most sophisticated pacemaker to cover all clinical eventualities, but this would expose the patient to additional procedural risks (more complex implant procedure) and is an unnecessary expense. The other extreme strategy is to give all patients the simplest pacemaker sufficient to guarantee effective treatment of bradycardia, but this would deny many patients optimal therapy and expose them to complications such as pacemaker syndrome. Use of single chamber pacemakers to treat cardioinhibition in vasovagal syndrome is contraindicated as VVI pacing may exacerbate the condition through reflex mechanisms.

In the UK there has been delay compared to other European countries in the uptake of sophisticated pacemaker systems. Pacemaker choice is summarized in Box 9.4.

## Choice of pacing electrode

Pacemaker leads and pacemaker programming output may be either bipolar or unipolar.
• Unipolar leads have a terminal electrode and use the pacemaker generator box as the other pole of the circuit.

---

**Box 9.3  Non-Bradycardia Indications for Pacemaker Therapy**

• Antitachycardia pacing
• Atrial stabilizing pacing (multisite atrial pacing)
• Pacing to optimize ventricular function

---

**Box 9.4  Pacemaker Choice**

• Single chamber
• Dual chamber
• Single or dual chamber plus rate response

• Bipolar electrodes detect the electrical activity of depolarizing cells located close to the electrodes, which helps to minimize inappropriate detection of far-field signals. This configuration may allow non-cardiac electrical events to be inappropriately sensed (e.g. see below).

## Pacemaker implantation

Almost all pacemakers are implanted in a prepectoral pouch under local anaesthetic, often with additional sedation. A small cavity in the subcutaneous tissue is fashioned a short distance below the clavicle, sufficiently medial to avoid interference with arm movement. Pacemaker generators sometimes produce minor discomforts with ipsilateral arm movement and so most insertions are in the left prepectoral region, because most patients are right handed. Muscle activity (see below for complications) can interfere on rare occasions with pacemaker function (myoinhibition) and so attention to details of location are important. Pacemaker cans weigh about 20 g. Pacemaker leads (electrodes) are passed into the cardiac chambers (RA and/or RV) via the great veins. Venous access is obtained using a Seldinger technique via the subclavian vein or under direct vision with the cephalic vein. Single chamber pacemakers require only a single pacing wire; most dual chamber pacemakers require two pacing wires although in some recent devices both atrial and ventricular pacing electrodes are mounted on a single lead. Under fluoroscopic control the pacing leads are advanced into the cardiac chambers and positioned at anatomically satisfactory sites at which electrode testing gives satisfactory pacing parameters. Testing of pacemaker electrodes is performed at the time of implantation (Box 9.5).

## Pacing wire and electrode construction

Wires are fixed into the RV trabeculations or RA appendage, either by the anchoring action of tines (terminal plastic flanges) or extendable screw mechanisms (active fixation lead) at the tip of the electrode. Most electrodes are constructed of titanium with an outer surface of polyurethane. The tip electrode is metal but

> ### Box 9.5  Parameters Tested at Pacemaker Implantation
>
> • Sensed R or P wave amplitude
> • Pacing threshold (in mV or mA at 0.05 ms pulse width)
> • Pacing lead impedance
> • Pacing lead stability on deep inspiration/coughing
> • Muscle stimulation/diaphragm stimulation at maximum device output

may have steroid eluting tip properties to help reduce the inflammatory response to wire implantation on the endocardial surface which would otherwise interfere with pacing characteristics.

## Pacemaker complications

### Pacemaker syndrome

When, during VVI pacing, spontaneous P wave rate and ventricular paced rate are the same or similar, simultaneous native atrial and paced ventricular contraction may occur, atrial contraction occurring when the AV valves are closed by ventricular systole. Reflux of atrial blood into the vena cavae can be symptomatic causing malaise, bloating, dyspnoea and chest discomfort.

### Pacemaker-mediated tachycardia

Poor programming of a pacemaker can lead to tachycardia. Retrograde conduction from ventricle to atrium through the AV node (which may occur in the presence of SN disease or rarely anterograde AV block) may lead to atrial depolarization prior to SN depolarization/atrial pacing. If the pacemaker is able to sense this early atrial depolarization it will generate a paced ventricular beat with repetition of the cycle and hence tachycardia.

### Pacemaker follow-up

Pacemaker longevity varies between types of pacemakers and how much it is used. Generator battery life may be up to 10 years. After implant it is customary practice to check pacemaker function at 1 month and thereafter annually. The interval is determined both by the battery capacity and the electrical properties of the pacemaker. Deterioration may also occur in the pacing leads, either due to a gradual degradation of the lead structure or to alteration of the lead/endocardial interface so that lead electrical properties or pacing thresholds may change and become unacceptable in terms of the pacemaker's capabilities. Infrequently, lead breaks may occur due to fracture of the pacing wire, usually at points of frequent stress such as under the clavicle or across the tricuspid valve.

*Driving after pacemaker implantation*
The Driving and Vehicle Licensing Agency (DVLA) is responsible for regulation of driving licence holders in the UK. At present pacemaker recipients are required to notify the DVLA of their therapy and they are not allowed to drive for a period of 1 week from device implant. After a satisfactory pacemaker check they may return to driving with a 3-yearly renewable driving licence.

## Tachycardia

### Sinus tachycardia
This may be a physiological response to exercise or stress but abnormal automaticity, either of the SN or an ectopic focus in either atrium or ventricle, or a re-entry excitation mechanism may cause non-physiological tachycardia.

**Automatic tachycardias** are due to abnormal pacemaker properties in either diseased specialized pacemaker tissue or ordinary cardiac tissue which develops pacemaker properties as a consequence of disease. Examples are ectopic atrial tachycardias occurring in children with congenital heart disease or VT complicating acute myocardial ischaemia.

**A re-entry circuit** is illustrated in Fig. 9.6. For re-entry to occur a circuit must have an anatomical barrier to electrical conduction and a zone of slowed conduction, so that the refractory period (time to recovery of excitability after depolarization) is shorter than the total

conduction time around the re-entry circuit. In this way myocardium is again available for depolarization by the time the circular excitation wave front completes the circuit. Re-entry circuits may be the tachycardia mechanism for either supraventricular (SVT) or ventricular tachycardias (VT).

Tachycardias may be classified as SVT or VT (Box 9.6).
• SVT either originate or require participation in the re-entry circuit of cardiac tissue above the AV rings.
• Ventricular arrhythmias originate in ventricular myocardium and maintenance of the tachycardia does not require the involvement of conducting tissue in the AV rings.

### Treatments for tachycardia
Treatments include anti-arrhythmic drug therapy, device therapy (antitachycardia pacemaker, implantable defibrillator) and curative ablative therapy (either surgical or using catheter fulguration techniques).

### Anti-arrhythmic drug therapy
The use of anti-arrhythmic drugs is discussed in relation to each type of tachycardia in subsequent sections. A classification of anti-arrhythmic drugs by Vaughan-Williams (Table 9.2) has been the cornerstone of the clinical ap-

---

**Box 9.6 Classification of Tachycardias**

*Supraventricular*
• Triggered: ectopic atrial tachycardia/focal AF
• Re-entry: AF/macro re-entrant atrial tachycardia
• A-V re-entrant tachycardia
• A-V nodal re-entrant tachycardia

*Ventricular*
• Triggered: idiopathic left VT/right ventricular outflow tachycardia/ventricular ectopic activity/torsades de pointes
• Micro re-entrant: fascicular tachycardia
• Macro re-entrant: VT (monomorphic or polymorphic)/ventricular fibrillation

## WOLFF–PARKINSON–WHITE SYNDROME

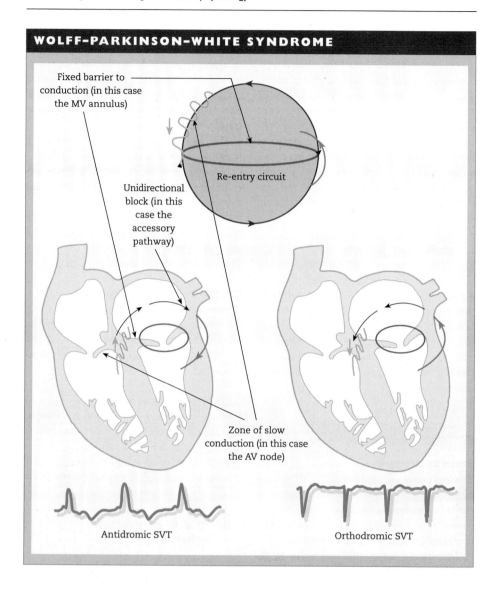

Fixed barrier to conduction (in this case the MV annulus)

Re-entry circuit

Unidirectional block (in this case the accessory pathway)

Zone of slow conduction (in this case the AV node)

Antidromic SVT

Orthodromic SVT

**Fig. 9.6** Re-entry circuit demonstrating antidromic and orthodromic tachycardias in Wolff–Parkinson–White syndrome.

proach to anti-arrhythmic drug choice, although this classification does have its limitations and has been recently reinforced by the 'Sicilian Gambit' classification (Table 9.3). In many conditions, anti-arrhythmic drug therapy is secondary or adjunctive to ablative or device therapy.

### Catheter ablation techniques

Following accidental induction of complete heart block during a cardiac catheterization procedure, the therapeutic possibilities of minimally destructive ablative procedures were appreciated. **Ablation** procedures damage a small area of myocardium, critical to an arrhythmia mechanism using an endocardial percutaneous catheter approach. The target tissue is either critical to an arrhythmia substrate or part of the conduction system.

## THE VAUGHAN-WILLIAMS CLASSIFICATION

| Class | Action | Prototype agent |
|---|---|---|
| I | Local anaesthetic action reducing Na current | Quinidine |
| II | β-blockade | Propanolol |
| III | Action potential prolongation | Amiodarone |
| IV | Calcium channel blockade | Verapamil |

**Table 9.2** The Vaughan-Williams anti-arrhythmic drug classification.

## DRUG ANTI-ARRHYTHMIC CLASSIFICATION

| Mechanism of arrhythmia | Anti-arrhythmic effect | Ionic current targeted |
|---|---|---|
| **1 Abnormal impulse initiation automaticity** | | |
| A Enhanced normal | Decrease in phase 4 depolarization | $I_f$, $I_{ca-T}$ (block) |
| B Abnormal | Decrease in phase 4 depolarization or maximum diastolic potential | $I_{KAch}$ (activate) $I_K$, $I_{KAch}$ (activate) $I_{Ca-L}$, $I_{Na}$ (block) |
| Triggered activity due to | | |
| A Early after-depolarization (EAD) | Shorten action potential or suppress EAD | IK (activate) |
| B Delayed after-depolarization (DAD) | Decrease calcium overload or suppress DAD | $I_{Ca-L}$, $I_{Na}$ (block) $I_{Ca-L}$ (block) $I_{Ca-L}$, $I_{Na}$ (block) |
| **2 Abnormal conduction** Re-entry dependent on Na channels | | |
| A Primary impaired conduction (long excitable gap) | Decrease excitability and conduction | $I_{Na}$ (block) |
| B Conduction encroaching on refractoriness (short excitable gap) | Prolong effective refractory period | $I_K$ (block) |
| Re-entry dependent on CA channels | Decrease excitability and conduction | $I_{Ca-L}$ (block) $I_{Ca-L}$ (block) |
| **3 Other mechanisms** Reflection | Decrease excitability | $I_{Ca-L}$, $I_{Na}$ (block) $I_{Ca-L}$, $I{Na}$ (block) |
| Parasystole | Decrease phase 4 depolarization | $I_f$ (block if MDP high) |

**Table 9.3** Drug anti-arrhythmic classification based on mechanism of action at the ion channel level: the 'Sicilian Gambit'.

• Damage to AV node and specialized conduction system tissue reduces ventricular response rate to atrial activity or, in the case of AV nodal ablation, creates iatrogenic complete heart block. An implanted pacemaker is required to maintain an adequate ventricular rate, because an escape ventricular rhythm is usually slow or may be absent.

Early procedures used high-energy electrical shocks delivered at an endocardial site to ablate myocardium. These energy systems produced lesions by the creation of a voltage gradient. Though effective, they had unacceptable disadvantages:
• large, uncontrolled lesion size;
• late ventricular dysfunction due to shock-related barotrauma;
• procedural discomfort necessitated general anaesthesia.

Low-energy direct current (DC) shock systems cause less barotrauma and have a lower complication risk, but it is still difficult to titrate the level of energy against lesion size, and the technique requires general anaesthesia.

Radiofrequency (RF) energy requires low-voltage, high-frequency current to ablate myocardium via a steerable catheter with a tip-mounted electrode. Discrete and accurately targeted lesions can be achieved. Myocardium is damaged by a combination of resistive and conductive heating. It is currently the energy system of choice for catheter ablation procedures.

## Device implantation for tachycardia

Antitachycardia pacemakers are able to pace-terminate certain types of SVT and VT. Ablation procedures have superseded the use of anti-tachycardia pacemakers in the treatment of supraventricular tachycardia and antitachycardia pacing, for VT carries the risk of tachycardia acceleration, or even the induction of ventricular fibrillation. Thus, antitachycardia pacing devices for pace-termination of VT are usually combined with the ability to deliver defibrillation shocks — the automatic implantable cardiac defibrillator (AICD).

## Supraventricular tachycardias

### Sinus node re-entry, intra-atrial re-entry, and ectopic atrial tachycardias

With the exception of 'common' atrial flutter, these are all rare tachycardias. Intra-atrial re-entrant circuits can be located anywhere in the atrium. Generally circuits can be divided into those which generate an atrial depolarization pattern which is very close, and sometimes identical, to that generated by the SN (SN re-entry) and those which do not (intra-atrial re-entry). It is uncertain whether the SN itself is capable of functioning as part of the re-entry circuit. Distinction between these tachycardias rests entirely on the atrial activation pattern mapped at electrophysiology study.

**SN re-entry** usually generates a tachycardia of around 130 b.p.m. and has the following diagnostic features:
• initiated by atrial or ventricular pacing, and by atrial or ventricular premature extrastimuli;
• the same atrial activation pattern as sinus rhythm;
• unaffected by AV nodal blocking manoeuvres but slows in response to vagal tone. Pharmacological treatment usually fails. SN 'modification' or ablation using catheter techniques can abolish the re-entry circuit and therefore the tachycardia, but SN damage may necessitate subsequent pacemaker insertion. These procedures are rarely required.

**Intra-atrial re-entry tachycardia** involves atrial myocardium distant from the SN. It is:
• rarely induced by ventricular extra-stimulation;
• associated with intra-atrial conduction delay (unlike SN re-entry), necessary for the induction of intra-atrial re-entry;
• different in atrial activation pattern to that in sinus rhythm;
• usually faster than SN re-entry (around 140–240 b.p.m.);
• less responsive to vagal manoeuvres than SN re-entry.

Pharmacological treatment usually fails, although verapamil and adenosine can sometimes be successful in terminating an episode. Catheter ablation techniques have been used to interrupt re-entry but experience is limited.

**Ectopic atrial tachycardia** is:
- usually associated with organic heart disease or metabolic derangement;
- more common in children;
- not reliably initiated by pacing techniques;
- different in atrial activation patterns from sinus rhythm;
- not responsive to vagal manoeuvres;
- sometimes suppressed by overdrive pacing.

Drug therapy often fails. Surgical and catheter ablation of tachycardias may be the treatment of choice, especially for children. The tachycardia substrate may 'burn' itself out during the teenage years. Impairment of ventricular function has been documented in association with incessant tachycardia, but often returns to normal on abolition of tachycardia. Deteriorating ventricular function is the principal indication for invasive treatment.

## Atrial fibrillation

AF may be the consequence of primary electrical disease of the atrium (in particular, 'focal' AF is thought to be the consequence of abnormal 'triggering' ectopic foci), secondary to structural heart disease causing atriopathy, or complicating systemic conditions such as hyperthyroidism.

AF is classified as:
- paroxysmal (spontaneous return to sinus rhythm);
- persistent (sinus rhythm achievable with intervention);
- permanent (sinus rhythm not achieveable even with intervention).

In general, paroxysms of AF become more frequent, and ultimately established, as atrial disease progresses. Atrial hypertrophy and dilatation secondary to structural heart disease is often the substrate for AF, but it may occur in structurally normal hearts. Micro re-entry circuits or focal triggering sites in the atria

cause repetitive excitation of atrial myocardium. The atria cease to contract in a co-ordinated fashion. Frequent and irregular atrial activation result in bombardment of the AVN by depolarization wavelets. Due to its specialized conduction the AV node cannot depolarize in response to each wave of excitation, and so the ventricular response rate to AF is determined by its conduction properties.

The causes of AF include:
- triggering foci (idiopathic);
- atrial myopathy;
- atrial pressure or volume overload due to structural hear disease.

Anti-arrhythmic drug therapy may be directed to control of the ventricular response rate to AF by impairing the conduction properties of the AV node (digoxin, verapamil, β-blockers), or to stabilization of the atrium to prevent AF occurring—amongst other properties, sotalol, amiodarone and dofetilide all prolong the action potential and thus increase refractoriness in the atrial myocardium, making atrial re-entry circuits less sustainable. Class 1 drugs slow intra-atrial conduction and by this mechanism may also help maintain sinus rhythm. If the ventricular response rate to AF cannot be controlled by AV nodal blocking agents, drug side-effects are unacceptable or the subjective sensation of AF is unacceptable to the patient, then AV node conduction can be permanently interrupted by ablation. Permanent pacing is then required to maintain an adequate ventricular rate, and there is a long-term risk of morbidity or death associated with the procedure. AV nodal 'modification' may reduce ventricular response rate to AF without complete interruption of AV conduction, and so avoid the need for permanent pacing, but may still leave the patient with the sensation of palpitation due to the persistence of an irregular ventricular beat.

### Anticoagulation and antiplatelet drugs

AF renders the atria and particularly the left atrial appendage susceptible to intra-atrial thrombus formation. This can give rise to

embolism, the most dangerous consequence of which is a cerebrovascular accident (stroke). The risk is greatest in patients with:
• accompanying mitral valve disease;
• enlargement of the LA or other structural heart disease; and
• a history of previous systemic embolism, diabetes mellitus or hypertension, and in those over 65 years old.

In these high-risk groups, anticoagulation with warfarin (INR 2–4) reduces stroke risk five-fold. In other low-risk patient groups (paroxysmal AF in the structurally normal heart), treatment with aspirin alone may be sufficient. Transoesophageal echocardiography may have a role in identifying patients with intra-atrial thrombus, although its value in guiding management of patients in whom atrial thrombus is not seen, is undecided.

## Cardioversion

External DC countershock is used to convert persistent AF to sinus rhythm when it is felt likely that the patient will remain in sinus rhythm for the long term, with or without additional drugs to stabilize the atrium and reduce likelihood of reversion to AF. This is performed under general anaesthesia and shocks of between 50 and 360J are delivered. High energy levels (>300J) are often required to terminate AF. The use of digoxin is not a contraindication to cardioversion, although in the presence of digoxin toxicity, DC shock is said to increase the risk of ventricular fibrillation. Because of the risk of embolization, patients are anticoagulated for 6 weeks prior to attempted cardioversion. Even if cardioversion successfully restores sinus rhythm, anticoagulation should be continued for a further 2 weeks as atrial 'stunning' leaves even patients in sinus rhythm susceptible to further intra-atrial thrombus formation during this time. Implantable endocardial atrial defibrillators which can be patient activated are currently under assessment. Internal cardioversion using pervenous techniques to place defibrillation catheter electrodes in the RA or coronary sinus and low-energy shock waveforms, has become an alternative to external cardiover-

sion. It is limited by the need to gain vascular access and place intracardiac electrodes, but can be performed under sedation without the need for general anaesthesia and has a higher success rate in patients refractory to external cardioversion.

## Atrial fibrillation ablation

Surgical creation of linear scars within atrial myocardium to prevent sustenance of re-entry circuits by atrial compartmentalization can abolish AF, and it is a well established but little used therapy because of concomitant patient morbidity. Techniques for catheter ablation of triggering foci for AF or to create long linear lesions to emulate surgical compartmentalization are under evaluation.

## Atrial flutter

Atrial flutter has recently been reclassified (Box 9.7). Typically the atrial flutter rate is 300 b.p.m.; 2:1 conduction through the AVN will give a ventricular response rate of 150 b.p.m. Antiarrhythmic drug therapy may modify either the ventricular response or the atrial flutter rate. Counterclockwise macro re-entrant atrial tachycardia (CCMAT) or **'common flutter'** constitutes about 90% of atrial flutter cases, the typical 'saw tooth' atrial flutter pattern being apparent in the inferiorly orientated standard and augmented leads (II, III and aVF) on the ECG (Fig. 9.7a). The re-entry circuit involves an isthmus of tissue in low-RA between the ostium of the coronary sinus and septal leaflet of the tricuspid valve. Otherwise atrial flutter (10% cases) is termed 'uncommon', and differently

---

**Box 9.7  Classification of Macro Re-Entrant Atrial Tachycardia**

• Typical atrial flutter:
  Counterclockwise typical atrial flutter;
  Clockwise typical atrial flutter
• True atypical flutter
• Surgical scar re-entrant atrial tachycardia

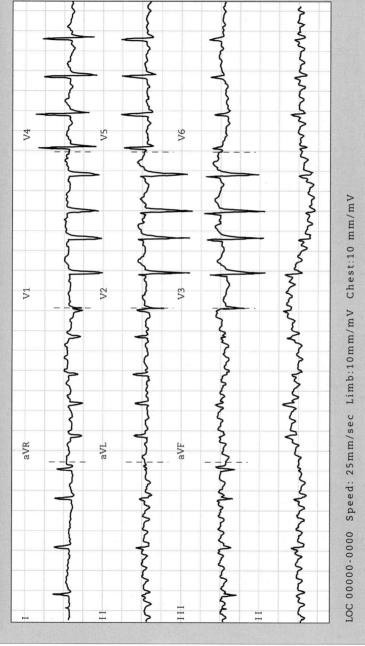

(a)

**Fig. 9.7** (a) Atrial flutter ECG. Note the characteristic 'saw-tooth' pattern in inferior leads. (b) Pre-excitation on surface ECG of patient with Wolff–Parkinson–White syndrome. The pathway is located on the right free wall. Note the slurred upstroke of the QRS (so-called delta wave of pre-excitation) which is exaggerated after the atrial premature beat indicated by the arrow due to the greater proportion of the ventricular mass activated via the connection (slowed AV node/His-Purkinje conduction after premature extrastimulation).

**PRE-EXCITATION**

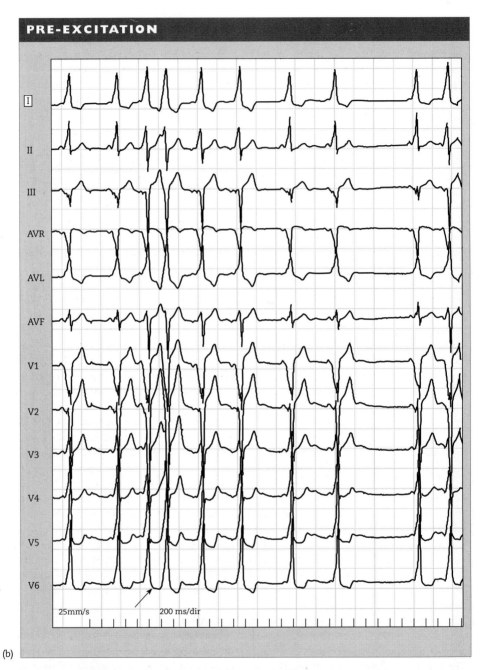

25mm/s          200 ms/dir

(b)

Fig. 9.7 *continued*.

orientated circuits are used which do not give the typical saw-tooth ECG appearance.

'Incisional tachycardia' is a macro re-entry atrial circuit that revolves around scar tissue created by surgical entry to the atrium, and may be amenable to ablation treatment. It most commonly manifests as a type of atrial flutter in patients with congenital heart disease after palliative surgery.

Atrial flutter is usually paroxysmal but may become 'incessant'. When this occurs, reduction of the ventricular response rate by AV nodal blocking drugs is often ineffective because even reduction to 3:1 block may give a tachycardia of 100 b.p.m. Patients usually undergo DC cardioversion, and atrial stabilizing drugs (sotalol/dofetilide/amiodarone) may prevent or reduce the frequency of recurrence. For incessant or frequent paroxysmal CCMAT, when drug therapy is unsatisfactory, ablation of the re-entry circuit is rapidly becoming the treatment of choice by creation of a linear lesion at a critical location in the atrial flutter circuit, usually at the tricuspid valve/inferior vena cava isthmus. An alternative is AV node ablation, as for AF, with pacemaker implantation.

## Atrioventricular re-entry tachycardia

Accessory AV connections are muscle bundles connecting atrial and ventricular myocardium across the AV ring. Though they develop during embryogenesis and are present from birth, paroxysms of tachycardia may not occur until late childhood, teenage years or even adulthood. Although present in as many as 1 in 3000 individuals, estimates vary widely as to the proportion (10–95%) of such individuals who will experience symptomatic AVRT. Pathways that are able to conduct anterogradely (atrium to ventricle) are usually evident on the resting surface ECG (pre-excitation) (Fig. 9.7b). A portion of the ventricular mass is excited by the excitation front traversing the accessory pathway. This portion of the ventricular mass depolarizes early relative to the remaining ventricular mass,

which is depolarized via the normal conduction system, because unlike the AV node there has been no delayed conduction in the accessory pathway. Thus in sinus rhythm the PR interval is short. However, this pre-excited portion of the ventricle spreads the excitation wavefront via slowly conducting myocardium, giving rise to a slurred deflection at the beginning of the QRS complex (the delta wave). Pathway conduction during tachycardia may be from atrium to ventricle (antidromic AVRT) with retrograde conduction through the AV node (Fig. 9.8). This is uncommon and produces a broad complex tachycardia. More usually, conduction is retrograde in the accessory pathway and anterograde through the AV node, resulting in a narrow complex tachycardia.

Some patients can display both types of AVRT, and approximately 10% of patients with AVRT have multiple pathways with complex mechanisms of tachycardia. In addition to re-entry tachycardia, the presence of an accessory pathway predisposes to AF. This may be due to retrograde conduction from ventricle to atrium during the atrial vulnerable period. AF can be life threatening in some patients with pre-excitation if the accessory pathway has rapid anterograde conduction characteristics which allow very rapid ventricular response rates to AF (the ventricle losing its usual protection from the slow conduction properties of the AV node) and ventricular fibrillation can ensue. Although uncommon, this is the mechanism where sudden death occurs in patients with accessory pathways. Mahaim pathways are uncommon connections between AV nodal tissue and RV. Tachycardia mechanisms are similar. Accessory pathways are common in Ebstein's anomaly.

### Treatment

Anti-arrhythmic drugs can be used to modify the conduction properties of the AV node or accessory pathway so as to render the re-entry circuit unsustainable. Thus, drugs which slow AV nodal or accessory connection conduction (β-blockers, calcium antagonists, class I drugs or amiodarone), may reduce the ventricular rate when paroxysms of tachycardia occur, or the

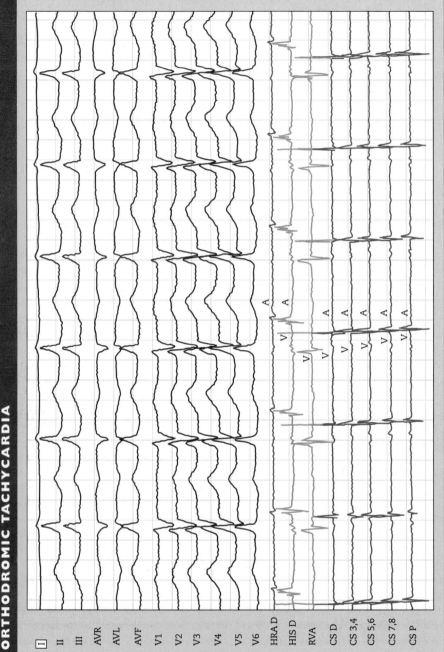

**Fig. 9.8** Orthodromic tachycardia. Retrograde atrial activation (A) in coronary sinus leads (ESP→CSD) shows atrial activation occurs earliest in left atrium in SVT (compare to A in high right atrium HRAD) and area of the His bundle (HISD). This confirms a left-sided accessory pathway.

frequency of attacks. Complete freedom from paroxysms of tachycardia is difficult to achieve using drug therapy. Catheter ablation of accessory pathways is now the treatment of choice in symptomatic patients and has a high primary success rate (about 95%) and a low associated morbidity.

## Atrioventricular nodal re-entry tachycardia

The substrate for this re-entry tachycardia is again present from birth but may not cause symptomatic tachycardia until adult life. It is more common in young females and is a more common tachycardia than AVRT. The re-entry circuit exists within, or is intimately related to, the AV node and its associated tissues but is independent of the ventricle. AV conduction during normal rhythm occurs through two 'pathways' which have differing conduction characteristics:
• one 'pathway' has a slow conduction velocity but short refractory period;
• the other 'pathway' has a faster conduction velocity but longer refractory period.

The precise location and tissue character of these 'pathways' is debated and in part inferred from the results of catheter ablation procedures. The re-entry circuit uses these fast and slow conduction limbs (Fig. 9.9). Two types of AVNRT are recognized: common and uncommon. In the common type (90%) retrograde conduction is via the fast pathway and in the remainder the circuit is reversed.

### Treatment
Drugs which influence AV nodal conduction may modify the properties of the re-entry circuit (principally calcium antagonists, β-blockers and class 1 drugs), but complete freedom from tachycardia is difficult to achieve. Ablation procedures are now the treatment of choice. Catheter ablation of either the slow or fast pathway (both termed AV nodal 'modification') can be achieved by selective destruction of a portion of the AV node or tissues adjacent to it.

• 'Slow pathway' ablation maintains normal AV nodal anterograde conduction.
• 'Fast pathway' ablation leads to PR interval prolongation reflecting damage to the normal properties of the AV node.

Thus, slow pathway ablation is the most commonly used ablation procedure. Complete heart block occurs in up to 1% of cases and requires permanent pacing.

## Sudden cardiac death

Sudden cardiac death is defined as death from a cardiac cause within 1 hour of the onset of symptoms. It is a major cause of mortality in the Western world, being responsible for up 60 000 deaths per annum in the UK. Although a proportion of such deaths follow acute myocardial infarction, some die of a primary arrhythmia unrelated to infarction. As many as two-thirds of sudden cardiac deaths may be due to ventricular arrhythmia, the substrate being a scarred myocardium which generates VT, which may then degenerate to ventricular fibrillation. Risk stratification for those considered susceptible to ventricular arrhythmias involves Holter monitoring, a signal-averaged ECG, electrophysiological study, and assessments of ventricular function. The signal-averaged ECG is a technique involving computer analysis of surface ECG lead recordings to identify depolarization in the later portion of the QRS (late potentials) which are thought to be indicative of slowed myocardial conduction and the presence of an arrhythmia substrate. All the above investigations have relatively low sensitivity and specificity. Patients rescued from sudden cardiac death have a poor prognosis, with a 30% 2-year mortality. They should be investigated for possible underlying coronary artery disease and considered for treatment with an AICD.

## Ventricular ectopics

Although a common and largely benign phenomenon, frequent ventricular ectopic activity

## AV NODAL RE-ENTRY TACHYCARDIA

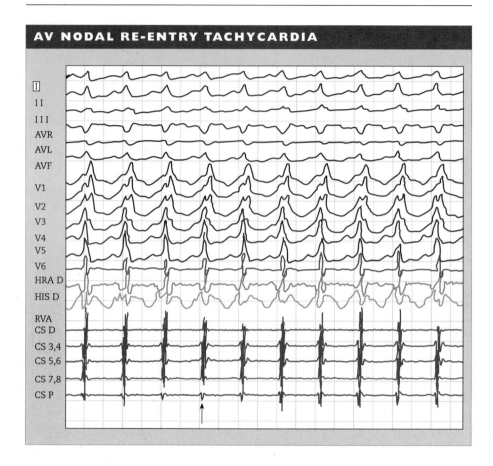

Fig.9.9 Re-entry circuit in AV nodal re-entry tachycardia. Arrow indicates simultaneous nature of atrial activation (from atrial electrogram pattern) in both right and left atria due to spread of activation from the AVRNT re-entry circuit in the AV node/triangle of Koch. Note also rate related right bundle branch aberrancy in the surface ECG in this patient.

may indicate underlying structural heart disease. There is no evidence that suppression of ventricular ectopic activity by anti-arrhythmic drug treatment improves the prognosis of the underlying disease or reduces the risk of sudden death. Indeed drug trials to assess the impact of ectopic activity suppression by Class Ic drugs after myocardial infarction have shown an increased sudden death rate in 'successfully' treated groups. This may reflect the proarrhythmic potential of some anti-arrhythmic drugs.

### Ventricular tachycardia

Monomorphic VT has a constant QRS morphology (Fig. 9.10) but polymorphic VT has continuous variation in the QRS morphology. Sustained tachycardia continues for a minimum of 30 s and non-sustained tachycardia self terminates within 30 s. ECG differentiation from other broad complex tachycardias is illustrated in Fig. 9.11.

### Mechanisms

Re-entry (see Fig. 9.6) in and around scarred myocardium is the commonest mechanism of recurrent monomorphic sustained VT. How-

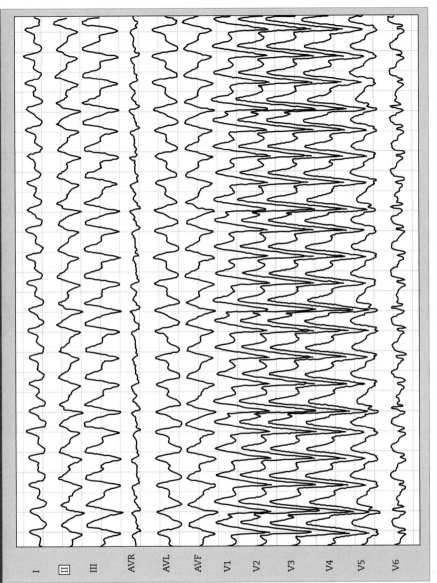

**MONOMORPHIC VENTRICULAR TACHYCARDIA**

I

II

III

AVR

AVL

AVF

V1

V2

V3

V4

V5

V6

**Fig. 9.10** 12 lead ECG of monomorphic ventricular tachycardia, showing monomorphic (QRS of constant configuration in a given ECG lead other than for occasional complexes when there is fusion with activation via the His Purkinje system) sustained (lasting longer than 30 s) VT at 25 mm/s paper speed. Tachycardia rate is 190 b.p.m.

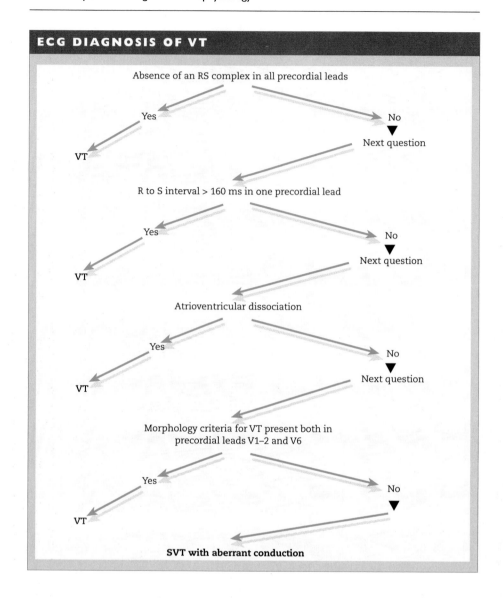

**ECG DIAGNOSIS OF VT**

Absence of an RS complex in all precordial leads

Yes                                                    No

▼
Next question

VT

R to S interval > 160 ms in one precordial lead

Yes                                                    No

▼
Next question

VT

Atrioventricular dissociation

Yes                                                    No

▼
Next question

VT

Morphology criteria for VT present both in
precordial leads V1–2 and V6

Yes                                                    No

▼
VT

**SVT with aberrant conduction**

**Fig. 9.11** ECG diagnosis of VT.

ever, acute severe metabolic changes in myo-cardium, including those caused by acute is-chaemia, can cause spontaneous cell membrane depolarization. Thus, 'early after depolariza-tions' are caused by abnormality of ionic flux during the repolarization phase which may then generate polymorphic VT.

## Electrophysiology study of VT
(Fig. 9.12)

Standard electrophysiological 'induction pro-tocols' have been shown reliably to initiate VT in patients who have the necessary arrhythmia substrate. However, the reproducibility, sensi-tivity and specificity of ventricular extrastimula-tion studies has been best characterized in patients with ventricular arrhythmias compli-cating healed myocardial infarction. Their value

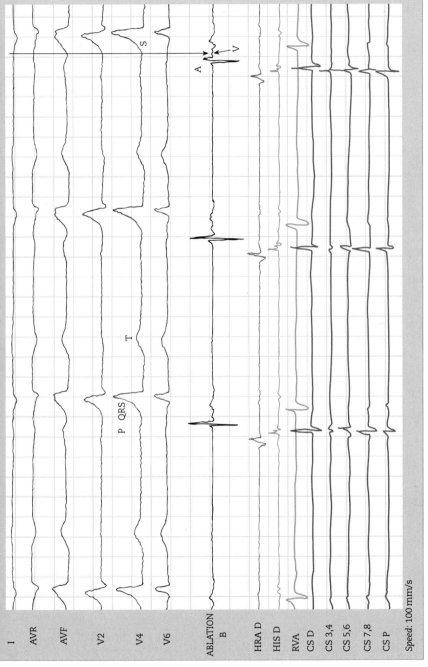

**Fig. 9.12** Electrograms recorded at site of successful accessory pathway ablation. (a) The arrow is drawn at the outset of the surface ECG (QRS) delta wave. Note its timing relative to the ventricular electrogram recorded from the tip of the ablation catheter (ablation B). The sites of origin of the electrograms are indicated by the labelling of the traces on the left of the illustration. CSD to CSP represent five sites in coronary sinus; RVA, right ventricular apex; HIS D, the region of the His bundle; HRA D, high right atrium. (b) Arrow indicates loss of pre-excitation (accessory pathway ablated) 1 s after onset of RF current delivery.

(a)

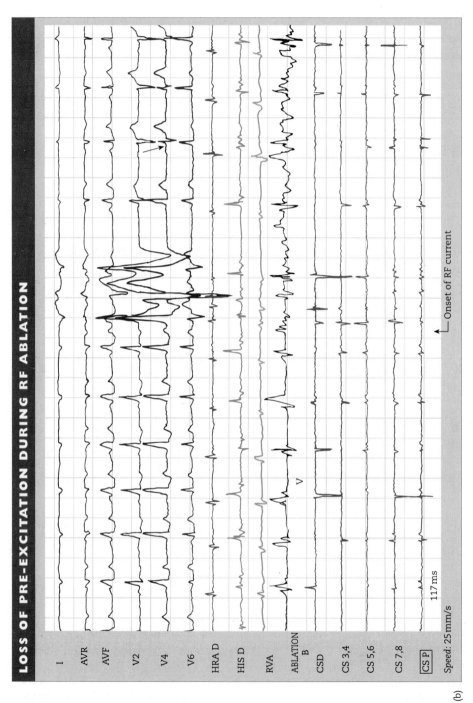

**Fig. 9.12** continued.

in assessing prognosis or symptomatic efficacy of drug or other therapies in dilated, arrhythmogenic or hypertrophic cardiomyopathies is uncertain. A typical induction protocol uses constant ventricular pacing at the right ventricular apex at a drive rate of 100 b.p.m. for seven beats (drive train), with delivery of a single premature extrastimulus following each drive train. The intervals between the last beat of the drive train and the premature extrastimulus is decrementally decreased in small steps (usually 10ms) until the extrastimulus fails to generate a QRS complex, indicating failure to capture local ventricular myocardium. A second, and subsequently a third, extrastimulus is introduced and then the process is repeated at a faster drive rate (usually 150 b.p.m). This scheme is used at both right ventricular apical and right outflow tract pacing sites. Some protocols also involve the use of isoprenaline or other proarrhythmic drugs. Study end-points are the induction of ventricular arrhythmia or completion of the study protocol without arrhythmia induction.

However, induction of polymorphic VT or ventricular fibrillation may be non-specific and not reproducible. Thus the relevance of these types of arrhythmia to a given clinical scenario is difficult to determine. Induction of monomorphic VT confirms the presence of a substrate for VT, whether or not the induced VT has the same QRS morphology as the clinically documented tachycardia. Inducibility can then be used as a guide to arrhythmia suppression by the drug(s), or the induced tachycardia can be 'mapped' to identify the re-entry circuit location with a view to either catheter ablation or surgical resection. The choice of therapy will in part be determined by the underlying disease. Most ventricular arrhythmias are the consequence of myocardial scarring complicating coronary artery disease and myocardial infarction. Anti-arrhythmic drugs and device therapy may be used whatever the aetiology of the arrhythmia substrate, while surgical and ablation treatments are limited in their application.

## Drug treatment

This is an area of rapidly changing opinion, but standard practice is to perform a baseline electrophysiological study in patients with either documented monomorphic VT or a high clinical suspicion of the arrhythmia. Subsequent non-inducibility after the patient has been established on a selected oral anti-arrhythmic drug treatment indicates likely improvement of prognosis, compared with clinically guided empirical drug therapy or no therapy, and a reduction in the frequency of symptomatic palpitation. Holter monitoring in highly selected patients may be as accurate as electrophysiology study in predicting anti-arrhythmic drug efficacy.

Amiodarone may improve prognosis in some particular patient groups (e.g. hypertrophic cardiomyopathy) but for most patients with ventricular arrhythmias, confers no prognostic benefit although it is commonly prescribed empirically in UK practice. The data with respect to prognostic benefit conferred by amiodarone therapy for all disease substrates giving rise to ventricular arrhythmia is complex and unclear. However, drug manufacturers of anti-arrhythmic drugs in general and amiodarone in particular are unable to claim prognostic benefit as a drug therapy indication. Class I, II and III drugs (see Table 9.2) may all be used to reduce frequency of symptomatic palpitation.

The failure of drug therapy either to improve prognosis in carefully designed drug trials has stimulated the search for other treatments. These now include catheter ablation techniques, surgical resection of the arrhythmia substrate and AICD implantation. Anti-arrhythmic drug therapy still has an important role as an adjunct to these.

## AICD treatment

The AICD was conceived by Dr M Mirowski in the USA, with the first implant performed in a human in 1982. These are sophisticated devices which are able to sense and terminate VT or fibrillation. The devices are able to pace-terminate VT (Fig. 9.13), cardiovert VT or defibrillate from ventricular fibrillation. They offer tiered therapy and programmable, sophisticated arrhythmia sensing. First generation devices required the placement of epicardial defibrillation patch elec-

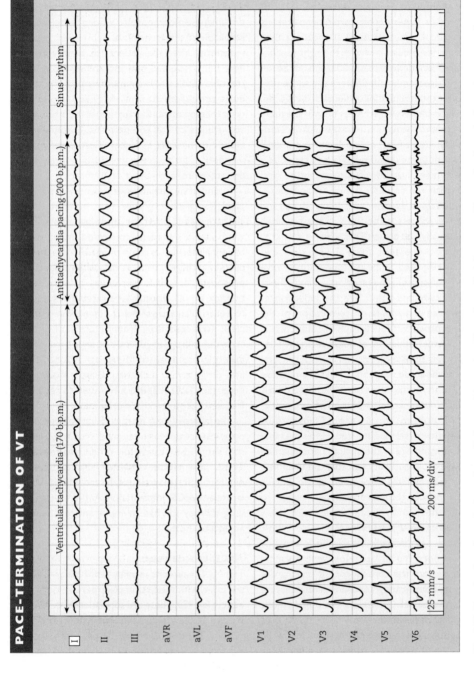

**Fig. 9.13** Termination of ventricular tachycardia by overdrive pacing. The tachycardia is interrupted by a train of ventricular pacing at a rate faster than the spontaneous ventricular tachycardia. Note the pacing spikes and changed QRS morphology during ventricular pacing.

trodes at formal thoracotomy but recent in-novations now allow endocardial placement of shock electrodes in a manner analogous to the implantation of a pacemaker device. Also, the devices were originally implanted in abdominal pouches with electrodes tunnelled subcuta-neously from the portal of venous entry (usually subclavian), whereas devices are now sufficient-ly small to allow routine prepectoral subcuta-neous implantation. Innovations include the combination of a full range of pacemaker func-tions for bradycardia within AICD units and in-creased capability for telemetry.

## Arrhythmia surgery

Surgical removal of scar tissue together with deeper endomyocardial incisions or application of cryoprobes to interrupt re-entry circuits can result in cure of VT complicating healed myo-cardial infarction. This approach requires open heart surgery and is associated with significant morbidity and mortality, and risks causing fur-ther impairment of ventricular function. Thus, to be a candidate for this therapy patients must have well-preserved ventricular function and the VT must be amenable to mapping tech-niques to allow the electrophysiologist to guide the surgical approach. Patients with multiple VT circuits, which are poorly tolerated haemody-namically, and with severe impairment of ven-tricular function will not be suitable for surgical therapy. Only a minority of patients with VT will be suitable for surgical intervention and most will have coronary artery disease.

## Catheter ablation of VT

Current technology offers only limited success (currently approximately 30% primary success rate in patients with coronary artery disease) in the ablation of the arrhythmia substrate of ven-tricular arrhythmias because ablation systems create lesions which are often too shallow to interrupt re-entry circuits. However, this is a rapidly developing area and it is likely that abla-tion techniques will be increasingly employed in the future, aided by rapid technological advancement in mapping and lesion creation techniques.

## Other ventricular arrhythmias

### Ventricular fibrillation

VF commonly complicates acute myocardial is-chaemia or infarction (reflecting electrical insta-bility caused by biochemical derangement in the myocardium). Monomorphic and polymorphic VT can degenerate into ventricular fibrillation leading to death. However, outside the context of acute myocardial ischaemia, VF is less com-mon than VT as a primary event. VF is likely to be the underlying arrhythmia in the majority of patients with sudden cardiac death.

### Right ventricular outflow tract tachycardia

The arrhythmia substrate is located in the right ventricular outflow tract and probably is a local-ized re-entry circuit. There is usually no obvious underlying structural heart disease on investiga-tion. It is a benign arrhythmia and amenable to catheter ablation.

### Fascicular tachycardia

This condition complicates some types of con-genital heart disease and coronary artery dis-ease. It is a relatively benign type of VT and is amenable to catheter ablation. The substrate is probably a micro re-entry circuit involving the left posterior hemifascicle, producing a charac-teristic surface ECG configuration during the tachycardia of right bundle branch morphology and superior axis (Fig. 9.14a).

### Bundle branch re-entry tachycardia

This tachycardia is caused by a re-entry circuit involving conduction bundle tissue as part of the re-entry circuit. Catheter ablation of the bundle branch limb of the circuit can abolish the arrhythmia.

### Torsades de pointes

*Long QT syndrome*

Sympathetic drive and variation in cardiac rhythm are known precipitants of torsades de pointes tachycardia in patients with the cell

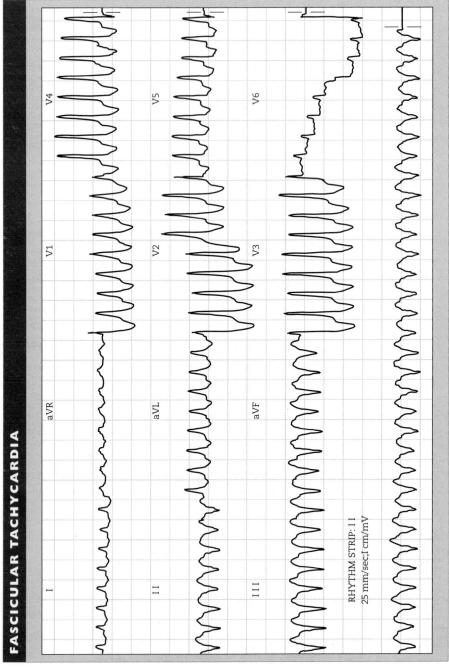

FASCICULAR TACHYCARDIA

I

aVR

V1

V4

II

aVL

V2

V5

III

aVF

V3

V6

RHYTHM STRIP: I I
25 mm/sec;1 cm/mV

(a)

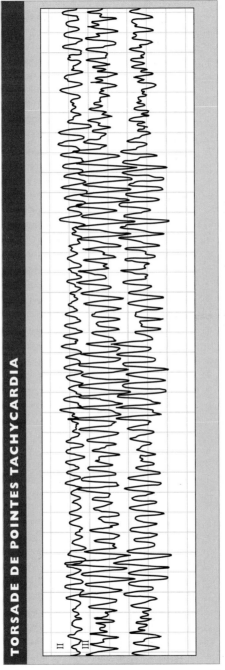

**Fig. 9.14** (a) Fascicular tachycardia. Note left axis deviation and right bundle branch block pattern. (b) Torsade de pointes tachycardia. Note characteristic 'complementary' and continuing axis change.

(b)

membrane ionic transport abnormalities that are thought to underlie long QT syndrome. The characteristic ECG features of this type of polymorphic VT (Fig. 9.14b) are associated with prolongation of the QT interval in sinus rhythm and are linked to abnormal repolarization mechanisms. The exact mechanism of the arrhythmia remains uncertain. It can be a component of a hereditary syndrome associated with deafness (Romano–Ward) but can complicate the use of anti-arrhythmic drugs which prolong myocardial repolarization (Class III action).

## Further reading

Benditt DG, Benson DW, eds. *Cardiac Pre-excitation Syndromes: Origins, Evaluation and Treatment*. Dordrecht: Kluwer Academic Publishers, 1986.

Ellenbogen KA, Kay GN, Wilkoff BL, eds. *Clinical Cardiac Pacing and Defibrillation*. London: WB Saunders Co, 2000.

Josephson ME. *Clinical Cardiac Electrophysiology: Techniques and Interpretation*, 2nd edn. London: Lea & Febiger, 1993.

Zipes DP, Jalife J, eds. *Cardiac Electrophysiology: from Cell to Bedside*, 3rd edn. London: WB Saunders Co, 1999.

# CHAPTER 10

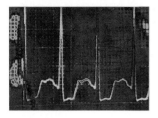

# Cardiopulmonary Resuscitation

## Introduction

A cardiac or circulatory arrest can occur under various circumstances. The patient may be in or out of hospital, there may be many or no trained personnel on the scene, and the facilities available may range from none to full cardiopulmonary bypass. An approach to resuscitation must be flexible enough to allow for these differing circumstances. Of all the deaths from myocardial infarction, 60% (60 000/year) occur before patients reach hospital and many are due to potentially correctable arrhythmias. The only two interventions that have ever been shown unequivocally to improve survival after a cardiac arrest are **basic life support** (BLS) and **defibrillation:** this supports the need to ensure that as many people as possible learn BLS techniques and that there is more widespread availability of defibrillators. Survival from cardiac arrest is greatest when:
• the event is witnessed;
• a bystander starts resuscitation;
• the arrhythmia is ventricular fibrillation (VF);
• defibrillation is undertaken as quickly as possible.

The need for resuscitation usually arises because of an acute inadequacy of blood supply to the vital organs. This is most often due to sudden ineffective or absent cardiac activity resulting from acute myocardial ischaemia. It may also arise following a major obstruction to blood flow through the central circulation (e.g. acute massive pulmonary embolus) or in the context of more chronic obstruction (e.g. valvular stenosis, pulmonary vascular disease). Less commonly, the blood supply to vital organs is maintained but oxygenation is inadequate, as may occur, for example, in sudden major airway obstruction. However, soon after the onset of inadequate oxygenation, the heart itself becomes ineffective and circulatory arrest is superimposed.

When a person collapses, or an 'arrest call' is broadcast in hospital, it does not necessarily mean that cardiac arrest has occurred. The patient may be unconscious for a variety of other reasons, such as head trauma, a cerebrovascular event, drug overdose or a simple faint. It is particularly worth considering hypoglycaemia as a potential cause of unconsciousness as it is so easily reversed. The remainder of this chapter, however, concerns mainly the management of cardiac arrest, and is based on the recommendations of the European Resuscitation Council (1998). Cardiopulmonary resuscitation (CPR) involves manoeuvres which are best learned by seeing them demonstrated rather than described. Those unfamiliar with these techniques should attend a suitable training course.

## Basic life support

BLS refers to the maintenance of an airway and

169

support of breathing and circulation without equipment (other than a simple airway device or protective shield). The algorithm describing the sequence of events in BLS is shown in Fig. 10.1.

## Airway and breathing

- Open the airway by tilting the head backwards and lifting the chin.
- Remove any obvious obstruction from the mouth, including loose fitting dentures but leave well fitting ones in place because their presence makes expired air rescue breaths (mouth-to-mouth) easier.
- Look for chest movement, listen, and feel for exhaled air with your cheek.
- Observe for 10s before deciding breathing is absent—if it is absent, give two effective rescue breaths.

## Choking

- Remove any obvious obstruction and if necessary slap the individual on the back five times.
- If this is unsuccessful consider the 'abdominal thrust' manoeuvre.
- If the subject becomes unconscious and the obstruction has not been dislodged, attempt expired air ventilation anyway because loss of consciousness may result in relaxation of the muscles around the larynx and allow air to pass.
- In hospital consider cricothyrotomy if obstruction continues.

## Recovery position

- If the patient is breathing, and unless it would aggravate an injury, remove any spectacles and turn the victim into the recovery position.
- This helps to ensure a good airway and avoids the tongue falling back in the mouth and obstructing the airway.
- It also minimizes the risk of inhalation of gastric contents.

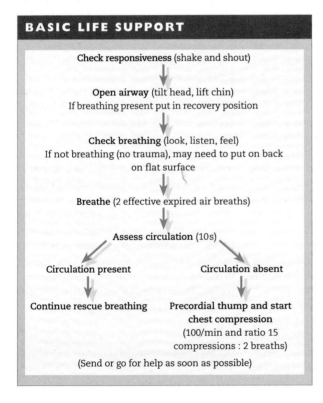

**BASIC LIFE SUPPORT**

Check responsiveness (shake and shout)
↓
Open airway (tilt head, lift chin)
If breathing present put in recovery position
↓
Check breathing (look, listen, feel)
If not breathing (no trauma), may need to put on back on flat surface
↓
Breathe (2 effective expired air breaths)
↓
Assess circulation (10s)
↓                    ↓
Circulation present        Circulation absent
↓                    ↓
Continue rescue breathing    Precordial thump and start
                chest compression
                (100/min and ratio 15
                compressions : 2 breaths)
(Send or go for help as soon as possible)

Fig. 10.1 Algorithm for basic life support.

## Expired air rescue breathing ('mouth-to-mouth')

- With the victim preferably lying flat on a firm surface, give 10 breaths per minute of expired air ventilation by mouth-to-mouth contact, pinching the soft part of the victim's nose to ensure your expired air fills their lungs and the chest wall rises and falls accordingly.
- This usually requires a tidal volume of around 400–600 mL in an adult.

## Circulation

- Look for any movement of the victim, including swallowing or breathing, and feel for the carotid pulse for 5 s before deciding if present or absent.
- Recheck for the presence of a pulse every 10 breaths during resuscitation.

## Precordial thump

- If no pulse is felt, a sudden firm blow to the front of the victim's chest should be given using a clenched fist.
- This may cardiovert early VF/ventricular tachycardia (VT) to sinus rhythm.

## Chest compression

This was previously termed 'cardiac massage', in the erroneous belief that cardiac compression resulted in expulsion of cardiac blood into the great arteries. This is now believed not to be the case because echocardiography has shown that the cardiac valves are regurgitant during cardiac arrest, and because coughing alone was shown to produce a life-sustaining circulation. The current 'thoracic pump' theory proposes that chest compression, by increasing intrathoracic pressure, propels blood out of the thorax, with forward flow occurring because the great veins inside the thorax collapse due to compression while the arteries remain expanded. Even when performed optimally, chest compressions do not achieve more than 30% of normal cardiac output.

- Locate the lower half of the sternum, interlock your fingers, and using the heel of both hands depress the sternum vertically 4–5 cm.

- The current recommendation is for 100 chest compressions per min to be performed.
- If you are the sole resuscitator, after 15 compressions give two effective breaths of expired air ventilation.
- If two or more resuscitators are present, give five compressions to each breath, stopping compression when ventilating.

### Advanced life support

When CPR is undertaken in hospital, BLS manoeuvres usually overlap with advanced life support (ALS). The management of ALS may broadly be divided into three stages.

1 **Revive** the patient by returning an adequate oxygenated blood supply to the vital organs using chest compression and expired air assisted ventilation.

2 **Restore** a spontaneous cardiac output, usually by early defibrillation.

3 **Review** the possible causes of the arrest and further measures that may be necessary (Box 10.1).

The algorithm for ALS is given in Fig. 10.2.

## Ventilation

The principles of ensuring and maintaining an airway and ventilation are the same as BLS, but the patient should be intubated with an endotracheal tube if possible.

- Intubation is the ideal but a laryngeal mask airway is an alternative that can be easily applied.
- Intubation should only be undertaken by those competent in its performance, otherwise vital time is lost and increasing hypoxaemia occurs whilst a less experienced person tries. Under these circumstances, the patient is much better served by effective expired air ventilation.
- If intubation is performed, adequate ventilation of both lungs should be confirmed using a stethoscope.
- During cardiac arrest and resuscitation, lung characteristics change because of an increase in dead space, and pulmonary oedema reduces lung compliance.

## Box 10.1  Review of Possible Causes

| Possible cause of arrest | Action |
| --- | --- |
| Acute myocardial infarct | ? Thrombolysis |
| Severe valvular disease | ? Urgent surgery |
| Aortic dissection | ? Refer to cardiothoracic unit |
| Tamponade | Pericardiocentesis |
| Acute massive pulmonary embolus | ? Thrombolysis or embolectomy |
| Pneumothorax | Chest drain |
| Airway obstruction | ? Bronchodilators/bronchoscopy |
| Haemorrhage | Blood transfusion, consider source of bleeding |
| Cerebrovascular event | ? Refer to neurosurgical unit |
| Septic shock | ? Vasoconstrictors/antibiotics |
| Anaphylactic shock | Andrenaline (epinephrine)/steroids |
| Addisonian crisis | Corticosteroids |
| Drug toxicity (e.g. β-blockers) | ? Antidotes/increase excretion (aminophyline or glucagon raise cAMP). |
| Electrolyte/glucose disorder | Correct as appropriate |

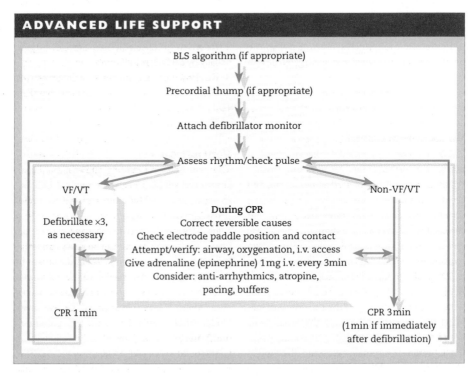

Fig. 10.2 Algorithm for advanced life support.

- Oxygenation is the primary objective and hence 100% inspired oxygen ($FiO_2$) should be used. $CO_2$ return to the lungs is limited during the initial period of an arrest so tidal volumes of 400–600 mL are sufficient. Adequate minute volume is also important to clear $CO_2$ and prevent hypercarbic acidosis, especially after the administration of $CO_2$ producing buffers such as sodium bicarbonate.
- Arterial blood sampling (femoral or radial), for estimation of blood gases and pH should be monitored periodically (every 5–10 min) and plasma electrolytes and glucose should be measured.

## Circulation

When cardiac arrest occurs in hospital, many staff are usually quickly on the scene so five chest compressions should be given for each lung expansion.

- The first person on the scene should check for the presence of a pulse and, if absent, give a precordial thump to the patient's chest.
- Effective chest compression and ventilation are the keys to maximizing the chances of a successful resuscitation, and their effective implementation should not be interrupted other than briefly for other procedures such as central venous cannulation.
- The best signs of restoration of oxygenated blood flow to the tissues are spontaneous movement by the patient, respiratory effort and small pupil size (although dilated pupils do not necessarily imply failure if atropine and catecholamines have been given during the arrest).
- Once effective BLS has been established, attention can be given to the treatment of arrhythmias.

## Arrhythmias

In adults, the commonest primary arrhythmia is **VF or pulseless VT**, and the great majority of those who will subsequently survive come from this group.

Survival rates depend crucially on the clinical situation in which VF/VT occurs. For instance, VF at the time of cardiac catheterization on low-risk patients can be successfully and quickly corrected in almost every case because of the immediacy of defibrillation. Conversely, successful resuscitation is often unsuccessful wherever it is performed if severe left ventricular dysfunction is present beforehand. Survival rates therefore need to be interpreted in the context of the clinical situation.

Prospects of survival with VF/VT diminish at 5% per min of delay to defibrillation, even if adequate BLS is being undertaken. The longer ventricular arrhythmia is allowed to persist the more degenerate it becomes, because of increasing myocardial ischaemia, and the more difficult it becomes to cardiovert. Prompt defibrillation improves survival.

**Electromechanical dissociation** (EMD) is a term used to imply absence of mechanical activity or undetectable activity in the presence of a continuing co-ordinated waveform on the electrocardiogram (ECG).

- It is usually caused by drug therapy, hypovolaemia or mechanical problems such as cardiac tamponade, massive pulmonary embolism, tension pneumothorax, intracardiac obstruction (tumour or thrombus) or myocardial rupture.
- It may also occur following myocardial infarction, especially of the inferior wall. The mechanism is uncertain but intracellular acidosis and autonomic effects are suspected.

Asystole and EMD are uncommon primary arrhythmias in out-of-hospital cardiac arrests (<10%) but occur in up to 25% of arrests in hospital. They have a much poorer prognosis than VF/VT, with survival rates of <5% when the arrhythmia is due to heart disease. Survival is better in the context of cardiac arrest due to drowning, hypothermia or drug overdose.

An **ECG** should be obtained as soon as possible.

- The paddles of a defibrillator will often act as monitoring electrodes, but standard limb lead electrodes should be used for more continuous recording.
- Ideally, standard electrodes should be attached to the defibrillator monitor so that synchronized cardioversion can be undertaken if appropriate (e.g. in ventricular tachycardia).

- If there is any doubt, the cardioverter should be switched to unsynchronized mode, as failure to detect the R wave of the ECG may prevent cardioversion and delay will ensue.
- It is important to remember that a straight line on the monitor may indicate faulty equipment or connections, rather than asystole.

When **defibrillation** is indicated the sequence should be:
- 200 joules (J), followed by 200 J and then 360 J given in quick succession if initially unsuccessful;
- any subsequent defibrillations should deliver 360 J. There is evidence that myocardial injury is greater with increasing energies, but in the context of resuscitation this is less relevant than the paramount importance of achieving successful cardioversion;
- only a small proportion of the delivered electrical energy traverses the myocardium during transthoracic defibrillation. It can be maximized by correct positioning of the paddles (just below the right clavicle and just lateral to the cardiac apex), by ensuring firm contact with the chest, and the use of couplants such as electrode pads between the paddles and the chest wall to improve electrical contact. If unsuccessful, an anteroposterior paddle position may be tried;
- when defibrillating, make sure all those attending keep clear and have no contact with the patient, bed or connected equipment.

## Drug therapy (see Table 10.1)

### Drug delivery

During a cardiac arrest many drugs will be used, although none has been proven to be of survival benefit. Venous administration is still the preferred route although the decision whether to insert a central venous line or give drugs by a peripheral venous cannula will depend on the experience of the person undertaking the insertion and the speed with which it can be inserted.
- Insertion must not delay defibrillation or interrupt BLS more than briefly.
- If drugs are given by a peripheral route, each injection should be followed by a 20 mL bolus of

saline to flush the agent closer to the central circulation.
- Intratracheal drug delivery is very much a second-line option because of unpredictable pharmacodynamics. Agents that can be given by this route if necessary include epinephrine (adrenaline), lidocaine (lignocaine) and atropine. Doses used should be two to three times the standard venous doses and agents should be diluted up to a volume of at least 10 mL with saline. After administering a drug into the trachea, give five ventilations to increase dispersion to the bronchial tree, which will assist absorption. Intracardiac drug delivery should only ever be undertaken by experienced staff in exceptional circumstances.

## Vasopressors

The most commonly used agent in cardiac arrest is epinephrine, although norepinephrine (noradrenaline) is sometimes used and vasopressin has been shown experimentally to have encouraging effects.
- The alpha-adrenergic vasoconstricting activity of epinephrine reduces the peripheral pooling of blood that occurs during the acidosis-induced vasoparalysis, and redirects the blood to the brain and heart.
- The beta-adrenergic effects of epinephrine increase sinus, A-V nodal and idioventricular activity and provide inotropic stimulation.
- Isoprenaline, through its unopposed beta-adrenergic effects, has similar activity to epinephrine but vasodilates rather than constricts.
- Be wary of using sympathomimetic agents where cardiac arrest is the result of solvent abuse, cocaine or other sympathomimetic drugs.

## Anti-arrhythmic agents

Incomplete evidence is available to make firm recommendations about the use of any of the multitude of anti-arrhythmic drugs available, although most clinical experience is available for lidocaine. Its effect on the defibrillation threshold of the heart and whether it is clinically beneficial during resuscitation are still debated. The use of atropine (3.0 mg intravenously) for

## CARDIOVASCULAR DRUGS

| Drug | Intravenous dose | Infusion dose* |
|---|---|---|
| Epinephrine (adrenaline) | 1 mg | 1–20 µg/min |
| Aminophylline | | 5 mg/kg over 20 min |
| Amiodarone | 5 mg/kg | 10–20 mg/kg/day |
| Atropine | 0.6–3.0 mg | |
| Bretylium tosylate | 200–400 mg | 1–2 mg/min |
| Calcium chloride (10%) | 5–10 mL | |
| Digoxin | 0.5 mg | 0.5–1.0 mg/day |
| Disopyramide | 50–150 mg | 0.4–1.0 mg/kg/h |
| Dobutamine | | 2.5–10.0 µg/kg/min |
| Dopamine | | 1–20 µg/kg/min |
| Flecainide | 100–150 mg | 0.15–0.25 mg/kg/h |
| Glucagon | | 2.5–7.5 mg/h |
| Glyceryl trinitrate | | 100–200 µg/min |
| Isoprenaline | 1–2 mg | 1–10 µg/min |
| Isosorbide dinitrate | | 1–10 mg/h |
| Labetalol | 50–200 mg | 15–50 mg/h |
| Lidocaine (lignocaine) | 100–200 mg | 1–4 mg/min |
| Methoxamine | 5–10 mg | |
| Metoprolol | 1–15 mg | |
| Mexiletine | 50–250 mg | 0.5–2 0 mg/kg/h |
| Norepinephrine (noradrenaline) | 100–200 µg | 1–20 µg/min |
| Ouabain | 0.25–1.0 mg | |
| Phenylephrine | 100–500 µg | 1–20 µg/min |
| Phenytoin | 50–500 mg | 400–600 mg/day |
| Procainamide | 50–200 mg | 2–6 mg/min |
| Propranolol | 1–10 mg | |
| Salbutamol | 250 µg | 3–20 µg/min |
| Sodium bicarbonate (8.4%) | | 50 mL or more according to pH |
| Sodium nitroprusside | | 10–300 µg/min |
| Streptokinase | | 1.5 million U over 1 h |
| Verapamil | 5–15 mg | |

*Infusion doses only apply to the first few hours and should be reviewed thereafter.

Table 10.1 Cardiovascular drugs.

bradyarrhythmias is well established, and results in complete vagal block for the normal duration of a resuscitation attempt.

### Buffers

In previously healthy people, arterial blood gas analysis does not show rapid or severe acidosis during a cardiac arrest, provided adequate BLS is given. Simply measuring arterial gas tensions may be misleading and bear little relationship to the internal milieu of myocardial or cerebral intracellular values. The role of buffer agents — most commonly 8.4% sodium bicarbonate — is still uncertain, and much of the recent adverse evidence against its use was derived from animal experiments; extrapolation to the situation of a human cardiac arrest is difficult. The consequent sodium load may be detrimental, and drugs may be inactivated (e.g. dopamine and catecholamines) or precipitated (e.g. calcium chloride and calcium gluconate) if given through the same intravenous line as sodium bicarbonate.

• Current advice is to give buffers only when acidosis is severe (arterial pH <7.1 and base excess <−10) or in certain situations such as cardiac arrest associated with hyperkalaemia or after tricyclic antidepressant overdose.
• Give 50 mL of 8.4% $NaHCO_3$ (= 50 mmol) and recheck arterial pH, giving more if necessary.

## Intravenous calcium

For many years, intravenous calcium was given with epinephrine in cardiac arrest, but opinion now is that it is contraindicated.
• Serum ionized calcium levels have been shown to be normal or elevated during arrests, and following calcium administration may rise to toxic levels.
• Some randomized trials, although open to criticism, have shown no additional benefit of calcium over saline.
• Nevertheless, additional calcium may be protective against arrhythmias in the presence of hyperkalaemia, and it should also be considered if the patient has recently been given a blood transfusion (calcium may be chelated by citrate in stored blood), or if the patient has been on high doses of calcium antagonists.
• However, as patients are often hyperkalaemic during an arrest and their prior drug therapy may be unknown, the indication for intravenous calcium may still be uncertain.
• When it is given, calcium chloride (5–10 mL of a 10% solution) is preferable to calcium gluconate because blood levels of ionized calcium are more predictable.

## Hyperkalaemia

This is best corrected by establishing an adequate circulation and tissue oxygenation, but if severe may require insulin (10 IU, i.v.) and glucose (10 g i.v.,= 20 mL of a 50% solution), followed by regular measurement of plasma pH, potassium and glucose.

## Management of arrhythmias

### Ventricular fibrillation
• Defibrillation (200 J) should be attempted as soon as possible.

• If unsuccessful, give a further 200 J, then 360 J if still in VF.
• After a shock the ECG monitor will often show an isoelectric straight line for a few seconds, so wait for a short interval before assessing its effect.

Over 80% of future survivors will have their VF cardioverted by one of these three initial shocks.
• If the arrhythmia persists, then identify and correct any reversible factors (hypoxaemia, hyperkalaemia, severe acidosis) and give **epinephrine** intravenously (1 mg = 1 mL of 1 : 1000 or 10 mL of 1 : 10 000 solution) every 2–3 min while VF/VT persists, to improve coronary and cerebral perfusion.
• Continue chest compression for 1 min, then attempt further defibrillation using up to three sequential 360 J shocks if necessary.
• Continue chest compression for 1 min and repeat the cycle until either successful, or attempts at resuscitation are abandoned.
• After two to three unsuccessful 1-min cycles, consider giving an anti-arrhythmic agent such as **lidocaine** (lignocaine) (100 mg i.v.).

There is no conclusive evidence that any drug can abolish VF, even if the circulation is maintained by BLS. **Bretylium tosylate** is an alternative to lidocaine and has been shown experimentally to have some favourable antifibrillatory properties, but it takes 20–30 min to reach its maximum effect. Other agents include **phenytoin** and **disopyramide**. All anti-arrhythmic drugs potentially have undesirable side-effects, such as negative inotropism. It is best to select a few drugs from different classes (Vaughan-Williams classification) and become familiar with their dose regimens and pharmacology, and to use well-established drugs until newer products are proven to be superior. Although **amiodarone** has become increasingly popular, its bioavailability and onset of action are unpredictable and its half-life is long. In the situation of a cardiac arrest, it is almost impossible to predict the success of any agent in an individual patient and there is bound to be a tendency towards last-resort polypharmacy.

Following successful cardioversion, frequent ventricular ectopics or runs of ventricular tachycardia may be indications for using a lidocaine infusion (1–4 mg/min). The benefit of this practice is unproven and routine use of a lidocaine infusion following successful cardioversion, in the absence of warning arrhythmias, is not indicated.

## Pulseless ventricular tachycardia

The management of pulseless VT is the same as VF. However, certain types of VT, especially the slower varieties, may give a better cardiac output than that achieved with chest compression.
• If one of these rhythms is established, it may be better to wait a short time for an improvement in tissue oxygenation and acidosis, which in turn may improve the chances of success of further defibrillation.
• It is important not to be obsessed with the ECG monitor and ignore the effect any arrhythmia may be having on the patient's circulation. Which VT rhythms produce a reasonable cardiac output and which ones do not depends on various factors, such as its rate, the state of the underlying myocardium, concomitant drug therapy, plasma electrolytes, pH and blood gases.

## Asystole

This may occur as the primary rhythm disturbance, especially when myocardial disease, antiarrhythmic drugs including β-blockers, hypoxia and electrolyte disturbance are present, but may also be the end result of protracted VF.
• If asystole is suspected, connections with the monitoring equipment should be checked, and a different ECG lead tried to ensure that it is not actually fine VF. If asystole is confirmed, **atropine** should be given (3.0 mg i.v.), to relieve the cholinergic depression which has been demonstrated experimentally to occur after myocardial infarction.
• This should be followed by epinephrine (1 mg i.v.) every 3 min.
   **Pacing** instituted soon after the onset of asystole in a patient with predominant nodal or conducting tissue disease is usually very successful, but has been more disappointing in the management of asystole in patients with myocardial disease.

• Transvenous flow directed or other temporary pacing wires can be inserted blind, but often fail to capture due to unrecognized incorrect positioning or myocardial scarring.
• Attempts at ventricular pacing via the oesophagus are usually unsuccessful.
• More recently, external pacing from skin electrode pads has proved effective for elective temporary pacing, but has been more disappointing when used during resuscitation.
• In persistent bradycardia, if atropine followed by isoprenaline fail to increase heart rate, then temporary pacing should be considered.

## Electromechanical dissociation

Management should be directed towards correction of any identifiable cause and the intravenous administration of epinephrine. Other vasoconstrictors, such as norepinephrine, may be tried as a last resort.

## Duration of resuscitation

There can be no hard and fast rules governing the duration of resuscitation attempts because individual circumstances differ markedly.
• Dilated pupils have been used as an indicator of cerebral damage but may be due to high endogenous or exogenously administered catecholamines, atropine therapy or ischaemia of the anterior chamber of the eye and therefore may not necessarily indicate poor prognosis.
• Before stopping attempts at resuscitation, the person leading the management of the arrest should be satisfied, as far as possible, that the likely cause of the arrest is known and that no further specific treatment is indicated.
• In the absence of a definite indication to stop earlier, such as associated terminal disease, attempts should continue for about 30 min, provided that there is good evidence of adequate tissue oxygenation (i.e. satisfactory pH and blood gases). If there is still no spontaneous cardiac activity after that time, further resuscitation is extremely unlikely to be beneficial.
• Exceptions to this are arrests associated with drowning, hypothermia and certain drug over-

doses, when survival may occur after even longer resuscitation periods.

• Without adequate oxygenation, irreversible brain damage begins after about 3 min and successful resuscitation attempts longer than 10 min are likely to result in a disabled individual.

The most helpful guide to the appropriate duration of CPR is a doctor or senior nurse who knows the patient, and informative case notes. Resuscitation attempts that are clearly inappropriate in light of the patient's age or underlying infirmity are not only frustrating to the CPR team, but are potentially damaging to patients, and may cause mental anguish to their relatives.

## Successful resuscitation

Unless specifically considered, the review stage after a successful resuscitation attempt may be overlooked in the congratulatory atmosphere

### Box 10.2 Post-Resuscitation Investigations

• **Chest radiograph**: consider pneumothorax, aspiration, pericardial effusion, position of endotracheal and nasogastric tubes, central venous line and pacing wire
• **ECG**: consider myocardial infarction, pulmonary embolism, rhythm disturbance, conduction disease
• **Echocardiogram**: consider tamponade, left ventricular dysfunction, valve disease
• **Arterial ph and gases**: confirm good oxygenation
• **Electrolytes**: consider hyperkalaemia, hypokalaemia, renal failure
• **Glucose**: consider hypoglycaemia, hyperglycaemia
• **Full blood count**: consider haemorrhage

that tends to occur. Once adequate spontaneous cardiac output has been achieved and the immediate therapeutic measures decided, the possible causes of the arrest, their management and other general measures should be considered. The investigations in Box 10.2 may be helpful.

## Neurological assessment

Neurological assessment after a successful resuscitation can be difficult. Hypoxia leads to cerebral oedema, which is worsened by hypercapnia, due to either inadequate ventilation or local release of carbon dioxide following bicarbonate administration. A fully conscious and communicative patient following a brief arrest obviously has a good prognosis, while a deeply unconscious patient who fails to respond to stimuli (in the absence of sedating or paralysing drugs) following protracted resuscitation has a poor prognosis. Between these two extremes, the prognosis is far less clear, especially in the early stages following resuscitation. In general, a 'watch and wait' policy should be employed and a neurological opinion should be requested before deciding the prognosis. Cerebral damage after a cardiac arrest may be minimized by meticulous attention to blood pH, gases and electrolytes. The possible beneficial effects of calcium antagonists and corticosteroids remain unproven.

## Further reading

The 1998 European Resuscitation Council guidelines for adult single rescuer basic life support. *BMJ* 1998; **316**: 1870–1876.
The 1998 European Resuscitation Council guidelines for adult life support. *BMJ* 1998; **316**: 1863–1869.

# CHAPTER 11

# Valvular Heart Disease

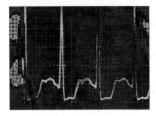

## Pathogenesis of valvular heart disease

In Europe and North America, degenerative valve disease is now more common than valvular heart disease, occurring as a consequence of previous infection (e.g. rheumatic fever, syphilis). In some patients there may be an underlying congenital abnormality of the valve (e.g. bicuspid aortic valve) or an abnormality of connective tissue (e.g. mitral valve prolapse). With the increasing age of the population, 'senile' calcification of a normal valve (e.g. calcific aortic stenosis) presenting in the 7th and 8th decades is a frequent indication for valve replacement. Surgical intervention has modified the 'natural' history of valvular heart disease. Whereas the myocardial component of valvular heart disease has, until recently, been a major cause of mortality, earlier valve repair or replacement at low risk has resulted in the preservation of myocardial function with superior long-term survival.

## Rheumatic fever

### Incidence

The incidence of rheumatic fever has decreased markedly in Western Europe and North America during the last few decades, due to an improvement in socioeconomic conditions, together with the introduction and widespread use of antibiotics. Nevertheless, worldwide there are 15–20 million new cases of rheumatic fever per year, and in developing countries the condition accounts for 25–50% of all cardiac admissions to hospital. There is recent evidence of an increase in the incidence of rheumatic fever in middle-class populations in both Europe and the USA.

Acute rheumatic fever is a disease of childhood with a peak incidence between the ages of 5 and 15 years; 20% of cases occur in adults.

### Pathogenesis

The pathogenesis of rheumatic fever is related to the immunological response to the cell membrane antigens of the Lancefield group A streptococcus. A number of factors can influence the susceptibility to cardiac damage including:

- age;
- socioeconomic conditions;
- ethnic origin;
- genetic factors;
- climate.

Rheumatic fever involves all layers of the heart (a pancarditis) with a pathognomonic lesion, the Aschoff body, which is a mass of cells, altered collagen and connective tissue components in the subendocardium that heals to form a fibrous scar. Other organs that may be affected by rheumatic fever include the skin, joints, lungs and central nervous system.

## Diagnosis

The diagnosis of rheumatic fever may be difficult. The revised Jones criteria (Table 11.1) act as a guide and reduce the chance of overdiagnosis. The presence of two major criteria, or one major and two minor criteria, together with evidence of preceding streptococcal infection are required to make a confident diagnosis of rheumatic fever. However, none of the manifestations are specific. As many of the criteria are clinical, the importance of careful and repeated examination of the patient cannot be overemphasized, particularly as some of the signs (e.g. heart murmurs) may be transient.

## Treatment

Treatment is aimed at eradicating the streptococcus, controlling pain and reducing the inflammatory process. In addition, the patient may require treatment for heart failure and the non-cardiac manifestations of the infection (e.g. chorea) and other complications.

## Prevention

There is general agreement that long-term prophylaxis following an attack of acute rheumatic

## REVISED JONES CRITERIA

*Major manifestations*
Carditis
Polyarthritis
Sydenham's chorea
Erythema marginatum
Subcutaneous nodules

*Minor manifestations*
Fever
Arthralgia
Previous rheumatic fever (or rheumatic heart disease)
Elevated acute-phase reactants (ESR, CRP)
Prolonged PR interval

CRP, C-reactive protein; ESR, erythrocyte sedimentation rate

Table 11.1 The revised Jones criteria for the diagnosis of rheumatic fever.

fever reduces both the late mortality and the chance of recurrent infection. In populations where compliance is a problem, intramuscular benzathine penicillin 1.2 MU every 4 weeks is recommended, but the usual regimen is oral penicillin G 0.25 MU twice daily. For patients allergic to penicillin, erythromycin 250 mg twice daily should be given. Antibiotic prophylaxis should be continued for 5 years after the acute attack or until the age of 30 years (whichever is the longer).

## Long-term follow-up

With the appropriate treatment, the 10-year mortality has fallen from 25% to 1% compared with the preantibiotic era. Furthermore, it can be expected that more than 90% of the hearts will be normal at 10-year follow-up.

## Aortic valve disease

### Aortic stenosis

#### Pathogenesis

The normal aortic valve consists of three semilunar cusps of similar size with a cross-sectional area of $3-4\,cm^2$. Obstruction (stenosis) at valve level may be either congenital or acquired. A bicuspid aortic valve is one of the most common congenital abnormalities (0.9–2.5% incidence) with a male preponderance (4:1). The pattern of acquired aortic stenosis in adults is changing because of the decreasing prevalence of rheumatic disease coupled with the increasing age of the population. Aortic stenosis as a consequence of rheumatic fever is uncommon in the UK (2% of cases) and in such cases the mitral valve is frequently involved.

Secondary calcification of a congenitally bicuspid aortic valve (Fig. 11.1) and primary degeneration of a normal valve (Fig. 11.2) account for the majority of cases of adult aortic stenosis. Only 40% of middle-aged patients with aortic stenosis have a bicuspid valve, but this type of aortic stenosis accounts for 70–80% of cases involving elderly patients. Calcification develops first in the free edges of the cusps and progresses towards the base. Approximately 50% of patients with a bicuspid aortic valve will develop significant aortic stenosis in later life.

In 'senile' calcification of normal valves, calcium is laid down first in the base of the valve and progresses to involve the free edges. 'Senile' calcification rarely ulcerates or embolizes but may be sufficient to cause the aortic systolic murmur, which reportedly occurs in 65% of normal subjects by the 9th decade.

Aortic stenosis in the adult progresses slowly. The restriction of the orifice produces resistance to left ventricular outflow and a reduction in cusp mobility. As the outflow gradient increases, cardiac output is augmented by compensatory left ventricular hypertrophy. Systolic function is maintained despite the increasing pressure overload but the ventricle eventually becomes stiff and non-compliant. The resulting impairment of diastolic function increases myocardial oxygen consumption, shortens the period of diastolic coronary artery filling and reduces myocardial perfusion pressure, which leads to subendocardial ischaemia.

## Symptoms (see Box 11.1)

Most patients remain asymptomatic until the aortic valve area is reduced to $1.0–1.5\,cm^2$. Chest pain, syncope and breathlessness are the classic triad of symptoms; once symptoms have developed, the prognosis is poor. The life expectancy for the patient with chest pain or syncope is 3 years and less than 2 years in those with breathlessness. Sudden death occurs in all age groups but most frequently in patients who were symptomatic.

## Physical signs (see Box 11.2)

The most important physical sign of aortic stenosis is the character of the pulse, best appreciated by palpating the carotid (or brachial)

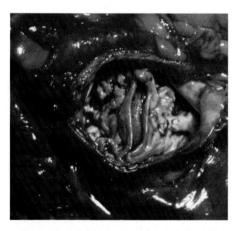

Fig. 11.1 Bicuspid aortic valve.

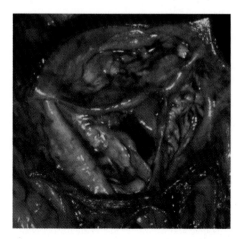

Fig. 11.2 Senile (tricuspid) aortic valve.

### Box 11.1 Symptoms in Aortic Stenosis

- Chest pain
- Exertional syncope
- Breathlessness
- Gastrointestinal bleeding may arise in patients with aortic stenosis in association with angiodysplasia of the colon
- Other complications include infective endocarditis, transient ischaemic attacks (classically amaurosis fugax) and stroke

### Box 11.2 Signs in Aortic Stenosis

- Small volume pulse
- Slow upstroke
- Single S2
- Ejection murmur (± EC)

arteries. The carotid pulse has a small pulse pressure with a slow upstroke caused by prolonged ejection. A palpable (anacrotic) notch in addition to a systolic thrill nearly always indicates severe aortic stenosis.

In the elderly, reduced elasticity of the peripheral arteries may mask pulse abnormalities when the lesion is severe. Calcification and rigidity of the aortic valve reduces the intensity of the aortic second heart sound (A2), and elevation of the left atrial pressure results in an audible fourth heart sound (S4). Because the valve is rigid, the systolic ejection click, so common in children, is rarely heard in the elderly.

The characteristic murmur of aortic stenosis is crescendo–decrescendo ('ejection'), beginning after the first heart sound (S1) and terminating prior to the second heart sound (S2) (Fig. 11.3). Neither the intensity nor the length of the murmur is related to the severity of the valve lesion. Occasionally, patients with critical aortic stenosis have no murmur because of low forward flow, allowing the diagnosis to be easily missed. Many patients with aortic stenosis (of any aetiology) have associated, often mild, aortic regurgitation

### Investigations

Although 70–80% of patients with aortic stenosis have an abnormal electrocardiogram (ECG), a normal ECG does not exclude important aortic stenosis. Left ventricular hypertrophy on voltage criteria may be associated with the so-called 'strain' pattern (Fig. 11.4); T-wave inversion in isolation is an unreliable finding in the elderly.

In uncomplicated aortic stenosis, heart size is

normal on chest radiography but post-stenotic dilatation of the ascending aorta is present in 80% of patients (Fig. 11.5). Aortic valve calcification is often visible on the lateral chest radiograph (Fig. 11.6) without a significant gradient; conversely, aortic stenosis without valve calcification is very rare in the elderly.

M-mode and cross-sectional echocardiography are a useful means of assessing the consequences of aortic stenosis, such as left ventricular wall hypertrophy with a reduced cavity size and impaired diastolic function. Restricted leaflet motion on imaging may indicate aortic stenosis or low forward flow secondary to impaired ventricular function. Multiple echoes may arise from the valve in patients with valve calcification and do not necessarily indicate narrowing of the valve orifice.

Doppler echocardiography has proved invaluable in the assessment of aortic stenosis (see Chapter 3). The maximum systolic pressure difference across the valve (peak instantaneous pressure) can be calculated from the maximum velocity detected by Doppler as gradient $(mmHg) = 4v^2 \ ms^{-1}$. Estimates are unreliable in patients with a low cardiac output and, in this setting, a Doppler gradient of 40–50 mmHg may be significant.

Cardiac catheterization is undertaken predominantly in patients presenting with chest pain to delineate the coronary anatomy.

### Differential diagnosis

Other forms of left ventricular outflow obstruction, commonly hypertrophic obstructive cardiomyopathy, may mimic aortic stenosis. Echocardiography and a Doppler examination usually establish the diagnosis, although the presence of an asymmetrical pattern of hypertrophy in some patients with valvular aortic stenosis suggests a degree of overlap.

### Management

Medical therapy has little to offer once the patient has become symptomatic. Aortic stenosis is a mechanical problem and both diuretics and vasodilators may result in a reduction in either

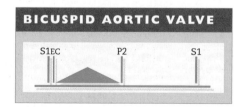

Fig. 11.3 Auscultatory findings in aortic stenosis.

## AORTIC STENOSIS

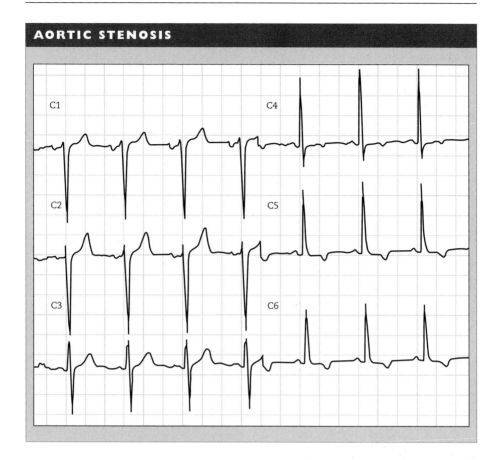

C1

C4

C2

C5

C3

C6

Fig. 11.4 Left ventricular hypertrophy and 'strain' in a patient with aortic stenosis.

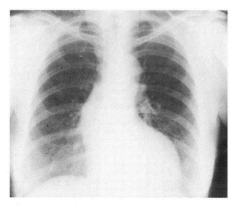

Fig. 11.5 Chest radiograph in aortic stenosis.

preload or afterload which effectively reduces left ventricular function or increases the gradient.

The asymptomatic patient with aortic stenosis should be followed up at 6- or 12-monthly intervals, using serial electrocardiography and echo-Doppler. When the patient becomes symptomatic, surgical referral becomes appropriate. A more difficult problem is the management of the patient who remains asymptomatic with a significant aortic gradient. As the aortic gradient is dependent on cardiac output, an absolute valve gradient should not determine the need for surgical intervention; however, a peak instantaneous gradient on Doppler of 70 mmHg or more (equivalent to a peak-to-peak withdrawal gradient of 50 mmHg measured invasively) usually indicates the need for surgery. If

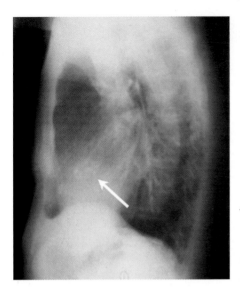

Fig. 11.6 Chest radiograph (lateral) in aortic stenosis.

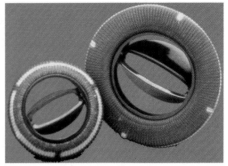

Fig. 11.7 A mechanical valve prosthesis.

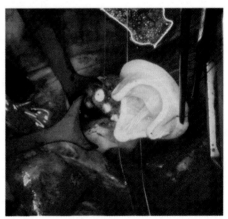

Fig. 11.8 A tissue (xenograft) valve.

ventricular function is compromised, a lower value may be significant.

### Aortic valve replacement

A mechanical prosthesis (either of the tilting disc or ball and cage type) is appropriate for the majority of patients (Fig. 11.7). A biological valve (porcine xenograft, homograft or pericardial) (Fig. 11.8) may be implanted in women of child-bearing age or the elderly (>70 years), in whom anticoagulants may be undesirable. Early mortality for aortic valve replacement is now less than 5%. Incremental risk factors include preoperative functional status and increasing age, although the latter does not appear to be a strong risk factor in experienced centres. Concomitant coronary artery bypass grafting should not increase the in-hospital mortality and indeed may reduce the early risk. Symptomatic results and late survival rates are excellent and superior to those following mitral valve replacement. Five-year actuarial survival rates of 70–90% with a 10-year survival of 70–75% are typical for reported series.

### Balloon aortic valvuloplasty

There has been recent interest in balloon dilata-tion of the aortic valve particularly in the elderly patient with aortic stenosis. Published experience suggests that the procedure is low in risk (<5%) with a worthwhile improvement in symptoms, particularly if the gradient can be reduced by 50% or more. However, in the majority of patients, the procedure is no more than palliative with recurrent stenosis occurring within 6–18 months after successful balloon dilatation. Furthermore, it appears that the natural history of untreated aortic stenosis is not modified by balloon valvuloplasty. The disappointing results with this technique are not surprising as the cause of flow reduction in the majority of patients is calcification of the valve cusps rather than commissural fusion.

Given the low operative risk and excellent

functional results of aortic valve replacement, aortic valvuloplasty should be restricted to symptomatic patients with other life-threatening conditions, such as carcinoma.

## Aortic regurgitation
### Pathogenesis

Several mechanisms may be responsible for the development of aortic regurgitation, depending on whether the disease process affects the valve cusps themselves or the aortic root.

Despite the reduction in the incidence of syphilis, aortic regurgitation as a consequence of an aortopathy appears to be increasing, accounting for one-third of patients coming to surgery.

Acute aortic regurgitation may be due to cusp rupture or perforation secondary to infection, aortic dissection and, rarely, closed chest trauma.

Connective tissue diseases (e.g. Marfan's syndrome) also occasionally cause acute aortic regurgitation.

Causes of chronic aortic regurgitation are listed in Table 11.2. In diseases of the aortic root, the cusps themselves may appear normal but an increase in root diameter causes a loss of the usual cusp overlap, leading to the development of a central regurgitant jet.

The severity of the condition depends on the aortic valve area, the heart rate and the diastolic pressure gradient between the left ventricle and the aorta. In early disease, the left ventricle maintains output by a degree of hypertrophy but eventually the diastolic overload produces left ventricular dilatation followed by a reduction in forward flow and pulmonary venous hypertension. Changes in heart rate or systemic vascular resistance may alter the regurgitant fraction.

### Symptoms (see Box 11.3)

As with mitral regurgitation, aortic regurgitation is well tolerated. The appropriate management is complicated by the late occurrence of symptoms, usually after considerable left ventricular damage has arisen that cannot be reversed by surgical intervention. Restriction of exercise tolerance due to breathlessness and fatigue is followed by orthopnoea and pulmonary oedema as a consequence of pulmonary venous hypertension.

### Physical signs (see Box 11.4)

Examination may reveal that the aortic regurgi-

---

**Box 11.3 Symptoms in Aortic Regurgitation**

- Fatigue
- Breathlessness
- Orthopnoea
- Nocturnal dyspnoea

---

## CHRONIC AORTIC REGURGITATION

| *Cusp abnormality* | |
|---|---|
| Perforation | Infective endocarditis |
| Reduction in area | Rheumatic disease |
| | Rheumatoid ankylosing spondylitis |
| | |
| *Aortic root disease* | |
| Root distortion | Rheumatoid ankylosing spondylitis |
| | Syphilis |
| | Non-specific urethritis |
| | Non-specific aortitis |
| Root dilatation | Syphilis |
| | Marfan's syndrome |
| | Ehlers–Danlos syndrome |
| | Pseudoxanthoma elasticum |

Table 11.2 Causes of chronic aortic regurgitation

## Box 11.4 Signs in Aortic Regurgitation

- Wide pulse pressure
- Hyperdynamic apex
- Early diastolic murmur
- ± Mid-diastolic murmur

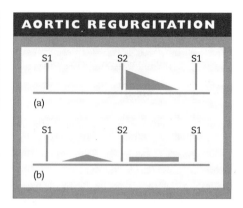

Fig. 11.9 Auscultatory findings in aortic regurgitation. (a) Early diastolic murmur. (b) Systolic flow murmur and mid-diastolic (Austin Flint) murmur.

tation is occurring as part of a systemic disorder (e.g. rheumatoid arthritis, ankylosing spondylitis and Marfan's syndrome). In acute aortic regurgitation, features of aortic dissection or endocarditis may also be present.

The wide pulse pressure and rapid diastolic run-off give rise to a number of clinical signs, which are reflected in the active, hyperdynamic and often laterally displaced apex beat. Typically, a high-pitched early diastolic murmur commences immediately after A2 and is audible at the left sternal edge and base; the length, rather than the loudness of the murmur, relates to severity. An additional systolic flow murmur is often audible and does not necessarily imply additional aortic stenosis. Similarly, a mid-diastolic flow murmur (Austin Flint murmur) may be present when aortic regurgitation is severe (Fig. 11.9). All these signs may be absent in acute aortic regurgitation because of equalization of the left ventricular end-diastolic and the aortic diastolic pressures. In these circumstances, the patient may appear breathless and unwell with a sinus tachycardia but otherwise quiet heart.

### Investigations

The ECG is rarely normal in chronic aortic regurgitation and often shows marked repolarization changes. In acute aortic regurgitation the ECG may be normal. Dilatation of the left ventricle leads to progressive cardiac enlargement on the chest radiograph. Although the ascending aorta is often prominent, the aetiology of the valve lesion cannot be determined. On echocardiography, the left ventricular dimensions in early aortic regurgitation are normal, often in association with mild left ventricular hypertrophy. Contractility is well preserved and may be exaggerated. If aortic regurgitation is neglected,

left ventricular dilatation ensues with a progressive reduction in systolic function, leading to a left ventricle similar in appearance to that seen in dilated cardiomyopathy. Abnormalities of the aortic root (such as in Marfan's syndrome) can also be demonstrated by echocardiography.

Doppler echocardiography, particularly colour-flow mapping, is very sensitive and can detect minor degrees of aortic regurgitation, and map the direction of the jet which may give additional information regarding the severity of the lesion. Most surgeons require the patient to undergo aortography before considering operative intervention. Conventional transthoracic echocardiography (TTE) in adults demonstrates the proximal part of the aortic root on imaging, whereas transoesophageal echocardiography (TOE) visualizes the entire aorta. Similarly, magnetic resonance imaging (MRI) may give the surgeon sufficient information to avoid the need for cardiac catheterization.

### Medical management

More than 50% of patients with untreated aortic regurgitation are alive after 10 years, therefore a conservative policy is usually followed. The asymptomatic patient with mild aortic regurgitation should be followed up at 6- or 12-monthly intervals by serial echo-Doppler. Evidence of left ventricular dilatation with or without a reduction in function suggests surgical intervention is appropriate. Diuretic and vasodilator therapy (e.g. angiotensin-converting enzyme (ACE) inhibitors) may be used as a holding manoeuvre. As these lesions are also prone to infective endocarditis, good dental hygiene is important and all patients should be given antibiotic cover for dental and other minor operative procedures.

## Surgical intervention

The early and late mortality following aortic valve replacement for aortic regurgitation is similar to the results of valve replacement in aortic stenosis (see p. 184). In the current era of cardiac surgery, aortic root replacement is no longer a risk factor for early mortality.

## Mitral valve disease

### Rheumatic mitral valve disease
#### Pathogenesis

Mitral stenosis is the most common late consequence of rheumatic carditis. A latency period of 20 years between the acute infection and symptomatic valvular dysfunction is not uncommon with the typical patient presenting in the 4th or 5th decade. In patients from the Far East and South America, severe valvular disease may present in their early twenties.

Pathological abnormalities of the valve include commissural fusion, fibrous scarring and obliteration of the normally layered valvular architecture as a result of healed acute valvulitis and superimposed fibrosis. Progressive fibrous bridging across the valvular commissures may produce a rigid 'fishmouth' deformity resulting in a fixed orifice, which is both stenosed, and regurgitant. The valve leaflets become calcified and the chordae tendineae thickened, fused and shortened.

#### Symptoms (see Box 11.5)

The clinical features of mitral stenosis are determined by the left atrial pressure, cardiac output and pulmonary vascular resistance. As the left atrial pressure increases, pulmonary compliance is reduced making breathing more laboured. Initially, breathlessness only arises when the heart rate is increased, for example during exercise, stress and fever. As the severity of the lesion increases the patient becomes orthopnoeic. Prior to the onset of paroxysmal dyspnoea, nocturnal coughing may be the only symptom of an elevated left atrial pressure. Nowadays, haemoptysis is rarely seen. Palpitation due to atrial fibrillation becomes more common with increasing age; 80% of patients over the age of 50 years have this complication.

Pulmonary arterial pressure rises in parallel with an increase in left atrial pressure, in most patients becoming 10–12 mmHg greater than left atrial pressure. In some patients, particularly those with severe mitral stenosis, pulmonary arterial pressure rises disproportionately, so-called reactive pulmonary hypertension. Right-sided symptoms may predominate in these patients (see p. 193).

#### Physical signs (see Box 11.6)

The most important and often neglected physical sign in mitral stenosis is accentuation of S1. Sudden tensing of the mitral leaflets by the subvalve apparatus and the halting of the downward movement of the mitral valve causes a high-pitched opening snap in early diastole, 40–120 ms after S2 (Fig. 11.10). If the valve is still

---

**Box 11.5 Symptoms in Mitral Stenosis**

- Fatigue
- Breathlessness
- Orthopnoea
- Nocturnal dyspnoea
- ± Palpitation (atrial fibrillation)

---

**Box 11.6 Signs in Mitral Stenosis**

- Loud S1
- Mid-diastolic murmur
- ± Opening snap
- ± Pulmonary oedema

## MITRAL STENOSIS

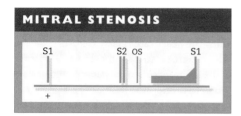

**Fig. 11.10** Auscultatory findings in mitral stenosis.

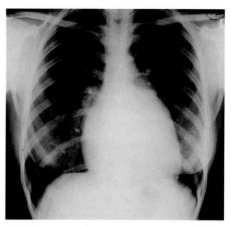

**Fig. 11.11** Chest radiograph (PA) in mitral stenosis.

mobile, the interval between S2 and the opening snap will vary inversely with the mean left atrial pressure. The classical low-pitched rumbling diastolic murmur is often localized to the apex or axilla; it is short in duration when the valve lesion is mild. The duration, not the loudness of the murmurs relates to lesion severity.

Mitral facies are usually indicative of long-standing mitral stenosis associated with pulmonary hypertension. Other physical features include the signs of pulmonary oedema (basal lung crackles), together with fluid retention, hepatic congestion and tricuspid regurgitation.

### Investigations

In the majority of patients, mitral valve disease is adequately assessed non-invasively but occasionally cardiac catheterization and haemodynamic investigation are necessary. The features of mitral stenosis on the ECG are non-specific; if the patient is in sinus rhythm, a broad biphasic P wave is present in 90% of patients with mitral stenosis. P-wave morphology is related to left atrial dilatation rather than hypertrophy.

In pure mitral stenosis, the size of the heart on chest radiography is normal unless long-standing pulmonary hypertension has caused dilatation of the right-sided chambers. The left atrium is selectively enlarged, causing dilatation of the left main bronchus, which may be more easily seen on a penetrated film (Fig. 11.11). In the elderly, mitral valve calcification (visible on the lateral view) must be differentiated from mitral annulus calcification. When left atrial pressure rises, there is pulmonary venous dis-

tension followed by upper lobe blood diversion and the radiographic signs of interstitial and alveolar oedema.

Echocardiography combined with Doppler examination is the single most useful investigation in the patient with mitral valve disease. Suitability for a conservative procedure (e.g. valvotomy or valve repair) is best determined by echocardiography. Both M-mode and cross-sectional echocardiography show valve thickening and a reduction in the mid-diastolic closure rate of the anterior leaflet. The posterior leaflet may also be tethered and move anteriorly (instead of posteriorly) during diastole. The left atrial dimension is increased and occasionally thrombus may be visible in the left atrial appendage. TOE is more reliable in the identification of intracavity thrombus. The pressure drop across the mitral valve using continuous-wave Doppler correlates well with the haemodynamic gradient measured at cardiac catheterization but, as with direct measurement of the gradient, the Doppler gradient is very much dependent on heart rate. The pressure half-time may be a more reliable index of the severity of mitral stenosis (see Chapter 3).

Invasive assessment by cardiac catheterization is limited to certain subgroups of patients, for example, to define the coronary anatomy, and is no longer a prerequisite to mitral valve surgery.

## Medical management

The objective of drug therapy for mitral stenosis is to control the ventricular rate, reduce left atrial pressure and prevent systemic thromboembolism.

The onset of atrial fibrillation, which usually occurs in the 6th decade, is often associated with rapid symptomatic deterioration. Digoxin is the drug of choice at a dose sufficient to maintain the resting ventricular rate between 60 and 70 b.p.m., usually 0.125–0.25 mg/day depending on age, body weight and renal function. Although effective at rest, digoxin is often disappointing in controlling the ventricular rate during exertion. Toxicity may occur if the patient is hypokalaemic. Difficulty with rate control may require a small dose of an additional β-blocker (e.g. atenolol 25 mg once daily) or a calcium antagonist (e.g. verapamil 40 mg twice daily). Alternative agents include a β-blocker alone or amiodarone.

Electrical or chemical cardioversion rarely restores sinus rhythm long term in the patient with significant mitral stenosis.

Fluid retention responds well to diuretic therapy, however, pulmonary oedema occurs as a consequence of an anatomical obstruction and overvigorous diuretic therapy may result in hypovolaemia, hypokalaemia and prerenal azotaemia. Large doses of loop diuretics should be avoided in favour of a thiazide or combination diuretic.

In the patient with atrial fibrillation due to rheumatic mitral valve disease, there is a 15–20-fold increase in the risk of stroke from systemic thromboembolism, highest at the time of onset of atrial fibrillation. Patients with significant mitral stenosis, especially if there is evidence on echocardiography of left atrial enlargement, require anticoagulation with warfarin aiming to maintain the international normalized ratio (INR) between 2.0 and 2.5. The exception is the patient over the age of 70 years, presenting for the first time without a previous history of thromboembolism, in whom the risks of anticoagulation probably exceed the potential benefits.

## Mitral valve surgery

If the patient remains significantly limited despite diuretic therapy and control of the ventricular rate, surgical intervention or balloon valvuloplasty should be considered. Occasionally, patients with recurrent thromboembolism, despite adequate anticoagulation, may also require operation. However, it should be borne in mind that the long-term results of mitral valve surgery are less favourable than those of aortic valve replacement, especially as symptomatic deterioration may be very slow in mitral valve disease.

A conservative procedure on the mitral valve is possible in a small minority of patients. Usually they are young, in sinus rhythm and without evidence of involvement of the subvalve apparatus by the rheumatic process on echocardiography. Most of these patients in whom open mitral valvotomy is considered are suitable for balloon mitral valvuloplasty (see below).

Replacement of the mitral valve with a mechanical prosthesis is usually appropriate, as the patient will require anticoagulation in any case for the atrial fibrillation. A tissue valve may be considered for the very elderly or women of childbearing age in whom anticoagulation may be a problem. Early mortality for mitral valve replacement is 6–8% with a late valve related mortality of 3–5% per annum, which is not related to valve type. Thromboembolic complications with mechanical valves occur at a rate of 3–5% per patient-year follow up.

## Balloon mitral valvuloplasty

Balloon dilatation of the mitral valve appears to be a suitable alternative to surgery in selected patients. Left atrial thrombus must be excluded by TOE, mitral regurgitation should be minimal, and the results are more favourable if the valve is non-calcified without evidence of chordal fusion and shortening. An Inoue balloon is introduced under local anaesthesia from the right femoral vein and via a trans-septal approach from the right to the left atrium; the balloon is dilated sufficiently to cause splitting of the fused commissures (Fig. 11.12). Early mortality is low at less than 1% with a morbidity of 2–4%. Early experience suggests that the results match those from mitral valvotomy, even in the elderly.

## Degenerative mitral valve disease
### Acute mitral regurgitation
Within 14 days of an acute myocardial infarct, 0.4–0.5% of patients die from acute mitral regurgitation secondary to papillary muscle rupture. Sudden, severe mitral regurgitation results in early acute pulmonary oedema and cardiogenic shock; without immediate mitral valve replacement, 75% of patients die within 24 hours. Unlike chronic mitral regurgitation, there is insufficient time for compensatory mechanism of left atrial and left ventricular dilatation to adapt to the volume load. Other causes of acute mitral regurgitation include valve destruction (cusp perforation or chordal rupture) by infective endocarditis, partial papillary muscle rupture and spontaneous chordal rupture.

## Chronic non-rheumatic mitral regurgitation
### Pathogenesis
Myxomatous degeneration of the mitral valve leads to a spectrum of valve abnormalities ranging from minor degrees of cusp prolapse, present in up to 5% of the population, to a 'floppy valve' due to chordal elongation or rupture causing significant mitral regurgitation.

### Symptoms (see Box 11.7)
Many patients remain asymptomatic until the insidious onset of fatigue, breathlessness and palpitation, the latter presenting as a hyperdynamic heartbeat, extrasystoles or atrial fibrillation.

---

**Box 11.7 Symptoms in Mitral Regurgitation**

- Fatigue
- Breathlessness
- Orthopnoea
- Nocturnal dyspnoea
- Palpitation (atrial fibrillation)

---

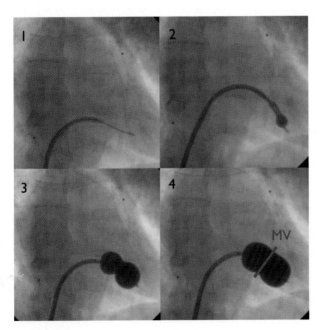

Fig. 11.12 Balloon mitral valvuloplasty.

## Physical signs (see Box 11.8)

The pulse and venous pressure appear normal in isolated mitral regurgitation, unless there is secondary pulmonary hypertension. Palpation of the precordium is an important means of assessing the severity of mitral regurgitation. If mild, the precordial impulse is quiet but, as the severity increases, the cardiac apex becomes hyperdynamic and displaced laterally, often in association with a systolic thrill.

Mild degrees of mitral regurgitation due to mitral valve prolapse are characterized by a quiet, late systolic murmur, associated with one or more systolic clicks. As the regurgitation becomes more severe, the murmur lengthens, obscuring S2 and the systolic clicks (Fig. 11.13). Murmur location, typically at the apex, may be unreliable because a jet directed anteriorly can be heard at the base and radiates to the neck.

## Investigations

The ECG may be normal in mild to moderate mitral regurgitation. As the left atrium enlarges, the P waves become biphasic. Later still, when the left ventricle dilates the anterior, voltages become prominent, often in association with T-wave inversion.

In moderate to severe mitral regurgitation, there is evidence of both left atrial and left ventricular dilatation on chest radiography. Left atrial enlargement may reach aneurysmal proportions. Pulmonary venous congestion and interstitial oedema arise late in the course of the disease.

Serial echo-Doppler examinations have largely replaced radiography in the follow-up of the patient with mitral regurgitation. Prolapse of one or both leaflets may be visible as well as the redundant cusp tissue typical of a 'floppy' valve. Similarly, ruptured chordae can be seen,

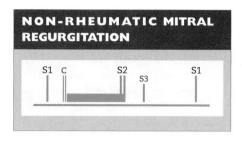

**NON-RHEUMATIC MITRAL REGURGITATION**

Fig. 11.13 Auscultatory findings in non-rheumatic mitral regurgitation.

although there may be difficulty in differentiating between a vegetation and the rolled-up cusp margin seen in partial chordal rupture. In mild disease, the left ventricular and left atrial dimensions are normal but, as the regurgitation increases in severity, left ventricular and septal movement become more vigorous; eventually the left ventricle dilates with a reduction in systolic function.

Doppler ultrasound is an accurate and sensitive method of detecting mitral regurgitation. Both the direction and the magnitude of the regurgitant jet(s) can be mapped using colour-flow techniques, allowing a semi-quantitative assessment of the severity of the lesion (see Chapter 3).

Haemodynamic assessment is usually only necessary prior to mitral valve surgery, when cardiac catheterization is required to document the coronary anatomy.

## Medical management

Patients with mild mitral regurgitation may only require antibiotic prophylaxis (see p. 201). As the severity of the disease progresses, a mild diuretic or vasodilators (e.g. angiotensin converting enzyme (ACE) inhibitor) are equally effective. Only if these measures fail to provide symptomatic relief, or if there is echocardiographic evidence of progressive cavity dilatation, should surgical intervention be considered.

Atrial fibrillation should be treated as for mitral stenosis (see p. 189). The incidence of systemic thromboembolism is said to be low in isolated mitral regurgitation, but in the patient

---

**Box 11.8 Signs in Mitral Regurgitation**

- Hyperdynamic apex
- ± Systolic thrill
- Pansystolic murmur
- ± Systolic click(s)

with atrial fibrillation treatment with warfarin is recommended.

## Surgical intervention

Progressive symptoms of fatigue or breathlessness, or echocardiographic evidence of left ventricular dilatation (even without symptoms) indicate the need for surgical intervention. Reconstruction of the mitral valve has superior long-term results compared with valve replacement with a similar early mortality of 0–2%. Results are particularly good for repair of posterior leaflet prolapse. Cusp resection is often combined with chordal shortening, reinforced with some type of annuloplasty. Late complications associated with thromboembolism or anticoagulation are avoided with repair. Patients with mitral regurgitation as a consequence of myocardial ischaemia or infarction form a high-risk subgroup, with an early mortality of 10–20% reflecting the associated impairment of ventricular function in these patients.

### Mitral valve prolapse syndrome

Mitral valve prolapse, which is a normal variant occurring in 5–10% of the population at large, may be associated with a more widespread spectrum of cardiac and extra-cardiac symptoms. These include:

- chest pain;
- palpitation;
- anxiety;
- fatigue;
- lethargy;
- an inability to concentrate;
- exercise intolerance;
- postural giddiness.

Because of the diverse nature of the symptoms, there is a tendency for the physician to dismiss the symptoms as having no organic basis. It is important to take a careful history and to confirm the diagnosis of mitral valve prolapse on echocardiography. Evidence of pre-excitation or variable inferior repolarization changes may be present on the resting ECG and a 'false-positive' exercise response is not un-

common. Atrial and ventricular ectopics may be documented by Holter monitoring.

The mainstay of treatment is careful explanation and reassurance. Avoidance of stimulants (e.g. tea and coffee) may be helpful and, in occasional patients, a small dose of a β-blocker (e.g. atenolol 25 mg once daily) may be beneficial. Investigations should usually stop short of invasive testing unless there is concern that there may be additional coronary artery disease.

### Mitral annulus calcification

This is a condition of the elderly in which calcium is laid down in the mitral annulus and may occasionally spread to involve the conducting tissue, causing heart block, or the mitral leaflets themselves causing mitral regurgitation. Females are affected more frequently than males and there is an association with hypercalcaemia, diabetes mellitus and systemic hypertension. Symptoms are unusual although calcification may act as a source of systemic thromboembolism or be the substrate for infective endocarditis. The diagnosis can be confirmed by echocardiography or on the lateral chest radiograph, the calcified annulus appearing as a curved J- or U-shaped shadow (see Fig. 19.5).

### Infective endocarditis

See Chapter 12.

### Pulmonary valve disease

See Chapter 18.

### Tricuspid valve disease

## Pathogenesis and aetiology

The tricuspid valve consists of three leaflets of differing size. The annulus of the valve is a dynamic structure that changes size during the cardiac cycle. Most commonly, tricuspid regurgitation is 'functional', that is the valve leaks as a consequence of right ventricular dilatation secondary to pressure overload, for example, from mitral or aortic valve disease, or cor pulmonale. Other rare causes of tricuspid regurgitation include right ventricular infarction, infective endocarditis, trauma, carcinoid or rheumatic fever. Tricuspid stenosis is very rare in Europe and North America and is nearly always associated with mitral valve disease.

## Symptoms

In most patients, the left-side symptoms predominate (breathlessness, orthopnoea, nocturnal dyspnoea). Patients may complain of visible neck pulsation from the raised venous pressure, fluid retention (abdominal and lower limb swelling), right upper quadrant pain (hepatic congestion), anorexia and weight loss.

## Physical signs

A raised venous pressure with a prominent systolic ('v') wave is characteristic, in association with a pansystolic murmur. The localization of the murmur and the increase in intensity with inspiration may not be useful in clinical practice. Late in the disease, hepatic pulsation may be present reflecting the severity of the regurgitation.

## Investigations

Atrial fibrillation on the ECG is the norm and the chest radiograph nearly always shows cardiac enlargement with additional features of left-sided disease. Echocardiography demonstrates dilatation of the right-sided chambers, often in association with paradoxical septal motion. Organic disease of the valve (e.g. vegetations) may be apparent. Doppler assessment allows a semi-quantitative assessment of the severity of the regurgitation, together with the calculation of right ventricular systolic pressure. Many normal subjects have mild tricuspid regurgitation on colour-flow mapping.

## Management

Tricuspid regurgitation is well tolerated. Management of the left-sided problem (e.g. mitral valve replacement) is appropriate, which will usually result in a fall in the right ventricular pressure thereby reducing the severity of the tricuspid regurgitation. An additional tricuspid annuloplasty may be required in severe cases. Tricuspid valve replacement is rarely undertaken today because of problems of valve thrombosis. In patients with infective endocarditis, a conservative approach (e.g. valve debridement and/or annuloplasty) may be required to restore valve competence.

## Innocent murmurs

A short innocent or physiological mid-systolic murmur can be heard in 8% of the normal population. Typically, a well-localized, quiet crescendo–decrescendo ('ejection') murmur is heard at the left sternal edge, and may be augmented by conditions that increase cardiac output (e.g. anaemia, fever, pregnancy). These murmurs are thought to arise from turbulence in the right ventricular outflow tract. The diagnosis is usually clear-cut on clinical examination alone; if necessary, echocardiography and a Doppler examination can confirm the absence of structural heart disease.

# CHAPTER 12

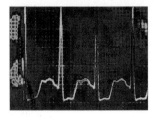

# The Endocardium

## Function and pathophysiology

The endocardium is a thin layer that invests the entire inner surface of the heart. The structure and thickness of the endocardium varies from one chamber to another and from one region to another within a given chamber. The endocardium is thicker in the atria than the ventricles and thicker in the left-sided chambers compared with the right. The endocardium is well developed in the left ventricular outflow tract, forming five distinct layers: (i) the endothelial layer; (ii) inner connective tissue; (iii) elastic tissue; (iv) smooth muscle; and (v) outer connective tissue layers. The total thickness of the endocardium in the left ventricular outflow tract is 200 μm, but as thin as 50 μm elsewhere in this chamber. The thickest endocardium is found in the left atrium where it may approach 900 μm. With increasing age, the endocardium increases in thickness and becomes more opaque due to a proliferation of elastic and collagen.

The endocardial connective tissue is continuous with that in the myocardial interstitium and valvular leaflets. Integrity of the endocardium is important as a means of reducing platelet deposition and thrombus formation, as well as reducing the likelihood of the deposition and multiplication of the microorganisms that cause infective endocarditis.

Localized thickening of the endocardium may result from haemodynamic derangement of the heart valves; 'jet' lesions may be seen as a result of aortic or mitral regurgitation, and ventricular friction lesions can occur in mitral valve prolapse or in patients with hypertrophic obstructive cardiomyopathy due to systolic anterior movement of the mitral valve.

## Carcinoid

### Pathology
Carcinoid tumours arise from cells originating in neural crest tissue (Kulchitsky cells). Most commonly, primary tumours arise in the small intestine, especially the terminal ileum and appendix, although carcinoid tumours have been described in the bronchi, pancreatic ducts, ovaries, testicle, rectum and stomach. Carcinoid tumours involving the appendix usually remain localized; the spread of tumour to regional lymph nodes or the liver may result in the carcinoid syndrome.

## Carcinoid syndrome

Symptoms of the carcinoid syndrome only occur when a primary tumour has metastasized to the regional lymph nodes or liver.

The classic symptom is flushing of the skin

that particularly affects the face, head and neck but may progress to involve the whole trunk.

Other features include bronchoconstriction, weight loss, profuse diarrhoea and abdominal pain. Carcinoid tumours metabolize the amino acid tryptophan, producing the vasoactive amine 5-hydroxytryptamine (serotonin) which is thought to be responsible for many of the clinical features of the syndrome. Urinary excretion of 5-hyroxyindole acetic acid (5-HIAA) is a useful marker for the condition, but high levels of this metabolite may occur from the ingestion of foods high in 5-hydroxtryptamine (5-HT) (e.g. bananas, pineapples and walnuts). If at all possible, histology confirmation of the diagnosis should be performed with biopsy of either the primary or secondary tumour. Treatment should include the control of diarrhoea (e.g. codeine phosphate, diphenoxylate), together with the administration of 5-HT antagonists (cyproheptadine, methysergide) and $\alpha$-blockers (e.g. phenoxybenzamine) for symptoms of flushing. The prognosis is variable. Many tumours are slow growing and metastasize late.

## Cardiac carcinoid

In carcinoid heart disease there is either focal or diffuse plaque-like thickening of the endocardium, which is nearly always limited to the right heart.

Inactivation of 5-HT by the lungs accounts for the relative sparing of the left-sided valves.

Cardiac involvement is only seen in patients with hepatic secondaries or when the venous drainage from the tumour bypasses the liver (e.g. bronchial and ovarian tumours). Deposition of fibrous tissue on the pulmonary valve results in predominant stenosis, although some additional regurgitation may occur. Adherence of the leaflets of the tricuspid valve to the ventricular septum causes tricuspid regurgitation, fibrous deposition of the plaque on the posterior and septal leaflets of the valve can result in tricuspid stenosis. The pathogenesis of the

carcinoid plaque is uncertain. Rarely, surgical debridement of the affected valve or valve replacement may be required.

## Endomyocardial fibrosis

Endomyocardial fibrosis (EMF) is a condition most frequently seen in the tropics with sporadic reports from temperate climates.

Progressive thickening and fibrosis of the endocardium affecting either the left or, more usually, both ventricles results in haemodynamics indistinguishable from a restrictive cardiomyopathy in association with atrioventricular valve regurgitation.

Apical obliteration of either ventricle by thrombus may result in systemic or pulmonary embolism. A moderate eosinophilia suggests an association with eosinophilic endomyocardial disease (see below) but may merely reflect concomitant parasitic infection found in the tropics. Treatment consists of diuretic therapy, with mitral or tricuspid repair or replacement, together with endocardial resection in selected patients.

## Eosinophilic endomyocardial disease

A rapidly progressive condition, first described by Loeffler, in which an eosinophilic endomyocarditis is associated with a systemic disorder including anorexia, weight loss, cough and wheezing.

Unlike EMF, the condition is seen more frequently in temperate climates.

Three stages of the condition are described: (i) the early necrotic stage; (ii) the thrombotic stage; and (iii) the fibrotic stage. The latter is pathologically indistinguishable from the histology seen in EMF. Endomyocardial biopsy may be diagnostic in the early necrotic stage, showing a combination of myocardial necrosis and an eosinophilic infiltrate. Typically, the peripheral blood eosinophils are degranulated with the suggestion that the proteins contained within the granules have been released and are cardiotoxic. Early treatment with steroids and immunosuppressive drugs may reduce the level of circulating eosinophils resulting in resolution of the myocarditis. Occasional patients require atrioventricular (AV) valve replacement or endocardial resection.

## Endocardial fibroelastosis

A condition of infancy and childhood of obscure aetiology, characterized by thickening of the endocardium by a white homogeneous glistening material usually involving the left atrium and ventricle.

Haemodynamics are similar to those found in a dilated cardiomyopathy with impaired systolic function, although occasional patients present with a restrictive defect. The differential diagnosis includes storage diseases (e.g. Pompe's), an idiopathic dilated cardiomyopathy, EMF and an anomalous coronary artery. The prognosis is poor.

## Infective endocarditis

### Clinical presentation

In the past, infective endocarditis was a disease of young adults but currently the average age is 50–60 years, with males affected more frequently than females (2:1). Approximately 300 new cases are notified annually in England and Wales. Factors responsible for the changing pattern of the disease include the widespread and early use of antibiotics, the increasing number of patients undergoing cardiac surgery and the increase in intravenous drug abuse. There is little evidence to suggest that the prognosis is improving, with an overall case fatality rate of approximately 30%. The widespread and indiscriminate use of antibiotics has resulted in an increase in the frequency of culture negative endocarditis, which is associated with a less favourable prognosis.

Although some forms of endocarditis are more virulent than others, antibiotic therapy

has modified the clinical course to such an extent that the terms 'acute' and 'subacute' are no longer applicable. 'Infective' rather than 'bacterial' is the preferred term as non-bacterial forms (e.g. marantic in advanced malignancy, Libman–Sachs in systemic lupus) may be seen infrequently.

### Portal of entry

Micro-organisms gain entry to the bloodstream by a variety of routes (Table 12.1), although the mode of access can only be determined in one-third of patients. Less than 15% of patients give a history of prior dental treatment.

### Pathogenesis

Endothelial damage results from turbulence (e.g. bicuspid aortic valve, pulmonary stenosis, mitral valve prolapse) and may also be associated with high-pressure interfaces (e.g. ventricular septal defect (VSD), patent ductus arteriosus (PDA), coarctation of the aorta, hypertrophic cardiomyopathy). Areas of endothelial injury may provide a focus for the formation of a platelet-fibrin aggregate within which a small focus of circulating bacteria become entrapped and multiply. A transient bacteraemia complicating, for example, a surgical procedure then leads to tissue destruction, septic emboli and immune complex deposition; the three

### INFECTIVE ENDOCARDITIS

| Portals of entry | % |
| --- | --- |
| Dental treatment | <15 |
| Genito-urinary tract | 4 |
| Gastro-intestinal | 4 |
| Respiratory | 3 |
| Skin | 3 |
| Cardiac surgery | 3 |
| Vascular surgery | 3 |
| Drug abuse | 1 |
| Pregnancy | <1 |
| Fractures | <1 |
| Unknown | 64 |

Table 12.1 Infective endocarditis: portals of entry.

mechanisms of tissue damage in the patient with infective endocarditis.

## Organisms

It is only with knowledge of the organisms responsible for infective endocarditis that the appropriate antibiotic treatment can be started. This is particularly important if therapy needs to be started early because of haemodynamic deterioration, before the organism is isolated. Table 12.2 lists the common organisms causing infective endocarditis. The spectrum of organisms may be different in some subgroups of patients. In recent years the HACEK (Haemophilus, Actinobacillus, Cardiobacterium, Eikenella, Kingella spp.) group of organisms has become an increasingly recognized cause of infection. Intravenous drug abusers are infected with staphylococcal spp. in 50% of cases, Pseudomonas spp. in 15% and fungi (frequently Candida spp.) in 5%. In patients with early prosthetic heart valves, infection with Staphylococcus spp. accounts for the majority of cases.

Culture-negative endocarditis occurs most frequently (>60% of cases) as a result of prior antibiotic treatment. Other causes include anaerobic (e.g. Bacteroides spp.) or other fastidious organisms (e.g. Brucella spp.), non-bacterial endocarditis (e.g. Coxiella burnetii or 'Q' fever), fungal infection (e.g. Candida, Aspergillus spp.) or non-infective (thrombotic) endocarditis. Endo-carditis in HIV-seropositive patients usually relates to intravenous drug abuse or infection of indwelling venous catheters and, therefore, is caused by staphylococcal spp. in the majority of patients.

## Symptoms (see Box 12.1)

Infective endocarditis is a diagnosis that is frequently missed due to the insidious nature of the disease.

General malaise, anorexia, weight loss, headache, sweats and rigors for a period of 4–8 weeks have often been attributed to a protracted 'viral illness'.

Other symptoms relate to systemic thromboembolism affecting any major vessel or immune complex deposition causing vascular injury in the skin, joints, kidney and the central nervous system (CNS).

Destruction of valve tissue can cause symptoms due to a raised pulmonary venous pressure including breathlessness, orthopnoea or nocturnal dyspnoea. Symptomatic deterioration may be particularly rapid when the aortic valve is infected.

## Physical signs (see Box 12.2)

General physical signs include asthenia, fever and anaemia.

**Box 12.1 Symptoms in Infective Endocarditis**

- Malaise
- Anorexia
- Weight loss
- Sweats
- Rigors

**Box 12.2 Signs in Infective Endocarditis**

- Fever
- Anaemia
- Clubbing (late)
- Heart murmur
- Splenomegaly
- Immune complex deposition
- Thromboembolism

**ORGANISMS CAUSING INFECTIVE ENDOCARDITIS**

| Organisms | % |
|---|---|
| Streptococcus spp. | 60 |
| Staphylococcus spp. | 20 |
| Bowel organisms (e.g. Strep. faecalis) | 15 |
| Other bacteria (inc. HACEK organisms) | 5 |
| Non-bacterial | <1 |
| Culture negative | 10 |

HACEK, Haemophilus, Actinobacillus, Cardiobacterium, Eikenella, Kingella spp.

Table 12.2 Common organisms causing infective endocarditis.

Many of the peripheral manifestations of the condition result from immune complex deposition in the skin (e.g. petechiae, subungal 'splinter' haemorrhages (Fig. 12.1), Osler's nodes, Roth spots and Janeway lesions).

Other classic features include finger clubbing (Fig. 12.2), splenic enlargement and haematuria.

Many of these clinical features may be absent, hence the late appreciation of the diagnosis in many patients. The clinical course in elderly patients may be very atypical and the patient may remain afebrile throughout the illness.

The cardiac manifestations include a tachycardia related to fever and anaemia, together with new or changing murmurs. Involvement of the mitral valve occurs in 30–45% of patients and the aortic valve in 15–25%. The characteristic signs of mitral and aortic regurgitation may not be obvious due to the rapid onset of tissue destruction. Occasionally, patients present with severe valve regurgitation with no detectable murmur. Other murmurs relate to the underlying heart lesion (e.g. PDA, VSD).

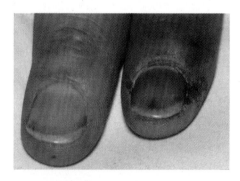

**Fig. 12.1** Splinter haemorrhages.

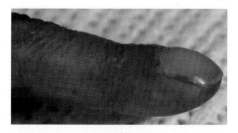

**Fig. 12.2** Finger clubbing.

In 10–15% of patients with infective endocarditis the presenting symptom is neurological and CNS complications occur in 15–30% of patients during the course of their illness. Mortality in this subgroup is double those without neurological complication. CNS complications of infective endocarditis include cerebral abscess, mycotic aneurysm, meningitis, cerebritis and subarachnoid haemorrhage.

### Investigations

A high erythrocyte sedimentation rate (ESR) (50–100 mm/1 hour) and C-reactive protein (CRP) are typical, in association with a mild leucocytosis and a normochromic normocytic anaemia. Rarely, a haemolytic anaemia or thrombocytopaenia may be seen.

Bacteraemia in infective endocarditis is continuous, therefore blood cultures timed to coincide with peaks of fever are unnecessary. Furthermore, there is no advantage in taking arterial blood, central venous blood or bone marrow for culture. Six sets of blood cultures taken over a 60 min period will suffice. Aerobic and anaerobic cultures are set up and additional cultures containing penicillinase, if penicillin has been administered within the previous 48 hours.

Close co-operation between the clinician and the hospital microbiology department is important for the optimum management of the patient with endocarditis. The microbiologist can offer advice regarding cultures, choice of antibiotic, monitoring antibiotic levels and the response of the organism *in vitro*. In a regional centre, the microbiologist will also liaise with the referring hospital and arrange for transfer of the organism if necessary.

In cases of culture positive endocarditis, the organism will be isolated from the first blood culture in 60–90% of cases within 48 hours.

Circulating immune complexes are present in 80–95% of patients and levels of haemolytic complement ($C_3$, $C_4$, $CH_{50}$) are reduced in 30% of patients.

Urine microscopy reveals microscopic haematuria (red cell casts) and proteinuria in at least 50% of patients.

Echocardiography is the mainstay of investigation, in the diagnosis of infective endocarditis, in the monitoring of treatment and in the timing of surgery. Echocardiography allows delineation of the anatomy including the presence of valvular regurgitation, chordal rupture and cusp perforation, vegetations, abscess formation, abnormal connections (shunts) and the overall haemodynamic effects on ventricular function. Transthoracic echocardiography should be supplemented by transoesophageal studies which increase both sensitivity and anatomic detail (see Chapter 3). The yield for visualization of

Table 12.3 Current recommendations for antibiotic treatment of infective endocarditis.

vegetations increases from approximately 65% to 95% using the transoesophageal approach.

## Antibiotic treatment

Antibiotic therapy should be tailored to the culprit organism (if known) (Tables 12.3 and 12.4). In general, combination intravenous antibiotics are used for a period of 4 weeks, with the monitoring of the antibiotic level against the organism *in vitro* in the laboratory. For sensitive organisms including *Streptococcus* spp., penicillin G 12–18 million U/24 hours in divided doses is combined with netilmicin 1 mg/kg every 8 hours, to maintain a trough concentration $<1 \mu g/mL$. The aminoglycoside can be discontinued after 2 weeks. Vancomycin 30 mg/kg per 24

## ANTIOBIOTICS FOR INFECTIVE ENDOCARDITIS

| Organism | Antibiotic regimen |
|---|---|
| Viridans streptococci<br>*Streptococcus oralis, mitis,*<br>*sanguis, mutans, salivarius* | **Fully sensitive to penicillin** (MIC ≤0.1 mg/L)<br>Benzylpenicillin 7.2 g daily i.v. in 6 divided doses for 2/52, **plus**<br>Netilmicin 80 mg i.v. in 2 doses (NB. monitor blood levels)<br><br>**Reduced sensitivity to penicillin** (MIC >100 mg/L)<br>Benzylpenicillin 7.2 g daily i.v. in 6 divided does for 4/52 **plus**<br>Netilmicin 80 mg i.v. in 2 doses for 4/52 (NB. monitor blood levels) |
| *Streptococcus bovis*<br>Enterococci<br>*Enterococcus faecalis,*<br>*faecium* | **As above**<br>**Netilmicin sensitive or low level resistant** (MIC <100 mg/L)<br>Ampicillin or amoxycillin 12 g daily i.v. in 6 divided doses for 4/52, **plus**<br>Netilmicin 80 mg i.v. in 2 doses for 4/52 (NB. monitor blood levels)<br><br>**Netilmicin highly resistant** (MIC ≥2000 mg/L)<br>Ampicillin or amoxycillin 12 g daily i.v. in 6 divided doses for 6/52, **plus**<br>Streptomycin (if strain is sensitive) |
| Staphylococci<br>*Staphylococcus aureus,*<br>*lagdunensis* | **Penicillin sensitive**<br>Benzylpenicillin 7.2 g daily i.v. in 6 divided doses for 4/52, **plus**<br>Netilmicin 80–120 mg i.v. in 3 doses for 1/52 (NB. monitor blood levels)<br><br>**Penicillin resistant, methicillin sensitive**<br>Flucloxacillin 12 g i.v. in 6 divided doses for 4/52, **plus**<br>Netilmicin 80–120 mg i.v. in 3 doses for 1/52 (NB. monitor blood levels)<br><br>**Penicillin and methicillin resistant**<br>Vancomycin initially 1 g i.v. over 100 min twice daily for 4/52<br>(NB. monitor blood levels to achieve a 1 h post infusion peak level of<br>30 mg/L and a trough level of 5–10 mg/L), **plus**<br>Netilmicin 80–120 mg i.v. in 3 doses for 1/52 (NB. monitor blood levels) |

MIC, minimum inhibitory concentration.

## TREATMENT IF PENICILLIN ALLERGIC

| Organism | Antibiotic regimen |
| --- | --- |
| Viridans streptococci<br>*Streptococcus oralis,*<br>*mitis, sanguis, mutans,*<br>*salivarius* | Vancomycin initially 1 g i.v. over 100 min twice daily for 4/52<br>(NB. monitor blood levels to achieve a 1 h post infusion peak level of<br>30 mg/L and a trough level of 5–10 mg/L), **or** |
| Streptococcus bovis | Teicoplanin 400 mg i.v. 12 hourly for 3 doses and then a maintenance<br>dose of 400 mg daily, **plus**<br>Netilmicin 80 mg i.v. in 2 doses for 2/52 (NB. monitor blood levels) |
| Enterococci<br>*Enterococcus faecalis,*<br>*faecium* | Vancomycin initially 1 g i.v. over 100 min twice daily for 4/52<br>(NB. monitor blood levels to achieve a 1 h post infusion peak level of<br>30 mg/L and a trough level of 5–10 mg/L), **plus**<br>Netilmicin 80 mg i.v. in 2 doses for 4/52 (NB. monitor blood levels) |
| Staphylococci<br>*Staphylococcus aureus,*<br>*lagdunensis* | Vancomycin initially 1 g i.v. over 100 min twice daily for 4/52<br>(NB. monitor blood levels to achieve a 1 h post infusion peak level of<br>30 mg/L and a trough level of 5–10 mg/L), **plus**<br>Netilmicin 80–120 mg i.v. in 3 doses for 1/52 (NB. monitor blood levels) |

Adapted from Working Party of the British Society of Antimicrobial Chemotherapy. Antibiotic treatment of streptococcal, enterococcal, and staphylococcal endocarditis. *Heart* 1998; *79*: 207–10.

**Table 12.4** Treatment regimens for adults allergic to penicillin.

hours in 2 equally divided doses is recommended for patients allergic to β-lactam antibiotics. For *Enterococci* spp., ampicillin 12 g/24 hours in divided doses is combined with netilmicin (dosing as above). *Staphylococcus* spp. should be treated with a combination of flucloxacillin 2 g every 4 hours combined with netilmicin (dosing as above). Methicillin-resistant *Staphylococci* spp. should be treated with vancomycin (dosing as above). In the presence of prosthetic material (e.g. heart valve), a combination of netilmicin, vancomycin and rifampicin 300 mg orally every 8 hours is recommended. HACEK organisms are best treated with a combination of cefotaxime 2 g i.v. once daily, together with ampicillin 12 g/24 hours in divided doses and netilmicin (dosing as above). Culture negative endocarditis should be treated with a combination of ampicillin, flucloxacillin and netilmicin (dosing as above). Antibiotic doses assume normal hepatic and renal func-

## ANTIBIOTIC PROPHYLAXIS

*Dental treatment*
Extractions, scaling or periodontal disease
(dental treatment likely to breach the gum
margin)

*Surgery or instrumentation of the upper
respiratory tract*
Bronchoscopy, laryngoscopy

*Genitourinary surgery or instrumentation*
Cystoscopy, prostatectomy

*Obstetric and gynaecological procedures*
Childbirth, Caesarean section, hysterectomy,
D & C

*Gastro-intestinal procedures*
Upper gastro-intestinal endoscopy,
colonoscopy

D & C, dilatation and curettage.

**Table 12.5** Indications for antibiotic prophylaxis.

## ANTIOBIOTIC PROPHYLAXIS AGAINST INFECTIVE ENDOCARDITIS

| Organism | Antibiotic regimen |
|---|---|
| Dental treatment | Amoxycillin 3 g single oral dose 1 h before treatment |
| Upper respiratory tract procedures | |
| Dental treatment (allergic to penicillin) | Erythromycin stearate 1.5 g orally 1–2 h before treatment, **plus** |
| Upper respiratory tract procedures (allergic to penicillin) | Erythromycin stearate 0.5 g orally 6 h later, **or** Clindamycin 600 mg single oral dose 1 h before treatment |
| Special risk patients | Amoxycillin 1 g i.m. just before induction, **plus** |
| 1 Patients with prosthetic valves who are to have a general anaesthetic | Netilmicin 120 mg i.m. just before induction, **then** |
| 2 Patients who are to have a general anaesthetic and who are allergic to penicillin or who have penicillin in the previous month | Amoxycillin 0.5 g orally 6 h later |
| 3 Patients who have had a previous attack of infective endocarditis | |
| 4 Patients undergoing genito-urinary procedures | |
| 5 Patients undergoing obstetric and gynaecological procedures | |
| 6 Patients undergoing gastro-intestinal procedures | |
| Special risk patients (as above) (allergic to penicillin) | Vancomycin 1 g by slow i.v. infusion over 1 h, **plus** Netilmicin 120 mg i.m. just before induction |

*NB. Reduce doses proportionately for children.

Table 12.6 Current recommendations for antibiotic prophylaxis against infective endocarditis*.

tion. Doses may be reduced in the elderly and according to lean body mass.

### Surgical intervention
Surgical intervention should be considered in high-risk groups of patients. High risks include:
- infection on prosthetic heart valves;
- haemodynamically significant aortic or mitral regurgitation;
- infection with *Staphylococcus* spp.;
- fungal endocarditis;
- shunts;
- abscess formation;
- atrioventricular block;
- large (>10 mm diameter) vegetations.

The timing of surgery is crucial and depends on clinical judgement, which should include the assessment of the whole patient. In general, surgical intervention should be undertaken early, before the advent of renal impairment, antibiotic resistance/toxicity and intracardiac extension of infection. Aortic regurgitation, in particular, should be treated with valve replacement prior to haemodynamic deterioration. In the setting of infective endocarditis, aortic valve replacement is associated with a perioperative mortality of 4–8%, mitral valve replacement with a mortality of 5–10%, and a reoperation rate of 5–10%. There is some evidence that valve replacement using tissue valves is superior to prosthetic valves in the setting of active infection. Patients operated on early after a cerebral complication (abscess, thromboembolic stroke, cerebritis) do particularly poorly.

## Prognosis

In the majority of patients, fever and constitutional upset resolves within 1 week of the commencement of antibiotics. Fevers persisting more than 2 weeks may indicate resistant organisms, an inappropriate antibiotic regimen, ongoing immune complex deposition or focal sepsis. Persistent fever is associated with a poor prognosis and may be an indication for surgical intervention. A fever that settles and then recurs after 2–3 weeks usually indicates a reaction to an antibiotic; the fever may be associated with a second elevation in ESR or CRP. Both the temperature and the abnormal inflammatory markers normalize promptly once the antibiotic has been discontinued.

There is little evidence that the prognosis in infective endocarditis has improved over the last 25 years, with an overall mortality of 15–30% in reported series. An adverse prognosis is associated with *Staphylococcus* spp., *Enterococcus* spp. and culture-negative endocarditis. Other significant factors include increasing age, renal impairment, involvement of the aortic valve and cerebral complications.

## Antibiotic prophylaxis

The British Society of Antimicrobial Chemotherapy has produced a set of guidelines relating to the appropriate use of antibiotic prophylaxis for patients at risk from infective endocarditis. Table 12.5 lists the indications for endocarditis prophylaxis and Table 12.6 lists the current drug regimen.

# CHAPTER 13

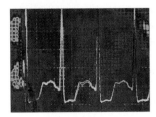

# The Pericardium

## Anatomy and function

The pericardial sac surrounds the heart in the mediastinum. It encloses:
- the aortic root;
- the main pulmonary artery;
- the origin of the pulmonary veins and the venae cavae.

These vessels' adventitia is anchored by the pericardium and its ligamentous extensions into the sternum, vertebral column and diaphragm, also anchoring the heart during changes in body position.

The pericardium also has visceral and parietal aspects. The visceral pericardium is a serous membrane, applied to the surface of the heart and composed of a single layer of mesothelial cells. It reflects on itself so lining the inner surface of the parietal pericardium, which is fibrous tissue made up of collagen and elastin fibres. A thin film of fluid is secreted into the space between the two pericardial layers, lubricating the epicardial surface of the heart, facilitating motion within the pericardial sac and reducing friction with the surrounding organs. The pericardial attachments may anchor the heart during changes in body position. Absence of pericardium (congenital or after surgical removal) does not significantly impair cardiac function.

## Acute pericarditis

### Aetiology
- Idiopathic
- Viral infection (especially Coxsackie)
- Bacterial infection (especially tuberculosis)
- Myocardial infarction
- Autoimmune disease (systemic lupus erythematosus (SLE), rheumatoid, systemic sclerosis)
- Uraemia
- Neoplasia
- Trauma.

An autoimmune process can be triggered by exposure of cardiac antigens to the immune system, as may occur after cardiac surgery (postcardiotomy syndrome) or myocardial infarction (Dressler's syndrome).

### Clinical features
*Symptoms*
1 Left precordial pain:
- persistent;
- usually positional (relieved by sitting forward and exacerbated by lying supine);
- usually sharp and radiating to neck or shoulders.

2 Dyspnoea (often the consequence of shallow breathing or may indicate the development of a pericardial effusion).

3 Systemic features of inflammation (such as fever, malaise and arthralgia).

*Physical signs*
- May be none

• Auscultation of a 'pericardial rub' (high-pitched, scratching sound) with audible components throughout the cardiac cycle, intensity varying with position, and often evanescent.

Clinical features of cardiac tamponade may appear if a pericardial effusion significantly elevates the intrapericardial pressure.

## Investigations

The electrocardiogram (ECG) may show the characteristic change of convex upward elevation of the ST-segment in all leads (Fig. 13.1). In the absence of a significant pericardial effusion the chest radiograph and echocardiogram are unhelpful. Virology or autoimmune screening may demonstrate an underlying cause. ASO titres are elevated in rheumatic fever and cold agglutinins in mycoplasma infection. Thyroid function tests should be performed to exclude hypothyroidism and an estimation made of renal function (uraemic pericarditis). If there has been recent cardiac surgery or myocardial infarction, cardiac-specific antibodies may be detected. Aspiration of pericardial fluid, when present in sufficient amount, may sometimes be undertaken in order to diagnose a bacterial or fungal aetiology.

## Management

Treatment is directed to the underlying condition and for control of symptoms. Response to non-steroidal anti-inflammatory drugs is usually dramatic. The illness usually subsides over the course of 7–14 days, although in a small minority chronic or relapsing pericarditis may follow. If pain is not rapidly controlled steroid therapy should be considered.

## Complications

Haemorrhage into the pericardial sac may occur, particularly in patients on anticoagulants.

Fig. 13.1 ECG in acute pericarditis.

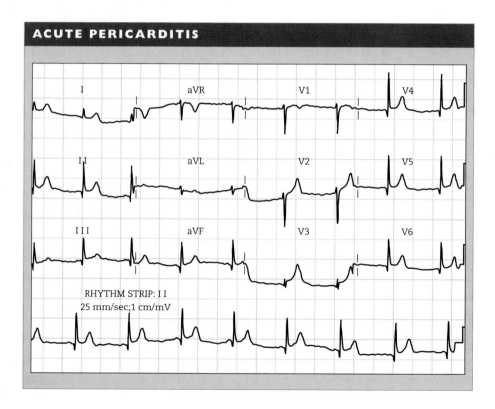

**ACUTE PERICARDITIS**

I    aVR    V1    V4

II    aVL    V2    V5

III    aVF    V3    V6

RHYTHM STRIP: II
25 mm/sec; 1 cm/mV

An acute haemorrhagic episode may progress to pericardial tamponade, constrictive pericarditis or chronic (relapsing) pericarditis. The latter may recur over months and years and may require long-term steroid or immunosuppressive therapy.

## Constrictive pericarditis

### Pathophysiology

Constrictive pericarditis usually begins with an episode of acute pericarditis. Fibrotic thickening of the pericardial sac impairs filling of the cardiac chambers during diastole. Calcification or fibrosis of the pericardium may limit diastolic filling which abruptly terminates during early diastole at the volume set by non-compliant pericardium. Impaired diastolic filling results in a reduced cardiac output together with high, usually equal, diastolic pressures in all four cardiac chambers.

### Aetiology

• Idiopathic (probably following an episode of unrecognized acute pericarditis)
• Tuberculosis (silent acute pericarditis with silent progression to constriction)
• Autoimmune causes of acute pericarditis and systemic sclerosis
• Malignant disease (malignant infiltrations or radiotherapy).

### Clinical features

1 Those of the underlying condition
2 Those related to elevation of right and left atrial filling that produce symptoms of:
• abdominal discomfort (with hepatic and gut engorgement);
• head muzziness;
• dyspnoea;
• reduced exercise tolerance.

The venous pressure may be elevated well above the jaw and, unless the patient is examined sitting up, this clinical sign may be missed. There is a rapid early phase of diastolic filling followed by its sudden cessation due to the inability of the cardiac chambers to dilate further,

producing a rapid 'x' and 'y' descent and positive Kussmaul's sign when examining the jugular venous pressure. A diastolic pericardial knock (filling sound), occurring earlier than the third heart sound (S3), may be heard.

> **Box 13.1  Clinical Findings in Constrictive Pericarditis**
>
> • Rapid 'x' and 'y' descent in venous pressure
> • Positive Kussmaul's sign
> • Pericardial knock

### Investigations

The chest radiograph may be normal but pericardial calcification or an increased heart size may be apparent. ECG changes are non-specific and include atrial fibrillation, low voltage complexes and ST/T wave abnormalities. Echocardiography may show abnormal diastolic function. Visualization of thickened pericardium is unreliable. Computerized tomographic (CT) scanning is usually the best means of imaging the pericardium but magnetic resonance imaging (MRI) is a good alternative and may better demonstrate cardiac function.

On cardiac catheterization simultaneous intracavitary pressure recordings during diastole show equilibrium of pressure in all four cardiac chambers. There is a **rapid 'x' and 'y' descent** of the right atrial waveform, and ventricular diastolic filling may show the 'square root' sign (Fig. 13.2). There may be modest elevation of pulmonary artery pressure and pulmonary venous (pulmonary capillary wedge) pressures. Infusion of intravenous saline may be necessary to demonstrate these haemodynamic features.

### Management

Most symptomatic patients become progressively more disabled without surgical resection of the parietal pericardium. This is a major and often difficult surgical procedure. The alternative of palliation with diuretic therapy is short lived.

## CONSTRICTIVE PERICARDITIS

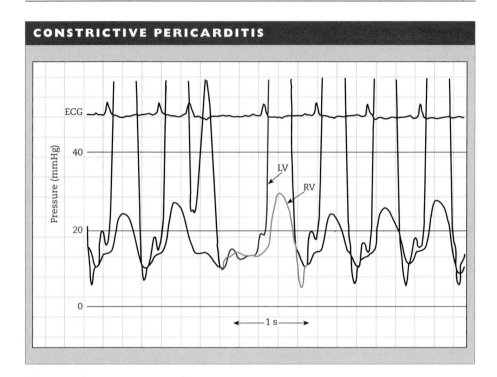

**Fig. 13.2** Square root sign in constrictive pericarditis.

### Pericardial effusion and cardiac tamponade

#### Aetiology

Pericardial effusion may develop in response to any parietal pericardial inflammation. When pericardial fluid accumulates under pressure (due to large volume or indistensible pericardium, or both), the right atrial and right ventricular diastolic pressures may be exceeded by the intrapericardial sac pressure. The transmural pressure gradient declines to zero and tamponade occurs, causing:

- a fall in diastolic filling;
- a fall in stroke volume;
- a fall in cardiac output;
- impairment of venous return.

Often a pericardial effusion is not clinically apparent but, as it enlarges, cardiac tamponade ensues. Symptoms occur if the volume of the effusion is large or if a more moderate volume accumulates sufficiently rapidly, without there being time for distension of the pericardial sac, or if the pericardium is abnormal and indistensible. The normal pericardial sac contains 15–30 mL of fluid. Up to 2 L of effusion may be present without haemodynamic features of tamponade if the effusion accumulates gradually, but as little as 250 mL of rapidly accumulated fluid may have haemodynamic consequence. After cardiac surgery there may be blood and clot in the pericardial space. The osmotic effects of clotted blood may cause rapid filling of the pericardial sac.

#### Clinical features

Moderate effusions, especially when chronic, may produce no signs but, as the volume accumulates, the patient will become breathless, have a reduced exercise tolerance and may notice venous neck engorgement. Systemic arterial pressure falls, the venous pressure is elevated, **the 'y' descent is abolished and the 'x' descent exaggerated**. The heart sounds are quiet, the respiratory rate and pulse rate are increased and pulsus paradoxus may be present.

---

### Box 13.2 Clinical Findings in Cardiac Tamponade

- No 'y' descent and exaggerated 'v' descent in venous pressure
- Quiet heart sounds
- Pulsus paradoxus

---

### Investigations

- The chest radiograph may show an increased heart size if >250 mL of pericardial fluid is present, often giving a rather globular appearance to the heart.
- The ECG may have features of pericarditis or, when the effusion is large, electrical alternans of the QRS may occur (due to beat-to-beat alteration of the right and left ventricular filling) and the voltages may be small.
- Echocardiography shows diastolic collapse of the right ventricle and right atrium early in tamponade. The absence of an effusion excludes the diagnosis but a loculated posterior pericardial effusion may be difficult to image on transthoracic echocardiography, particularly in the postoperative patient.
- Cardiac catheterization has little role, although it can quantify haemodynamic impairment. If the diagnosis of effusion is made on echocardiographic findings and clinical features

of tamponade are present then pericardiocentesis is required.

### Management

Pericardiocentesis (tapping of pericardial fluid) relieves the haemodynamic embarrassment. This is performed usually as a percutaneous technique, a needle passing into the pericardial space under fluoroscopic or ultrasound control, and the Seldinger technique, adapted for passage of a drainage catheter into the pericardial space over a guide wire using either a sub-xiphoid or transthoracic approach. Recurrent effusions, as occur with malignant tumour involvement of the pericardium, may require a window to be created between the pericardial and pleural or abdominal space, using a formal surgical approach with a mini-thoracotomy. Laceration of the pericardial sac by a balloon inflated in the pericardial space and then avulsed into the pleural space has recently become accepted as an alternative to formal surgery and is performed in the catheter laboratory under sedation. Injection of sclerosing agents into the pericardial space after drainage is of limited value in preventing reaccumulation.

### Further reading

Baue AE, ed. *Glenn's Thoracic and Cardiovascular Surgery.* Appleton and Lange, Tsamford, Connecticut, 1996.

Grossman W, Baim DS, eds. *Cardiac Catheterization, Angiography, and Intervention.* London: Lea & Febiger, 1991.

Soler-Soler J, Permanyer-Miralda G, Sagrista-Sauleda J, eds. *Pericardial Disease: New Insights and Old Dilemmas.* London: Kluwer Academic, 1990.

# CHAPTER 14

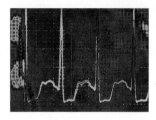

# *Cardiac Tumours*

## Myxoma

Myxomas are tumours which usually appear as pedunculated intracardiac masses, the stem often arising from the atrial septum (atrial myxomas). They are:

- the commonest form of cardiac tumour but are rarely malignant;
- found most commonly in the left atrium (approximately 90% of cases), then right atrium and then ventricles, but infrequently are present in more than one chamber;
- neoplastic in origin but the precise cell of origin remains undefined;
- histologically a mucoid stroma with stellate shaped cells and pleomorphic nuclei;
- commoner in near relatives of affected individuals.

Myxomas may directly interfere with the blood flow through the cardiac chambers and give rise to symptoms from the haemodynamic consequences (which depend on the chamber involved). When the tumour mass is in the left atrium, it may give rise to clinical signs which mimic mitral stenosis. On clinical examination, auscultatory features are:

- a 'tumour plop', analogous to the opening snap of a stenosed mitral valve (pathognomonic);
- splitting of the first heart sound (S1);
- accentuation of the pulmonary component of the second heart sound (S2);
- accompanying mitral flow murmurs (commonly a diastolic murmur but also a regurgitant systolic murmur).

Right atrial murmurs may mimic tricuspid valve stenosis while ventricular myxomas may block outflow of blood from the ventricles. Very rarely they can grow so large as to occupy an entire cardiac chamber.

The consequences of tumour embolization are generally obvious (cerebrovascular accident, occlusion of arterial flow to a limb). Noteworthy is the possibility of pulmonary hypertension, complicating obstruction of the pulmonary arterial bed. Systemic features include arthralgia, anaemia, fever, constitutional malaise and weight loss. A raised erythrocyte sedimentation rate (ESR) is common but a normal ESR does not exclude the diagnosis. Coupled with the cardiac murmurs, these clinical features may suggest a differential diagnosis of bacterial endocarditis.

Echocardiography is the investigation of choice. Myxomas are usually visible on transthoracic views but better images are obtained by transoesophageal echocardiography. Urgent surgical intervention is mandatory. Surgical excision requires removal of the tumour pedicle and a surrounding lip of tissue. It is usually curative but long-term follow up is advisable as late recurrences are possible.

## Sarcoma

These are:
- rare in the heart;
- arise most commonly in the right atrium;
- commonly present with symptoms related to obstruction to venous flow.

Definition of the tumour type depends on the primary cellular component and includes angiosarcoma, fibrosarcoma or rhabdomyosarcoma. Treatment is palliative. Surgical excision can be attempted but is usually limited by the extent of surgical damage that would be involved.

## Rhabdomyoma

These are:
- the commonest cardiac tumours of infants and children;
- derived from cardiac embryonic tissue;
- found equally frequently in both ventricles, and nearly all are multiple;
- found in both atria (about 30%);
- strongly associated with tuberous sclerosis (a familial syndrome characterized by hamartomas of various organs, epilepsy, mental deficiency and adenoma sebaceum).

Although benign, surgical management may require extensive resection.

## Metastatic disease

Metastasis of cancer tissue to the heart is a rare primary presentation of malignant disease but does occur occasionally in established neoplasms, most commonly:
- bronchial carcinoma;
- breast carcinoma;
- malignant melanoma;
- leukaemia;
- lymphoma.

Commonest cardiac consequences of metastatic disease are:
- arrhythmias (usually atrial fibrillation or heart block);
- malignant pericardial effusion (forms slowly and may reach large volumes before presentation with haemodynamic effects).

# CHAPTER 15

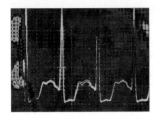

# Diseases of the Aorta

## Introduction

The aorta is the principal artery connecting the heart to the systemic vascular system. Its wall has three layers:
1 tunica intima (thin layer of endothelial cells);
2 tunica media (spirally arranged laminated elastic tissue);
3 tunica adventitia (principally collagen but also containing the adventitial vessels and lymphatics).

In the media elastic tissue predominates with little smooth muscle so that contractile force is stored in the aortic wall as systole develops which is then dissipated during diastole. In this way, the aorta plays an important role in the maintenance of diastolic circulatory force. There are specialized sensory cellular structures in the ascending aorta and the aortic arch which contribute to the regulation of systemic vascular resistance via the central vasomotor centre and the vagus nerve.

The aortic root is approximately 3 cm in diameter and gives off the coronary sinuses near the aortic valve ring. It gives rise to the ascending aorta which then becomes the aortic arch and gives off the brachiocephalic vessels (innominate, left carotid and left subclavian arteries). In the superior mediastinum it turns 180° from a cranial to caudal direction, in an anteroposterior and slightly leftwards direction. The descending thoracic aorta runs caudally in the posterior mediastinum from the aortic arch, and becomes the abdominal aorta at the diaphragm.

## Acute aortic dissection

This is a catastrophic disorder often leading to sudden death. A tear in the aortic intima allows it to be dissected or stripped of its subintimal layers, destroying the media. The process may be initiated either by spontaneous haemorrhage within a diseased area of aortic wall with subsequent intimal tearing, or the tear may be caused by shear forces from within the aortic lumen.

### Classification
The Stanford classification (Fig. 15.1) divides dissections into:
• **type A** (involves the ascending aorta);
• **type B** (ascending aorta is spared).

Prognosis and management are related to involvement of the ascending aorta in dissection and, for this reason, the authors recommend the use of this simple classification.

### Aetiology
There is weakness of the aortic media with breakdown of elastic and collagen tissues (cystic degeneration). Age-related degeneration, perhaps accelerated by hypertension, is the com-

## AORTIC DISSECTION

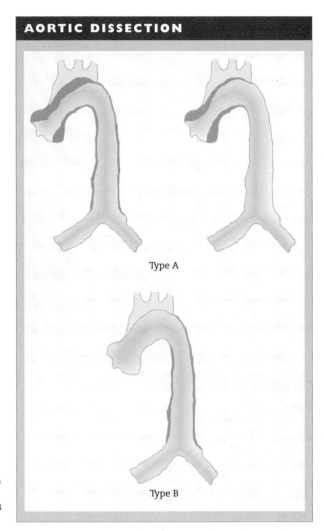

Type A

Type B

**Fig. 15.1** Stanford classification of aortic dissection. Type A involves ascending aorta, type B involves only descending aorta.

monest process but Marfan's, Ehlers–Danlos and Noonan syndromes are complicated by aortic dissection because of their involvement of connective tissue. Occasionally, dissection follows disruption of atheromatous plaque or aortic arteritis.

### Clinical features

Patients are most commonly (66%) males in the 6th and 7th decades of life. Symptoms are:
• sudden, severe pain (tearing in character, interscapular or front of the chest in location);
• nausea;
• vomiting;
• diaphoresis;
• syncope.

Dissection involving a coronary artery may cause myocardial ischaemia, and when a dissection ruptures into the pericardium acute tamponade occurs.

### Physical findings

• On examination, hypertension is a common finding in the absence of tamponade.

• Absence or diminution of pulses is common (mainly in head, neck and arm vessels). **Aortic regurgitation** is also common (indicates that a type A dissection has occurred with either dilatation of the aortic root or disruption of the aortic ring causing aortic regurgitation (AR), although type A dissection may occur without AR. If the AR is severe, left ventricular failure may be present.

• Pleural effusion may indicate rupture into a pleural space.

Occasionally, an acute aortic dissection may go unrecognized and, if the patient survives the diagnosis, may only be made some years later because of increasing AR or as an incidental observation on a chest radiograph or other investigation.

### Investigations

• Routine laboratory investigations are often unhelpful. An elevated creatinine may be due to pre-existing renal disease, often due to chronic hypertension, but also occurs acutely due to renal ischaemia as a consequence of the dissection extending to and involving the renal arteries.

• A chest radiograph will often show a widened mediastinum, although an anteroposterior portable film will tend to exaggerate its dimension.

• Contrast **aortography** was, until recently, the investigation of choice but has now been surpassed by non-invasive imaging techniques. Coronary angiography is rarely attempted when the diagnosis of aortic dissection has been made as it tends not to alter management.

• Transthoracic **echocardiography** may demonstrate an abnormal aortic root or the presence of an intimal flap. Image definition is excellent and the risk of a false-positive or false-negative diagnosis is very low and comparable to angiographic imaging. It has the advantage of being relatively non-invasive and can be undertaken in the operating theatre if surgery is felt to be needed urgently.

• In less extreme situations, magnetic resonance imaging (MRI) or computerized tomographic (CT) scanning (Fig. 15.2) are probably the investigations of choice, and can often

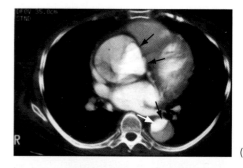

(a)

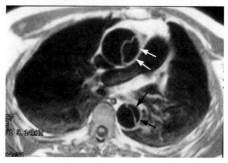

(b)

**Fig. 15.2** Type A aortic dissection: (a) CT scan; (b) MRI scan. Arrows indicate 'false' lumen in ascending and descending thoracic aorta.

demonstrate both the entry and exit points of the dissection. Their disadvantages are that they require a degree of patient co-operation to achieve good images and access to the patient is difficult at a time when haemodynamic support and resuscitation may be needed.

### Management

• The patient should be given adequate analgesia.

• Any hypertension must be strenuously controlled.

Prescribe:

• a combination of β-blockers to lower blood pressure and reduce the rate of rise of aortic blood flow velocity — dV/dT); or

• the α- and β-blocker labetalol or vasodilators such as prazosin, hydralazine and some of the calcium antagonists;

• or the centrally acting agent methyldopa.

Intravenous sodium nitroprusside is frequently used as a short-term measure. Avoid angiotensin-converting enzyme (ACE) inhibitors because of possible extension of the dissection to involve the renal arteries.

## Surgical management

Surgical management of type A dissection is associated with improved survival and should be performed as an emergency procedure as the mortality is high within the first 24 hours from diagnosis. A variety of surgical procedures may be undertaken, including aortic valve replacement, aortic root replacement with coronary reimplantation and aortic reconstruction using wrap around or replacement grafts. When thoracic aortic surgery is required, damage to the spinal cord vasculature may result in neurological damage and even paraparesis. For patients in whom medical therapy is initially chosen, surgery may be necessary if there are complications such as vital organ compromise (e.g. kidneys, intestines), haemorrhage or evidence of further dissection. Long-term antihypertensive therapy is indicated for all patients.

## Aneurysms of the aorta

A **'true' aneurysm** is a localized dilatation of the aorta where the walls of the aneurysm have all the normal layers of the aortic wall. A 'false' aneurysm is really a contained rupture, with the wall of the aneurysm being made up of adventitia and periaortic fibrous tissue. This may result from previous trauma (aortic transection) or chronic dissection. Atherosclerotic aortic degeneration is the commonest cause of thoracic aortic aneurysms. Localized aortic root dilatation is also common and although often idiopathic, as opposed to being due to a recognized syndrome such as **Marfan's**, is assumed to be due to an abnormality of medial connective tissue. Aortitis is now an uncommon cause of aneurysm formation in developed countries due to the fall in the prevalence of syphilis but may be associated with **rheumatoid disease, Reiter's syndrome** and **giant cell arteritis**.

Aortic aneurysms gradually enlarge and will eventually rupture. The larger the aneurysm, the greater the risk of rupture. The commonest locations for aneurysms are ascending aorta (45%), descending thoracic aorta (35%), arch (10%) and thoracoabdominal (10%).

## Clinical features

Patients with true aneurysms are often asymptomatic. When symptoms do occur, pain is the commonest manifestation and may be acute or chronic. Its position depends on the location of the aneurysm but is frequently precordial and may radiate to neck and jaw when the thoracic aorta is involved or between the scapulae if the aneurysm is in descending aorta. Symptoms may follow compression of adjacent structures and stretching of the recurrent laryngeal nerve in aneurysms of the arch may cause hoarseness. Frequently, there are no physical signs but coexisting hypertension is common. When the ascending aorta is involved, aortic root dilatation may result in aortic regurgitation.

## Imaging techniques

A plain chest radiograph may suggest the diagnosis but more detailed assessment of the aneurysm's location, size and the involvement of major vessel branches are all critical to the management of these conditions. Contrast aortography was the investigation of choice but this has now been superseded by MRI and CT scanning, which are also used for follow-up after surgical intervention.

## Management

Surgical techniques vary but include replacement of the aortic vessel by synthetic graft. Surgery carries a high post-operative risk of mortality or morbidity. Depending on the site of the aneurysm and the experience of the surgeon, mortality varies from 5% to around 50%, with the greatest risk being for aneurysms of the aortic arch. The commonest causes of morbidity are neurological sequelae, particularly paraplegia and paraparesis when aneurysms involve the descending thoracic aorta, cerebral damage with aneurysms of the aortic arch, and renal failure after repair of descending thoracic or thoracoabdominal aorta. Ten-year survival is around 40% and there is need for reoperation during follow-up, due to aneurysmal dilatation at the site of anastomosis between synthetic graft and native aorta. Recent advances offer the possibility of new surgical and interventional approaches using grafts which can be deployed endovascularly to stabilize the aortic wall.

Patients with asymptomatic dilatation of the aortic root >5 cm or thoracic aorta elsewhere of >6 cm, should be considered for surgery because rupture may occur.

## Marfan's syndrome

This is a genetic disorder of connective tissue which may be autosomal dominant but is not fully characterized. The nature of the connective tissue abnormality varies as does the phenotypic manifestation. The range of clinical features include:
- skeletal abnormalities;
- arachnodactyly;
- lens subluxation;
- aortic and mitral valvular disease;
- aortic disease.

Susceptibility to aneurysmal dilatation of the aorta, particularly of the aortic root, and aortic dissection are the principal features of aortic disease. Aortic root dilatation needs to be carefully monitored and aortic root replacement undertaken when dilatation progresses. Absolute aortic root dimensions may not be a particularly accurate guide to risk of aortic rupture, but wall tension is proportional to vessel diameter (Laplace's Law) and most clinicians would recommend surgery if the aortic root diameter exceeds 5 cm.

## Takayasu's aortitis

- This disease, although rare, occurs worldwide.
- It has a predominance in young Oriental females (male : female ratio is 1 : 9).

The aetiology is unknown but has been related to connective tissue disease and autoimmune disorders.

Aortic histological features are:
- pronounced intimal proliferation;
- fibrosis;
- elastic fibre degeneration in the media;
- round cell infiltration;
- thickened intima and adventitia;
- destruction of the vasa vasora.

Ultimately, the process leads to obliterative changes of the aorta and its branches with aneurysm formation, arterial stenoses and post-stenotic dilatations. The disease may be classified according to the pattern of aortic involvement. Initial presentation is often in the teenage years and, in the majority of patients, a systemic illness of malaise, fever, arthralgia, night sweats and pleuritic pain may mark its onset. The complications of the condition relate to the consequences of impaired arterial blood supply to vital organs which may be accompanied by systemic hypertension. These same features determine the morbidity and mortality of the condition. Treatments are directed towards suppression of its presumed immune aetiology with steroids or immunosuppressants, with symptomatic treatment of the arterial complications as they arise.

## Giant cell arteritis

This is an arteritis which predominantly occurs in the 6th decade onwards. Its cause is unknown but the disease mainly involves medium-sized arteries. The aorta and its main branches can be involved in a minority of cases. Characteristically, there is a granulomatous infiltration of the arterial media and often there is an accompanying inflammatory cell infiltrate of eosinophils. Weakening of the aorta can occasionally lead to aneurysm formation. Patients may have fever, malaise and headaches.

## Syphilitic aortitis

Syphilis is now a rare cause of aortitis. Spirochaetal infection of the aortic media, usually during the secondary phase of syphilitic infection, sets up a chronic inflammatory process. This results in weakening and destruction of the muscular and elastic components of the aortic wall, and aneurysmal dilatation, most commonly of the ascending aorta. Characteristically, the overlying intima becomes thickened and has a ridged appearance of 'tree bark'. The symptoms and signs are those of any aortic aneurysm. Tests for syphilitic serology should routinely be performed in patients with ascending aortic dilatation and, if positive, antibiotics (usually benzylpenicillin) is indicated. There is no evidence that this reverses or halts progression of the aortic disease. The indications for surgical intervention, either for resection of an expanding aneurysm or for aortic regurgitation, are as for the treatment of other aortic aneurysms.

## Traumatic injury of the aorta

Aortic rupture is seen with deceleration injuries, usually due to chest trauma. The diagnosis is usually suspected as a result of investigations undertaken for the patient's injuries. Mediastinal widening and distortion of the aorta may be apparent on the chest radiograph. If the diagnosis is suspected, thoracic aortography is the investigation of choice to demonstrate aortic transection. The commonest site for aortic transection is at its point of attachment to the ligamentum arteriosum, the remnant of the ductus arteriosus, and is usually just distal to the origin of the left subclavian. Immediate death is the commonest outcome of this injury, as a result of massive haemorrhage, but some survive due to containment of the rupture by the aorta's adventitia. Undiagnosed, this may lead to chronic false aneurysm formation. When diagnosed, immediate surgical repair is essential unless relatively contraindicated due to the extent of the patient's other injuries, particularly those involving the head.

## Aortic embolism

Most aortic emboli (90%) form within the left heart, precipitating conditions being recent myocardial infarction with formation of mural thrombus, severe ventricular impairment or ventricular aneurysm, atrial fibrillation with structural cardiac disease or prosthetic cardiac valves. The remaining 10% come from unknown sources, at least some of which are probably from atheromatous disease on the aortic wall. Although these emboli originating in the aorta are likely to be small, they may cause stroke, especially if the aorta has been cross-clamped during an operation.

When large emboli lodge in the aorta or its major branches, clinical features are those of sudden ischaemia affecting the tissues distal to the site of obstruction (pain, pallor, paraesthesia, pulselessness, paralysis or cerebrovascular). In as many as 25% of cases, the embolism lodges at the aortic bifurcation (saddle embolism). Embolectomy can usually be performed by using a Fogarty catheter. This is a balloon-tipped device which is introduced into the affected artery, the tip passed distal to the embolism and the balloon inflated prior to withdrawal of the catheter, so extracting the embolism by the pulling action of the balloon. Otherwise, removal under direct vision is necessary and may require extensive surgical dissection, and is associated with an operative mortality of 15–20%. Due to the risk of recurrent embolism, patients should receive long-term oral anticoagulants.

## Further reading

Baue, AE, ed. *Glenn's Thoracic and Cardiovascular Surgery,* 6th edn. Maidenhead: Appleton and Lange, 1996

Svensson LG, Crawford ES. *Cardiovascular and Vascular Diseases of the Aorta.* London: WB Saunders Co, 1996.

# CHAPTER 16

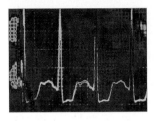

# Pulmonary Hypertension and Pulmonary Thromboembolism

## Pulmonary hypertension

### Introduction

The pulmonary circulation is a low pressure system with mean pulmonary artery pressure at rest being <20 mmHg. Pressures will be temporarily higher than this on exercise or at altitude but when consistently >20 mmHg under resting conditions pulmonary hypertension (PHT) exists. Whereas systemic arterioles respond to hypoxia by vasodilatation, pulmonary vessels vasoconstrict. When PHT occurs in the absence of any definable cause, it is termed 'primary' or idiopathic. When a cause is identified, PHT is termed 'secondary'.

### Aetiology

**Primary PHT** is a rare condition, affecting women at least twice as often as men and usually present in the 2nd or 3rd decades. Its aetiology is unknown but factors reported as potentially being implicated include:
- anorectic drugs (e.g. fenfluramine);
- cocaine;
- chemotherapeutic agents (e.g. mitomycin C, bleomycin, cyclophosphamide, carmustine);
- L-tryptophan;
- portal hypertension;
- connective tissue disorders (calcinosis, Raynaud's, oesophagus, sclerodactyly, telangiectasia (CREST) syndrome);
- HIV infection;
- toxic oil syndrome.

Extremely rarely, PHT may be due to progressive occlusion of the pulmonary venous rather than arterial vessels (**pulmonary veno-occlusive disease**), the aetiology of which is unknown.

Causes of **secondary PHT** include:
- chronic obstructive pulmonary disease (COPD);
- pulmonary fibrosis;
- ventilatory failure due to chest wall abnormalities;
- sleep apnoea;
- chronic pulmonary thromboembolic disease;
- connective tissue disease;
- living at altitude;
- left-heart disease (e.g. mitral valve, chronic left-ventricular failure);
- congenital heart disease with chronically high pulmonary blood flow (ventricular septal defect (VSD), atrial septal defect (ASD), patent ductus).

### Pathophysiology

The normal pulmonary circulation reacts to the increased blood flow associated with exercise by vasodilatation and recruitment of vessels which are not perfused at rest. This reduction in pulmonary vascular resistance (PVR) allows the normal right ventricle to accommodate large changes in venous return without increasing its pressure. A rise in PVR stimulates the development of right ventricular (RV) hypertrophy and, for some time, normal pulmonary blood flow can be maintained at the expense of PHT. The increasingly hypertrophied right ventricle demands higher myocardial blood flow which may not be met by coronary supply, resulting in myocardial ischaemia and chest pain. As the PHT worsens so the right ventricle dilates and fails to maintain normal pulmonary flow. Cardiac output falls and exercise tolerance deteriorates progressively until symptoms are present at rest. Advanced PHT, especially of the 'primary' type, may cause atrial (atrial fibrillation) and ventricular (ventricular tachycardia, ventricular fibrillation) arrhythmias, and patients are at risk of sudden death. Slow pulmonary blood flow and polycythaemia secondary to hypoxaemia increase the risk of pulmonary thrombosis *in situ*.

## Clinical features

Although the progression of primary PHT is very variable, patients usually do not become symptomatic until the condition is well advanced. Dyspnoea is common, and central angina-like chest discomfort and syncope may occur on exertion as the severity of PHT worsens. The patient may notice tissue cyanosis. Conversely, patients with secondary PHT usually present earlier with symptoms related to the underlying aetiology of their PHT (e.g. lung disease, congenital heart disease, venous thrombosis and pulmonary embolism (PE)). If PHT is advanced, then the symptoms will include those of primary PHT.

Whatever the aetiology, signs of PHT include:
- elevated jugular venous pressure (JVP);
- sinus tachycardia or AF;
- normal or low systemic blood pressure;
- poor peripheral circulation (cold extremities);
- central and/or peripheral cyanosis;
- RV third heart sound/fourth heart sound (S3/S4);
- loud pulmonary (P2) component of second heart sound (S2);
- tricuspid regurgitation;
- oedema;
- possibly hepatic enlargement and ascites.

Clubbing may be seen in certain chronic lung diseases and in cyanotic congenital heart disease, where additional signs specific to the underlying cardiac abnormality may be found. It is important to remember that in advanced PHT, due to long-standing left-to-right shunting (Eisenmenger's syndrome), cardiac murmurs may become absent because of equalization of pulmonary and systemic pressures. Hypoxaemia may be at least partially improved by inspiration of 100% oxygen ($FiO_2$), except in conditions of arteriovenous admixture (congenital cardiac shunts) where pulmonary venous blood is already maximally oxygenated. In children, this difference in response to an increase in $FiO_2$ may be used to help distinguish cardiac from pulmonary causes of hypoxaemia. Sleep apnoea, due to intermittent nasopharyngeal obstruction, occurs particularly in obese individuals, causing snoring and poor-quality sleep. Chronic nocturnal hypoxaemia results and may cause secondary PHT.

## Diagnosis

The **electrocardiogram** (Fig. 16.1) may show right axis deviation, right atrial or RV hypertrophy but will often be unremarkable. The presence of a barrel chest in chronic lung disease diminishes electrical voltages on the electrocardiogram (ECG) and may obscure evidence of hypertrophy.

The **chest radiograph** (Fig. 16.2) may show dilatation of the main pulmonary arteries in any cause of PHT, evidence of underlying lung disease or patchy pulmonary perfusion defects (chronic thromboembolic PHT).

**Pulmonary function tests** will be abnormal in patients with underlying lung disease. Carbon monoxide diffusing capacity is particularly low when PHT is present.

**Ventilation-perfusion (V/Q) lung scanning** may suggest previous pulmonary emboli (patchy perfusion).

**Computed tomography (CT) scanning**, especially the more modern spiral (helical) equipment, is increasingly being used both to image the pulmonary arteries and also to look for evidence of underlying lung parenchymal disease. Congenital cardiac abnormalities may also be demonstrable.

**Echocardiography** may show underlying cardiac disease (congenital or acquired) and the level of pulmonary artery pressure may be

## CHRONIC PHT

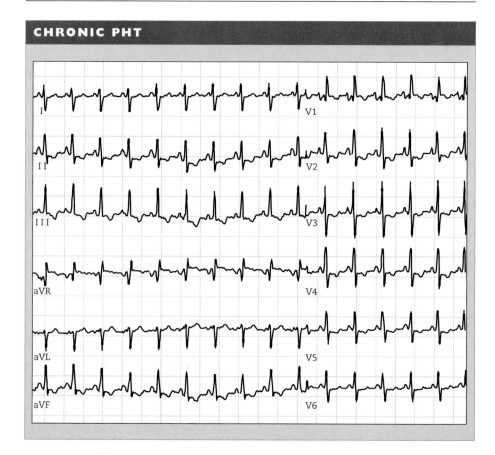

**Fig. 16.1** ECG taken from a patient with chronic PHT showing p pulmonale, RV hypertrophy with strain pattern and right-axis deviation.

estimated from a calculation of RV peak systolic pressure which can be made if tricuspid regurgitation is detectable.

**Right heart catheterization** can be undertaken to confirm a diagnosis of PHT, assess its severity and vasodilatory response to drugs or high concentration of inspired oxygen, and pulmonary arteriography may show evidence of thromboembolic disease.

### Treatment

For secondary causes of PHT, treatment should be directed towards the underlying aetiology.

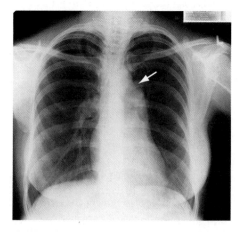

**Fig. 16.2** Chest radiograph from a patient with chronic PHT showing enlargement of the main pulmonary artery.

Lung diseases may respond to steroids, bronchodilators, domiciliary oxygen, antibiotics and congenital or acquired cardiac defects may be correctable surgically or ameliorated by a variety of pharmacological agents. PHT due to COPD may progress slowly (3 mmHg per year) but implies a poor prognosis. Sleep apnoea may respond to oxygen supplementation and continuous positive airway pressure (CPAP) via a close-fitting face mask.

Oxygen is a potent pulmonary vasodilator and, for any cause of PHT, supplementary domiciliary administration of oxygen, either using gas cylinders or an air concentrator, may improve symptoms. There is no evidence that supplementary oxygen alters prognosis.

In primary PHT, treatment is palliative because nothing has been shown convincingly to affect prognosis other than lung or heart–lung transplantation. Oral vasodilator drugs, particularly the calcium antagonist nifedipine, have been used to improve symptoms and may be required in high doses. They should be started with caution and under medical supervision because when PVR is markedly elevated the vasodilator drug may dilate the systemic but not the pulmonary vasculature, causing a marked fall in systemic blood pressure if a compensatory increase in cardiac output cannot be generated because of the fixed PVR. A beneficial symptomatic or haemodynamic response to vasodilators may indicate that the pulmonary vessels are still capable of some vasodilatation and may identify patients at an earlier stage in their disease process than those in whom the PVR is fixed.

Long-term vasodilatation with intravenous epoprostenol (prostacyclin) has been used whilst patients await transplantation. It is an expensive therapy but has been shown to help maintain patient stability. Surgical treatment for primary PHT has included a variety of procedures, such as single or double lung transplantation, with or without additional heart transplantation, and for chronic thromboembolic PHT has involved disobliteration of the proximal pulmonary arteries by thrombo-endarterectomy. The results of all these surgical procedures have been encouraging but case selection is particularly important.

There are some limited data to suggest that oral anticoagulation may improve survival in primary PHT but, because this condition is rare, the numbers of patients investigated in clinical trials of any therapy have been small and thus conclusions have had to be tentative. Nevertheless, current opinion is that patients with primary PHT should be anticoagulated with warfarin to achieve an international normalized ratio (INR) of 2.5–3.0. There is no evidence that anticoagulation benefits those with secondary PHT but this may be because it has been inadequately investigated to date.

## Pulmonary embolism

### Introduction

In the USA, there are about 600 000 symptomatic cases of PE each year, causing the death of 60 000 patients and contributing to the death of about 200 000 more. In the UK about 20 000 patients die each year in hospital as a consequence of PE and 40 000 have non-fatal episodes. Each year about 1 per 1000 of the UK population will have a PE, mainly during or soon after a period of hospitalization; the incidence rises with age. In an acute general hospital, PE may contribute to 1% of all admissions and to 15–20% of deaths.

### Aetiology

The classical clinical triad that predisposes to venous thromboembolism was described by Rudolph Virchow in 1856 as:

1 local trauma to a vessel wall;
2 hypercoagulability;
3 blood stasis.

Most patients with PE have clinical conditions associated with these predisposing factors, such as major trauma, recent surgery, obesity and immobility, smoking, increasing age, malignant disease, the oral contraceptive pill, pregnancy, hormone replacement therapy and other less common conditions (e.g. hyperviscosity syndromes, nephrotic syndrome).

Some patients with PE have an underlying primary clotting abnormality that renders them hypercoagulable, such as defective fibrinolysis, elevated levels of antiphospholipid antibodies and congenital deficiencies of antithrombin III, protein C, protein A, or plasminogen. These coagulation abnormalities are uncommon and routine screening is not cost effective, except for patients less than 50 years of age, those with a family history of thromboembolism and those with recurrent episodes of PE in the absence of an obvious cause. Resistance to activated protein C, caused by mutation of the factor V gene (Leiden mutation), has been identified. It may be present in up to 5% of the population, increases the risk of thromboses by 8–10 times in this group, and is found in 20% of those with thromboses.

## Pathophysiology

The clinical effects of PE depend on:
- the extent of pulmonary vascular obstruction;
- the release of vasoactive and broncho-constricting humoral agents from activated platelets (e.g. serotonin, thromboxane A2);
- the presence of pre-existing cardio-pulmonary disease;
- the age and general health of the patient.

RV afterload increases significantly when more than 25% of the pulmonary circulation is obstructed. This results initially in a rise in RV pressure, followed by RV dilatation and tri-cuspid regurgitation and, as the right ventricle begins to fail, a fall in RV pressure. An otherwise normal right ventricle is incapable of increasing pulmonary artery pressure much above 50–60 mmHg in response to sudden major obstruction of the pulmonary circulation, whereas in chronic thromboembolic or primary PHT RV pressure may rise gradually to suprasystemic (>100 mmHg) levels. A combination of reduced pulmonary blood flow, and displacement of the interventricular septum into the left ventricular cavity by a dilating right ventricle, both impair left ventricular filling. Thus, the dyspnoea of

patients with acute severe obstruction of the pulmonary circulation may be eased by ma-noeuvres that increase systemic venous return and left ventricular preload, such as lying flat, tilting with the head down and infusion of in-tavenous colloid. This contrasts with the dysp-noea of patients with left ventricular failure, which is eased by manoeuvres that reduce left ventricular preload, such as sitting upright and diuretic therapy.

## Clinical features

The clinical differences between the various presentations of PE are given in Table 16.1. The differential diagnosis of PE is broad and covers conditions as benign as minor anxiety states to more life-threatening diseases (Box 16.1). Many patients with PE have concomitant illnesses or are recovering from surgical procedures, which complicate the interpretation of physical findings. For instance, leg veins harvested for coronary bypass surgery result in swelling and tenderness of the operated leg, features com-patible with thrombosis, even in the absence of a deep-venous thrombosis (DVT). Cardiac surgery patients are often dyspnoeic and have chest pain post-operatively, making the diag-nosis of PE more difficult.

PE results in varying degrees of haemo-dynamic disturbance. A clinical classification has been suggested that describes the haemody-namic consequences of the embolus; however, many smaller emboli are not detected clinically.

**Acute minor PE** is a consequence of

---

### Box 16.1 Differential Diagnosis of PE

- Myocardial infarction
- Pneumonia
- Asthma
- Pneumothorax
- Acute pulmonary oedema
- Aortic dissection
- Pleurisy
- Fractured rib
- Musculoskeletal pain
- Right- or left-heart disease
- Cor pulmonale

## PE CLINICAL DIFFERENCES

|  | Acute minor PE | Acute major PE | Chronic PE |
|---|---|---|---|
| Dyspnoea | Mild | Severe | Chronic, progressive |
| Chest pain | Pleuritic | Acute, dull, central | Exertional, dull, central |
| Tachycardia | Mild | Usually marked | Variable |
| Blood pressure | Normal | Low | Normal until late |
| Cyanosis | No | Common | Common |
| Oedema | No | Not acutely | Common |
| JVP | Normal | Raised | Raised |
| Heart sounds | Normal | S3 | S3, S4, P2+ |
| Chest radiograph | Often normal | Usually abnormal | Abnormal |
| ECG | Usually normal | Usually abnormal | Abnormal |
| PA systolic BP | Normal | 30–50 mmHg | >70 mmHg |

BP, blood pressure; ECG, electrocardiogram; JVP, jugular venous pressure; P2, pulmonary second sound; PA, pulmonary artery; PE, pulmonary embolism; S3, third heart sound; S4, fourth heart sound.

Table 16.1 Clinical differences between the various presentations of PE.

obstruction of small distal pulmonary arteries, often resulting in parenchymal lung infarction. When symptoms occur, they include tachypnoea, pleuritic chest pain and haemoptysis. There is usually no haemodynamic disturbance and physical examination is often normal but may reveal a tachycardia, pleural rub and mild pyrexia.

**Acute major PE** results from significant obstruction to the proximal pulmonary arteries and usually causes severe dyspnoea, dull central chest pain, tachycardia, gallop rhythm, raised venous pressure and tachypnoea. When the degree of pulmonary arterial obstruction is sudden and severe, syncope or death may occur.

**Chronic thromboembolic** PHT is rare, occurring in approximately 0.1% of survivors of acute PE. It usually presents with a gradual onset of dyspnoea, with or without a history of previous venous thrombosis or pulmonary emboli. It is a result of chronically increasing pulmonary arterial obstruction, caused by unresolved or recurrent emboli, or thrombosis in situ. Exertional chest discomfort may occur and clinical findings are those of RV pressure overload.

## Investigations

**Electrocardiography** may show a sinus tachycardia or be normal in minor PE, but shows characteristic abnormalities in around 30% of patients with massive PE. These include the S1,Q3,T3 pattern (S wave in lead I, q wave and inverted T wave in lead III), right bundle branch block, p pulmonale and right-axis deviation. Non-specific changes, including sinus tachycardia, AF and T wave inversion in the anteroseptal leads (V1–V3), are seen in 80–90% of cases of proven PE.

**Echocardiography:** right-heart dilatation may be noted and an estimation of RV pressure may be possible if tricuspid regurgitation is detected. The presence of RV dysfunction is associated with a worse outcome. Occasionally, thrombus may be seen in the right heart. If a patent foramen ovale or ASD is seen, special consideration needs to be given to the management of possible paradoxical embolism from the venous to the systemic circulation.

**Chest radiography** changes are often non-specific. Dilatation of a major proximal pulmonary artery, and areas of pulmonary oligaemia may suggest major arterial obstruction. Wedge-shaped opacities in the peripheral lung fields due to pulmonary infarction, with or with-

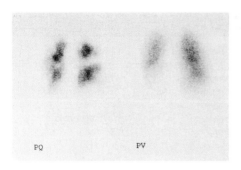

**Fig. 16.3** Radionuclide V/Q lung scan showing normal ventilation (PV) but patchy perfusion defects (PQ) due to PE.

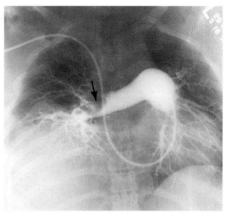

**Fig. 16.4** Pulmonary angiogram showing massive PE occupying most of the right main pulmonary artery.

out a small pleural effusion, may occur with minor PE. In chronic thromboembolic PHT, the cardiothoracic ratio may be increased and there may be features suggesting RV dilatation, patchy oligaemia and dilatation of the main pulmonary arteries. When PE is suspected, a normal chest radiograph in an acutely breathless, hypoxaemic patient increases the likelihood of PE. The chest radiograph is often more helpful when it suggests alternative diagnoses (e.g. lobar pneumonia).

**Isotope radionuclide V/Q lung scanning** (Fig. 16.3): a normal perfusion scan rules out significant PE. However, abnormal perfusion occurs in conditions other than PE, such as chronic lung disease and pneumonia and, when an assessment of ventilation is made simultaneously, evidence of V/Q mismatch greatly increases the likelihood of PE being the cause of reduced perfusion. Radionuclide scans are usually reported as representing a low, moderate or high likelihood of PE. When suggestive of PE, radionuclide scanning tends to underestimate the angiographic severity and haemodynamic disturbance of PE.

**Pulmonary angiography** (Fig. 16.4): patients with a normal isotope perfusion scan are extremely unlikely to have PE. The diagnosis of PE can be considered confirmed in patients in whom the index of clinical suspicion is high and whose isotope lung scan suggests PE is probable. These two groups of patients require angiography only exceptionally. However,

where the index of clinical suspicion is moderate or high and the isotope scan is equivocal, angiography should be considered.

**Magnetic resonance imaging (MRI)** and **CT scanning**, particularly spiral (helical) contrast enhanced CT, are increasingly used and may detect clinically unsuspected emboli. CT scanning is the investigation of choice in patients with suspected PE who also have pre-existing pulmonary disease because it allows an assessment of the co-existing lung disease, as well as helping determine whether PE is present.

**D-dimer**: in conditions where thrombus is formed, plasmin-mediated proteolysis of fibrin releases D-dimeric fragments. Increased levels of D-dimer have been found in 90% of patients with PE proved by V/Q lung scanning. However, although elevated levels are sensitive for the presence of PE, they are not specific. Levels are also elevated for up to 1 week post-operatively, in myocardial infarction, sepsis and other systemic illnesses. Used in conjunction with the clinical assessment, a normal D-dimer may have a negative predictive accuracy of 97% and may therefore be useful in excluding the presence of venous thrombosis

*Management* (Fig. 16.5)
A clear history of the patient's symptoms and

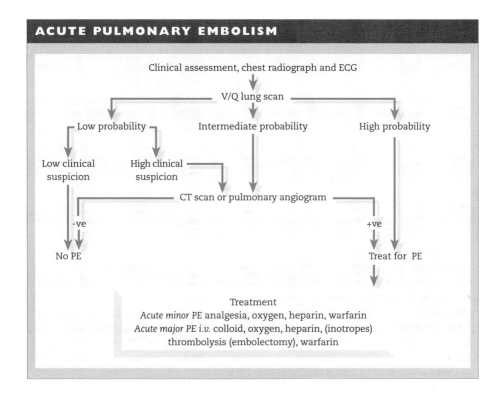

**Fig. 16.5** Management algorithm for suspected acute PE.

risk factors should be obtained. With few exceptions, patients suspected of having PE should have a chest radiograph and ECG, and be referred for V/Q lung scanning. Where the index of clinical suspicion is high, anticoagulation should be started, pending the results of investigations. Apart from supportive therapy (e.g. analgesia and oxygen), the three immediate treatment options for PE are anticoagulation with heparin, thrombolytic therapy and pulmonary embolectomy.

**Anticoagulation:** heparin accelerates the action of antithrombin III and prevents further fibrin deposition, allowing the body's fibrinolytic system to lyse an existing clot. There is a tendency to under-anticoagulate patients. Those with DVT and PE may require more unfractionated heparin to achieve adequate anticoagulation than those without active thrombosis, owing to the presence of high plasma concentrations of factor VII and heparin-binding proteins. Where high doses are required, monitoring of the plasma heparin level rather than the activated partial thromboplastin time (aPTT) is advisable. Low molecular weight (LMW) heparins are at least as effective as unfractionated heparin in the management of haemodynamically stable patients with PE and are less prone to binding than unfractionated heparin, so resistance is unlikely. Their half-lives are also longer, the dose response is more predictable and they may cause fewer bleeding side-effects. One randomized trial compared heparin with placebo in the management of PE; it concluded that heparin did not reduce the immediate mortality of PE but probably reduced deaths caused by further emboli. For those with significant haemodynamic disturbance caused by PE, heparin should be regarded as adjunctive rather than sole therapy.

**Thrombolysis:** controlled trials comparing thrombolytic agents with heparin have concluded that pulmonary emboli clear more rapidly with thrombolytic therapy. They also showed that mortality tended to be lower in those treated with thrombolysis rather than heparin. However, the sample populations were small and the results were not statistically significant. Achieving more rapid resolution of PE seems desirable because prolonged haemodynamic disturbance harms the patient and, if further emboli occur, they will have a smaller haemodynamic effect if previous ones have been partially lysed. Thrombolysis should be considered in patients with major PE who have had syncope, hypotension or severe hypoxaemia. A second advantage of thrombolysis is that potentially dangerous iliofemoral venous thrombi may be lysed, though this may result in detachment of thrombus from the vessel wall, resulting in further PE. There is no evidence that thrombolytic therapy results in better long-term restoration of pulmonary blood flow than does heparin treatment.

**Pulmonary embolectomy:** some patients are so severely compromised haemodynamically that they may not survive the 1 or 2 hours required to derive benefit from thrombolysis. Also, thrombolysis is contraindicated in some patients, and others deteriorate despite its administration. For the minority of patients with massive PE who fall into these groups, pulmonary embolectomy may be life saving. If embolectomy is considered, pulmonary angiography should be undertaken, to demonstrate the site and extent of pulmonary arterial obstruction and, most importantly, to ensure that the diagnosis is correct. Patients mistakenly undergoing surgical embolectomy for alternative diagnoses, such as myocardial infarction, have a high mortality.

Acute massive pulmonary emboli can sometimes be successfully disrupted using a catheter inserted into the pulmonary artery. The clot may be partially fragmented and improve pulmonary blood flow, and the smaller fragments may then respond more rapidly to thrombolysis.

**Procedures on the inferior vena cava (IVC):** once a PE has occurred, residual thrombus is almost always present in the deep veins, as has been demonstrated at autopsy in over 90% of cases. Attempts to prevent further emboli have been made by surgical interruption or plication of the IVC; however, percutaneous insertion of devices such as filters and umbrellas is more common. These techniques have been less widely used in the UK than in other European countries or the USA. The rate of recurrence of PE using treatment regimens not involving these devices is remarkably low (about 5%), and it is uncommon for treated patients to die from further embolism after hospital discharge or for them to progress to chronic thromboembolic PHT. For patients at high risk of further emboli, in whom anticoagulation is contraindicated, or in those who have recurrent emboli despite adequate anticoagulation, an IVC filter may be beneficial. In the acute phase of massive PE, any procedure on the IVC that reduces venous return is potentially detrimental.

## Acute minor PE

Patients with haemodynamic disturbance should be given analgesia, oxygen and heparin; this is superior to oral anticoagulation alone. The degree of anticoagulation required should be sufficient to keep the aPTT in the range 2.5–3.0 times control values. Loading with an oral anticoagulant is usually undertaken simultaneously. A reasonable strategy is to give 100 IU/kg of heparin as a loading dose, followed by an infusion of 1000–2000 IU/h. The risk of bleeding may be lower with a continuous intravenous infusion of heparin rather than intermittent intravenous bolus doses. LMW heparin may be used in haemodynamically stable patients (150–200 mg/kg body weight, once daily). When warfarin is started during active thrombosis, the levels of protein C and protein S fall, creating a thrombogenic potential. Oral loading with warfarin should therefore be covered by simultaneous heparin i.v. for 4–5 days. Oral anticoagulation is given to achieve an INR of 2.5–3.0 and is usually continued for 3–6 months, although the ideal duration of therapy is unknown. If a primary coagulopathy is identified, long-term treatment with warfarin should continue.

## Acute major PE

Where necessary, resuscitation should be undertaken before investigation. Patients should be tilted in the head-down position, given oxygen and moved to an intensive care unit (ICU) or high dependency unit (HDU) where haemodynamic and respiratory monitoring can be performed. A central venous line should be inserted to measure venous pressure and allow the judicious administration of intravenous colloid and inotropes and thrombolytic agents. If thrombolytic therapy is planned, a jugular rather than infraclavicular approach should be used. When central venous access is achieved, a thermodilution pulmonary artery catheter should be considered because this allows serial measurements of cardiac output and the monitoring of pulmonary artery pressure and mixed venous oxygen saturation, which help to assess the rate of resolution of the pulmonary arterial obstruction in response to treatment. If central venous monitoring is not available, transcutaneous arterial oximetry may provide an assessment of resolution. If possible, the insertion of arterial lines should be avoided when thrombolysis has been given.

Massive PE carries a high early mortality and vigorous therapy should be pursued. Unless contraindicated, give 1.5 million U of streptokinase over 2 hours, with or without hydrocortisone (100 mg), followed by streptokinase, 100 000 IU/h i.v. for 24–72 hours and then warfarin and heparin, until adequate oral anticoagulation is achieved. Urokinase has been used in the USA in preference to streptokinase and has been compared with tissue plasminogen activator (tPA). Trials suggest more rapid resolution of pulmonary thrombus with tPA i.v. 100 mg over 2 hours than with urokinase, but their effects are similar after 12–24 hours. Pulmonary arterial infusion of tPA has been shown to be no better than intravenous administration.

## Chronic thromboembolic PHT

Owing to its insidious nature, chronic thromboembolic PHT commonly presents late, at a stage when there is little alternative to pulmonary thromboendarterectomy or lung or heart–lung transplantation. Although vasodilators have been used to treat chronic PHT, they are ineffective if the primary abnormality is pulmonary arterial occlusion by fixed organized thrombus, although they may help recruit remaining pulmonary vessels. Domiciliary oxygen may help symptomatically.

## Deep-venous thrombosis

If a diagnosis of PE has been established, there is little to be gained by investigating the deep veins, because almost all these patients have DVT, although many are asymptomatic. In an autopsy study of patients who died of PE, 83% had a leg DVT but only 19% had shown symptoms. Similarly, PE may be asymptomatic in patients with DVT. In a treatment trial of proximal leg DVT, 40% of patients had asymptomatic PE, the diagnosis of PE being based on abnormal V/Q scans.

### Investigations

If the diagnosis of PE is less clear, or radionuclide lung scanning or pulmonary angiography are not available, investigations of the deep veins may be helpful. If the clinical suspicion of PE and radionuclide lung scanning are equivocal, investigations suggesting the presence of DVT, especially proximal to the calf, indicate the need for anticoagulation. About 75% of patients who present with clinically suspected DVT do not have the condition. Only 50% of patients with DVT show the classical symptoms of a tender, swollen calf with positive Homans' sign and these symptoms may be present in those without DVT. Thus, if DVT is suspected, further investigations are needed.

**Contrast venography** has been the gold standard investigation against which the newer techniques of impedance plethysmography, radiofibrinogen leg scanning and Duplex (Doppler flow assessment combined with ultrasound scanning) have been assessed. Their accuracy in detecting DVT depends on operator experience.

**Ultrasonography** is less invasive than venography and more accurate than impedance plethysmography. In experienced hands, and with the use of colour duplex Doppler, ultrasonography of the femoral, popliteal and calf trifurcation veins are highly sensitive (>90%) for detecting proximal vein thrombosis but are less sensitive (80% in symptomatic and 40–50% in asymptomatic patients) in detecting calf vein thrombosis. If the findings are normal but the clinical suspicion of venous thrombosis is high, the test should be repeated after 3–5 days. A normal investigation and normal plasma D-dimer value almost excludes thrombosis. Diagnosing recurrent venous thrombosis is often difficult because investigations may be abnormal as a result of previous episodes. In the absence of an obvious cause of DVT, occult malignancy should be sought, especially if the DVT is recurrent. Surgical procedures carrying the greatest risk of DVT include pelvic, hip and knee operations; without prophylaxis, 60–80% of these patients develop DVT. Patients suffering major trauma, myocardial infarction, stroke and thrombophilic disorders are also at risk. In these patients, low-dose subcutaneous heparin (5000 IU twice or three times a day), anti-embolism stockings and intermittent pneumatic leg compression are beneficial. The perioperative use of subcutaneous heparin can prevent about 66% of DVT, with significant reduction in fatal PE. LMW heparin is of particular benefit as prophylaxis in orthopaedic patients.

## Treatment

**Anticoagulation**: treatment for an established proximal DVT is intravenous heparin, given initially as a bolus of 5000 IU and followed by a continuous infusion of at least 30 000 IU/day for 4–7 days. The dose should be adjusted on the basis of laboratory tests. Patients receiving heparin who have subtherapeutic anticoagulation in the first 24 hours may have 15 times the rate of thrombotic recurrence of those who are adequately anticoagulated. Intermittent subcutaneous administration of heparin, 17 500 IU twice a day, especially with the LMW varieties, is also effective and may allow patients to be discharged earlier. Three meta-analyses of data from trials comparing LMW to unfractionated conventional heparin suggested that LMW heparins are more effective at preventing recurrence and cause fewer bleeding side-effects. Small falls in platelet levels are common in the early stages of unfractionated heparin treatment but only 3% of patients have an immune, immunoglobulin G- (IgG)-mediated, thrombocytopenia which can be profound and should be suspected when the platelet count falls below $100\,000/mm^3$ or less than 50% of baseline levels. The use of LMW heparin considerably reduces the occurrence of this complication.

Oral anticoagulation with warfarin should be started immediately, aiming for an INR of 2.5–3.0. The optimal duration of oral anticoagulant therapy is uncertain. The results of three randomized trials suggest that treatment should be for at least 3 months and possibly 6 months. Those with recurrent episodes should take warfarin in the long-term. Pregnant women requiring anticoagulation should be treated with unfractionated or LMW heparins, which do not cross the placenta and are safe for the fetus; warfarin can cause fetal bleeding and is potentially teratogenic. Heparin taken for more than 4 weeks may cause osteoporosis.

**Thrombolytic agents** can achieve more rapid resolution of DVT than heparin but have not been shown to lower recurrence or reduce post-thrombotic symptoms compared with standard anticoagulants. The post-thrombotic syndrome, caused by venous hypertension due to venous valvular incompetence and residual venous obstruction, is a chronic complication of DVT consisting of pain, swelling and occasionally ulceration of the lower legs. It occurs in over 50% of patients with proximal DVT and in about 33% of those with calf vein thrombosis.

**Treatment of calf DVT** is controversial.

Diagnostic studies suggest that only 20% of calf vein thrombi extend into proximal veins within 2 weeks of presentation. The remainder are probably small and resolve without consequence. One trial suggested the morbidity rate is lower in those who are anticoagulated for a calf DVT compared with those who are not but the number of patients studied was small. If anticoagulants are not given, the extension of the thrombus proximal to the calf can be assessed by ultrasonography.

## Further reading

American Thoracic Society. The diagnostic approach to acute venous thromboembolism. *Am J Respir Crit Care Med* 1999; **160**: 1043–66.

Arcosaoy S. Thrombolytic therapy for pulmonary embolism. A comprehensive review of current evidence. *Chest* 1999; **115**: 1695–707.

British Thoracic Society. Suspected pulmonary embolism: a practical approach. *Thorax* 1997; **52** (suppl 4): S1–S52.

Guidelines on diagnosis and management of acute pulmonary embolism. Task Force on Pulmonary Embolism, European Society of Cardiology. *Eur Heart J* 2000; **21**: 1301–1336.

Hirsh J, Hoak J. Management of deep vein thrombosis and pulmonary embolism. *Circulation* 1996; **93**: 1212–45.

Peacock AJ. *Pulmonary Circulation: a Handbook for Clinicians.* London: Chapman and Hall, 1996.

Rubin LJ. Primary pulmonary hypertension. *Chest* 1993; **104**: 236–50

# Pregnancy and the Heart

## Normal pregnancy

Pregnancy and the peripartum period are associated with many cardiovascular changes. Blood volume increases by an average of 50% and is greater than the increase in red-cell mass, leading to some dilution of haemoglobin. Haematocrit may fall by up to 35% and haemoglobin levels to around 110–120 g/L. Stroke volume and cardiac output increase by 30–50% but are usually lowest in the supine position due to caval compression by the gravid uterus causing reduced venous return. Systemic blood pressure falls to a nadir in the middle trimester due to vasodilatation but later increases towards term and especially with the pain and anxiety of labour. Diastolic pressure falls more than systolic causing an increase in pulse pressure. The heart rate normally increases by 10–20 b.p.m. in the last trimester. Vaginal delivery causes as much haemodynamic stress as a Caesarean section and should not be regarded necessarily as a safer option for the pregnant woman with pre-existing heart disease.

During normal pregnancy, **symptoms** include:
- tiredness;
- reduced exercise tolerance;
- dyspnoea;
- orthopnoea;
- lightheadedness;
- syncope occasionally.

On examination, **signs** include:
- tachycardia;
- wide pulse pressure;
- peripheral oedema;
- an elevated jugular venous pressure (JVP);
- palpable right ventricular impulse;
- loud first heart sound (S1);
- increased splitting of the second heart sound (S2);
- mid-systolic flow murmurs.

The **electrocardiogram** (ECG) may show QRS axis deviation and T-wave changes, and **echocardiography** reveals increased left- and right-ventricular dimensions, mild increases in atrial size, mild functional mitral and tricuspid regurgitation, and small pericardial effusion.

## Congenital heart disease

Most patients with non-cyanotic heart disease can be managed through a successful pregnancy although the associated haemodynamic changes usually result in worsening of symptoms. An unfavourable outcome can be anticipated in cyanotic heart disease, those with severe pulmonary hypertension and in patients with severe symptoms before pregnancy. Elective induction once the fetus is mature, with haemodynamic monitoring and specialized medical care can improve outcome. Caesarian section is considered in most women with anything other than simple congenital heart disease (e.g. atrial septal defect (ASD)). The need for antibiotic prophylaxis is disputed, but many feel that the risk of giving antibiotics is so small and the potential consequences of endocarditis so potentially catastrophic that, with the exception of a secundum ASD, all patients with congenital heart disease should be given prophylaxis.

## Primary pulmonary hypertension

This carries a high maternal mortality during pregnancy (40%), which should ideally be avoided or termination considered. Because oral contraceptives have been suggested as possible aetiological factors in this condition, sterilization by tubal ligation is the preferred form of birth control. If a pregnancy is continued for any reason, treatment is the same as for the underlying condition with spontaneous vaginal delivery being preferable to induction. If Caesarian section is considered, great care is required with anaesthetic agents which may cause profound hypotension (negative inotropism, systemic vasodilatation).

## Rheumatic heart disease

Progress through pregnancy depends on the nature and severity of the valvular disease. The most common lesion is mitral stenosis (MS), the haemodynamic effects of which can be expected to be much worse with the associated increase in blood volume. Unless the MS is severe (valve area $<1$ cm$^2$), patients can normally be managed through a vaginal delivery. Epidural anaesthesia is the preferred route, because this induces vasodilatation and a consequent beneficial fall in left atrial and pulmonary artery pressures. In severe MS with deteriorating haemodynamics, successful closed surgical mitral valvotomy or percutaneous balloon mitral valvuloplasty have been reported. Care must be taken to minimize any radiation exposure to the pregnant mother and, if procedures involving radiation are necessary, these should be delayed until as late in pregnancy as possible. Open mitral valve operations (valvotomy or replacement) carry a higher risk to mother and fetus. Patients with mitral or aortic regurgitation and those with anything other than severe aortic stenosis tolerate pregnancy fairly well. Most would recommend prophylactic antibiotics for vaginal or Caesarian delivery for all patients with valvular disease. Oral anticoagulants are potentially teratogenic and management in pregnant patients requiring anticoagulation for native or prosthetic valve reasons requires specialist cardiological and haematological involvement.

## Cardiomyopathies

The majority of patients with **hypertrophic cardiomyopathy** (HCM) can be managed successfully through pregnancy, although worsening of symptoms is common and the risk of ventricular arrhythmias increases. Treatment is similar to that of the non-pregnant female with the condition, taking care to avoid drugs that may be teratogenic or worsen fetal haemodynamics. The risk of endocarditis is increased in HCM, especially of the obstructive type, and most would recommend antibiotic prophylaxis for delivery. **Peripartum cardiomyopathy** is a rare but well-recognized occurrence of unknown aetiology, which occurs in approximately 1 : 10 000 pregnancies but with higher occurrence in Africa (up to 1%). The incidence is greater in women with twins, those over 30 years of age and in multiparas. It results in a dilated cardiomyopathy which can be severe and life threatening, with symptoms starting often in the last trimester but sometimes dismissed as being due to the later stages of normal pregnancy. Hence, the diagnosis may only be revealed after delivery. Treatment is similar to that of any patient with heart failure, hydralazine being a useful vasodilator which is safe in pregnancy. Some patients will be so severely affected that cardiac transplantation is occasionally indicated, although most will improve to a varying and unpredictable degree on delivery of the fetus. Further pregnancies should be discouraged because the condition can recur.

## Hypertension

See Chapter 4.

## Arrhythmias (see also Chapter 9)

Pregnancy is associated with an increased incidence of arrhythmias both in those with and those without known pre-existing cardiac disease. In healthy women, frequent atrial and ventricular ectopics may occur. Palpitations, dizziness and even syncope can occur in normal pregnancy and they are only uncommonly associated with a documented arrhythmia. Atrial flutter and fibrillation is rare, but re-entry tachycardias are commonly exacerbated in pregnancy. Anti-arrhythmic drugs should be avoided if at all possible, although digoxin, quinidine, lidocaine (lignocaine) and adenosine are thought to be safe. Direct current (DC) cardioversion can be performed if an arrhythmia is prolonged or haemodynamically compromising.

## Antibiotic prophylaxis in pregnancy

• Ampicillin i.v. or i.m. 2.0 g with gentamicin 1.5 mg/kg (not >80 mg) 30 min before procedure/delivery, with amoxycillin 1.5 g orally 6 hours later or i.v. 8 hours later.
• In those allergic to penicillin use vancomycin i.v. 1.0 g over 1 hour with gentamicin i.m. 1.5 mg/kg (not >80 mg) 1 hour before the procedure and again 8 hours after.
• For the low-risk patients 3.0 g of amoxycillin orally 1 hour before the procedure and 1.5 g 6 hours after, is sufficient.

# CHAPTER 18

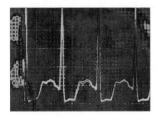

# Adult Congenital
# Heart Disease

## Introduction

Congenital heart disease is rare in adult practice but its frequency is changing due to improved survival following surgery and the greater tendency towards corrective rather than palliative surgery in early life. Long-term results of morbidity and mortality do not yet exist for many of the newer surgical procedures and the subsequent development of additional acquired cardiovascular diseases, such as systemic hypertension, coronary artery disease and degenerative valve disease, may further increase clinical complexity.

The incidence of congenital heart lesions is around 0.8% of live births. Not all patients will reach adult life. Further, many simple lesions are corrected by the time a patient reaches adulthood. For example, ventricular septal defects (VSDs) may close spontaneously and lesions such as atrial septal defects (ASDs) or patent ductus arteriosus (PDA) may be closed surgically or with percutaneously inserted devices in childhood, without the need for long-term follow up.

Traditionally, congenital heart lesions have been classified according to the presence or absence of cyanosis but this is no longer particularly helpful in the adult patient. It is more appropriate to separate common and uncommon lesions, and whether the patient has had previous surgery or not. Within this categorization, lesions may involve either shunts or obstruction to blood flow, or a combination of the two.

See Box 18.1 for a summary of common lesions and Box 18.2 for uncommon and complex lesions.

## Common lesions

### Shunt lesions

A shunt implies that there is direct communication between the left heart, or systemic arterial circuit (oxygenated blood), and the right heart, or pulmonary arterial circuit (deoxygenated blood). These communications most commonly occur between left- and right-sided structures at the same level within the circulation, such as between the atria (ASDs), ventricles (VSDs) or great vessels (aorto–pulmonary connections). Occasionally, shunting occurs between different levels, such as from aorta to right atrium or ventricle (sinus of Valsalva rupture) or between the left ventricle and right atrium (Gerbode defect of the membranous ventricular septum). Similarly, a coronary artery fistula to the right atrium or pulmonary artery can also cause a communication between the systemic and pulmonary circuits.

Initially, blood tends to flow predominantly from the left heart to the right heart because of their difference in pressures, although there may be a small amount of bidirectional flow in many cases. This 'left-to-right' shunting increases pulmonary blood flow so that more

## Box 18.1 Common Lesions

### Shunts

- Patent foramen ovale (PFO)
- ASD and aneurysms
- Anomalous pulmonary venous drainage
- VSD
- Patent (persistent) ductus arteriosus

### Obstructive lesions

- Pulmonary stenosis (PS)
- Aortic stenosis
- Coarctation of the aorta

### Others

- Marfan's syndrome

## Box 18.2 Uncommon and Complex Lesions

- Transposition of the great arteries (TGA)
- Corrected transposition
- Tricuspid atresia/absent right ventricle
- Sinus of Valsalva aneurysm
- Coronary artery fistula
- Tetralogy of Fallot
- Ebstein's anomaly
- Eisenmenger's and complications of cyanosis
- Right ventricular dysplasia

blood flows around the pulmonary compared to the systemic circuit. The ratio of blood flow between the two circuits (normally 1:1) can be measured at cardiac catheterization (see Chapter 3) with a pulmonary to systemic ratio (Qp:Qs) of 2:1 generally being regarded as being of haemodynamic significance. Uncorrected, a shunt of this magnitude will cause significant changes to the right heart, chronically increased pulmonary blood flow will cause increasing pulmonary hypertension, and, ultimately, the shunt will reverse and become predominantly 'right-to-left'. This causes cyanosis due to significant amounts of desaturated blood bypassing the lungs and entering the systemic circulation. As this point, the pulmonary hypertension is irreversible and an Eisenmenger's syndrome has developed. The term Eisenmenger's complex is generally re-

served for reversal of the shunt as a result of a large VSD as this was the original condition described. Once an Eisenmenger's syndrome has developed, surgical intervention to close the defect is inappropriate and would lead to worsening of the pulmonary hypertension, right heart failure and death.

The main complications of congenital cardiac defects are:

- pulmonary hypertension;
- infective endocarditis;
- cardiac failure;
- central cyanosis;
- atrial and ventricular arrhythmias;
- right ventricular failure;
- valve regurgitation.

### Patent foramen ovale

A patent forament ovale (PFO) is not really a congenital abnormality but a normal variation present in up to 25% of the adult population. It may be suspected in young patients with embolic stroke because paradoxical embolization of thrombus from the pelvic or leg veins can occur across the interatrial communication, into the left heart and thereafter to the brain. There are no clinical signs and electrocardiogram (ECG), chest radiograph and transthoracic echocardiography (TTE) are normal. The diagnosis is usually made by transoesophageal echocardiography (TOE) where flow can be seen between the layers of the atrial septum (Fig. 18.1) or contrast is seen to pass right-to-left through an otherwise intact atrial septum during a Valsalva manoeuvre which increases right atrial pressure. A PFO is also important in deep-sea divers because rapid decompression, as a result of surfacing too quickly, results in the formation of nitrogen bubbles in venous blood, which may then pass into the systemic circulation and cause neurological sequelae. In some cases, this may necessitate closure of the defect by a percutaneous device or surgery (see below).

### Atrial septal defect

There are three basic types of ASDs, classified according to their position:

1 secundum defects;

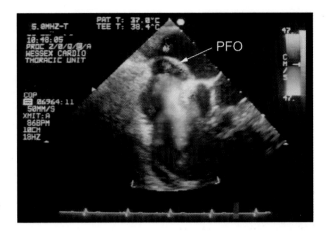

**Fig. 18.1** Transoesophageal echo of a patient with a PFO. Note the red colour between the layers of the atrial septum.

**2** sinus venosus defects; and

**3** ostium primum defects.

Secundum defects are the most common and most readily identified by echocardiography and are clearly visualized using TOE (Fig. 18.2). Sinus venosus defects can be difficult to image with conventional TTE and may only be seen using transoesophageal imaging (Fig. 18.3). The ostium primum defect is very rare in adults and, although it can occur in isolation, it is more often seen as the atrial component in a spectrum of atrioventricular septal defects (AV canal defect).

*Clinical features*

An ASD can present at almost any age. Symptoms are often minimal, being either mild exertional dyspnoea or palpitation due to atrial arrhythmias. Children often report that they are less able to play sports or keep up with their peers at school.

Clinical signs are also subtle and careful examination is required. The second heart sound (S2) is widely split and the separation of the two components (aortic second sound (A2)–pulmonic second sound (P2)) does not vary with respiration. The right ventricle may be palpable and there is usually a systolic flow murmur due to increased flow across the pulmonary valve. An ASD may be associated with mitral valve prolapse and some mitral regurgitation.

The **ECG** may show partial or complete right bundle branch block (RBBB), and the **chest radiograph** shows prominent pulmonary arteries and pulmonary plethora due to increased pulmonary blood flow. **Echocardiography**, especially transoesophageal, demonstrates the position of the defect and any dilatation of the right heart. Cardiac catheterization is now rarely performed for simple ASDs.

*Management*

Small defects which are not sufficient to cause significant dilatation of the right heart may not require any intervention. It is usually recommended that larger defects are closed unless the patient is elderly. Surgery carries a low morbidity and mortality but closure by percutaneously inserted devices is now an alternative in suitable patients, usually those with moderate-sized secundum defect.

Following successful surgical or device closure, long-term complications are rare and largely determined by the size of the left-to-right shunt before surgery and the age of intervention. The larger the shunt and the longer the defect exists prior to closure, then the greater chance of significant right-heart dilatation and the presence of pulmonary hypertension. The most common long-term problem is the development of atrial arrhythmias, particularly atrial fibrillation, which may require anti-arrhythmic medication and/or long-term anticoagulation. The risk of infective endocarditis in uncor-

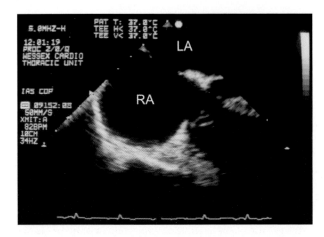

**Fig. 18.2** Transoesophageal echocardiograms from a patient with a typical secundum ASD, demonstrating a large hole between the left atrium (LA) and right atrium (RA) in the middle portion of the atrial septum.

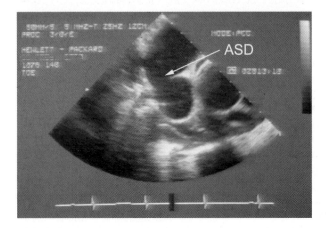

**Fig. 18.3** Transoesophageal echocardiography of a sinus venosus ASD.

rected ASD is so low that antibiotic prophylaxis is unnecessary unless there are other associated defects.

### Anomalous pulmonary venous drainage

Drainage of one or more pulmonary veins directly into the right atrium can occur as an isolated abnormality or in association with an ASD. As the haemodynamic effects are identical to those of an ASD, their presentation and clinical features are indistinguishable. TOE is the investigation of choice. When sufficient to cause right-heart dilatation, or where associated with a significant ASD, the abnormal vein or veins can be redirected into the left atrium at the time of surgery.

### Atrial septal aneurysm

This is due to the presence of excessive atrial septal tissue and is identified as a mobile, aneurysmal appearance to the septum on echocardiography. There is no shunt and treatment is not required. However, it has been identified as a possible cardiac source of embolism and in patients who present with a transient ischaemic attack or embolic stroke, the presence an atrial septal aneurysm may indicate the need for anticoagulation.

### Ventricular septal defect

VSDs can occur as isolated abnormalities or as part of more complex congenital heart disease. They can be single or multiple, affect the inlet, outlet or muscular portions of the ventricular septum and range in size from tiny to large, haemodynamically significant defects. VSDs are usually recognized in childhood. Initially the shunt is predominantly from left-to-right and the size of the shunt is dependent on the size of the defect and pulmonary vascular resistance. Large defects cause dyspnoea and failure to thrive and merit early surgical intervention. Left untreated, a large defect will cause severe pulmonary hypertension with a gradually reducing shunt volume, and eventually reversal of the shunt from right-to-left with the development of cyanosis. Small defects paradoxically cause loud pansystolic murmurs and small left-to-right shunts. Pulmonary hypertension does not develop and many small defects close spontaneously during childhood.

*Clinical features*

The diagnosis may have been made in childhood but some adults will present with dyspnoea or be diagnosed incidentally following a chest radiograph or routine medical examination. Occasionally, the first presentation is with infective endocarditis. On examination, there may be a loud pansystolic murmur at the lower left sternal edge, often associated with a palpable thrill. The heart sounds are normal unless there is developing pulmonary hypertension when P2 is loud. The right ventricle may be palpable, suggesting the VSD is haemodynamically significant.

The **ECG** and **chest radiograph** are normal in small defects but when abnormal in larger shunts they reflect the development of right ventricular dilatation and pulmonary hypertension. **Echocardiography** localizes the defect(s) and helps assess the size. Doppler velocity measurement can help predict the pulmonary artery pressure. It is now less common for cardiac catheterization to be required unless doubt exists over the severity of any pulmonary hypertension or the presence of associated congenital defects.

*Management*

Unlike ASDs, percutaneous device closure has not yet proven clinically useful and direct surgi-

cal closure of the defect is necessary. Surgery is performed for large defects, those of haemodynamic significance with evidence of pulmonary hypertension, or in patients who have previously developed infective endocarditis on a small VSD. Occasionally, defects which are located just below the aortic valve (subarterial defects) can affect the support of the valve and cause progressive aortic regurgitation, which may itself require surgical intervention. All patients with VSDs should be advised to have antibiotic prophylaxis for infective endocarditis.

## Patent ductus arteriosus

The ductus arteriosus connects the aorta to the main pulmonary artery and usually closes soon after birth. Persistent ductus arteriosus is a common congenital abnormality in children but rarely presents for the first time in adults. In complex congenital heart disease, the presence of a persistent duct may be valuable in allowing sufficient blood into the pulmonary circulation to maintain oxygenation prior to corrective surgical intervention. Large ducts are usually recognized in childhood and closed either by surgery or percutaneous device insertion. Small PDAs are closed to remove the risk of infective endocarditis.

*Clinical features*

When a PDA is detected in adult life, the patient is usually asymptomatic. A continuous murmur may be heard at the upper left sternal edge, the S2 is usually normal but single or even reversed splitting can occur. The **ECG** is usually normal, the **chest radiograph** may show pulmonary artery dilatation and pulmonary plethora, as well as dilatation of the left atrium and left ventricle in cases with a significant left-to-right shunt. **Echocardiography** demonstrates left atrial and occasionally left ventricular dilatation in the presence of a significant shunt and the ductile flow is easily visualized on Doppler ultrasound and colour-flow mapping within the pulmonary artery (Fig. 18.4).

*Management*

Closure of the PDA can either be undertaken

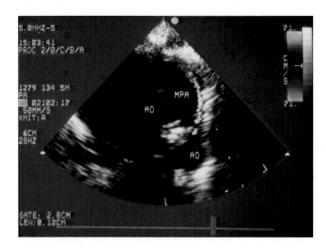

**Fig. 18.4** Doppler colour-flow map image of the main pulmonary artery demonstrating high velocity, turbulent flow from a persistent ductus arteriosus.

surgically or by percutaneous device insertion. Antibiotic prophylaxis against infective endocarditis is required unless the defect has been completely closed.

## Obstructive lesions

### Aortic stenosis

Congenital abnormalities of the aortic valve are common, if one includes bicuspid (rather than tricuspid) aortic valves which occur in up to 4% of the population. This does not mean that 4% of the population will develop aortic stenosis as many of these valves remain functionally adequate throughout life. However, congenital abnormalities of the aortic valve can predispose to the development of significant aortic stenosis due to progressive thickening of the valve, fusion of the cusps and calcification. The clinical presentation, diagnosis and management is detailed in Chapter 10. Timing of surgical intervention is based largely on a combination of symptoms, anatomical severity of aortic stenosis and the effect on the left ventricle. All patients with aortic stenosis of any severity should be advised to have antibiotic prophylaxis for infective endocarditis.

### Pulmonary stenosis

Unlike aortic stenosis, PS is almost always congenital in origin and may be part of a more generalized syndrome (e.g. Noonan's). Occasionally, carcinoid syndrome can affect the pulmonary valve but rheumatic involvement is virtually never seen in the Western world.

*Clinical features*

Patients are usually asymptomatic unless PS is severe. Occasionally, exertional dyspnoea, dizziness or even syncope can occur. A prominent ejection systolic murmur at the upper left sternal edge will be heard, often associated with a systolic ejection click. The pulmonary component of the S2 may be soft or absent. A palpable right ventricular heave may be present and there may be a raised jugular venous pressure (JVP) with dominant 'a' wave.

The **ECG** may suggest right ventricular hypertrophy and a tall peaked 'p' wave of right atrial dilatation may be present in severe cases. The **chest radiograph** may show post-stenotic dilatation of the pulmonary artery and evidence of right atrial dilatation. **Echocardiographic** abnormalities include:

• thickening and restricted opening of the pulmonary valve;

• right ventricular hypertrophy;

• right atrial dilatation;

• post-stenotic pulmonary artery dilatation.

Doppler ultrasound velocity measurements can estimate the gradient across the pulmonary valve and indicate the severity of PS. Occasionally, TOE is required to distinguish pulmonary valve stenosis from muscular infundibular narrowing of the right ventricular outflow tract, a distinction which is important as it affects management.

### Management

In cases of pure or predominant valve stenosis, as opposed to infundibular narrowing, it is often possible to relieve the obstruction with percutaneous balloon dilatation of the pulmonary valve. Here, the gradient across the valve can be measured directly and the effect of balloon dilatation assessed by both gradient measurement and angiography. In very distorted valves, or where there is significant infundibular stenosis, surgical intervention may be required to resect excess infundibular muscle. Surgical pulmonary valvotomy will relieve valve obstruction and can be performed at the same time. Long-term follow up of patients with previous surgical valvotomy or balloon valvuloplasty is advisable. Pulmonary regurgitation may be present and if progressive can result in right ventricular dilatation of failure. Early identification allows introduction of angiotensin-converting enzyme (ACE) inhibitors to off-load the right ventricle but reintervention with surgical repair may occasionally be required. Restenosis can occur and annual or biannual echocardiographic assessment should be undertaken. Patients with PS should receive antibiotic prophylaxis for infective endocarditis.

### Coarctation of the aorta

In adults with previously undiagnosed coarctation, the narrowed aortic segment is almost always at the upper part of the descending thoracic aorta, just distal to the origin of the left subclavian artery. It is rarely symptomatic and usually presents in a young adult because of the presence of systemic hypertension or an ejection systolic murmur. It is often associated with a congenitally bicuspid aortic valve.

### Clinical features

Clinical features include:
- weak femoral pulses;
- radiofemoral delay;
- systemic hypertension (see Chapter 4);
- an ejection systolic murmur over the left

precordium and over the third or fourth left intercostal space posteriorly.

A systolic murmur of associated bicuspid aortic stenosis may be present.

The **ECG** may demonstrate left ventricular hypertrophy. The **chest radiograph** may demonstrate rib notching on the underside of the ribs due to erosion from enlarged intercostal arteries which provide collateral flow. Post-stenotic dilatation of the upper descending aorta can cause a 3-sign with the '3' being made up of the aortic knuckle and the post-stenotic dilatation. **Echocardiography** may reveal left ventricular hypertrophy and a bicuspid aortic valve within the heart. Visualization of the coarctation is often difficult in adults. An increased velocity in the descending aorta may indicate the presence of coarctation but can significantly underestimate the true anatomical severity of the lesion if there is well developed collateral blood flow. Magnetic resonance imaging (MRI) is the investigation of choice (Fig. 18.5) and has reduced the need for cardiac catheterization. **Exercise testing** may be helpful in patients with only moderate narrowing and normal resting blood pressure where a hypertensive response to exercise indicates the need for repair of the coarctation.

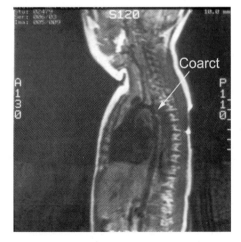

Fig. 18.5 MRI from a patient with coarctation of the aorta.

*Management*

Coarctation can be managed by balloon dilatation or by surgical repair. The increased risk of developing aortic aneurysm at the site of balloon dilatation has lead many centres to advise surgical repair for initial coarctation of the aorta, reserving balloon dilatation for patients who develop subsequent recoarctation. Early repair of significant coarctation is advisable. Some patients with hypertension will remain hypertensive post-operatively and, even if blood pressure and blood-pressure response to exercise return to normal after intervention, patients with coarctation are more likely to develop systemic hypertension in the future, with its associated long-term risks.

Recoarctation of the aorta can occur following successful surgical repair. If significant collateral flow is present, the clinical signs of recoarctation may be minimal, so serial imaging of the coarctation site with echocardiography or MRI is recommended.

## Other common congenital conditions

### Marfan's syndrome

Marfan's syndrome is an autosomal dominant condition involving mutations of the fibrillin gene on chromosome 15. It causes multisystem disorders involving musculoskeletal and ocular abnormalities but the cardiac manifestations are particularly important as these are the most common cause of death in these patients. Aortic root dilatation (see Chapter 12) predisposes to acute aortic dissection. Mitral valve prolapse is also associated with Marfan's syndrome and occasionally mitral valve repair or replacement is required if regurgitation is severe.

## Uncommon and complex lesions

There are a variety of other, uncommon congenital lesions that can reach adult life without surgical intervention in childhood and merit brief mention.

## Transposition of the great arteries

TGA is a congenital abnormality where the great vessels are transposed, resulting in oxygenated blood flowing from the left ventricle into the pulmonary artery, returning to the left ventricle through the lungs (Fig. 18.6). Deoxygenated venous blood from the right ventricle flows into the aorta, through the systemic circulation and back to the right heart. In the absence of any other associated defect such as ASD or VSD, survival in the early hours and days after birth is dependent on flow through the ductus arteriosus, which can be encouraged to remain patent by the infusion of prostacyclin.

Urgent neonatal intervention is required. Balloon atrial septostomy at cardiac catheterization creates an iatrogenic ASD allowing mixing of oxygenated and deoxygenated blood at atrial level. This is a temporary measure prior to definitive surgical intervention. Many patients who have reached adult life have undergone a Mustard or Senning operation. These are similar in nature, designed to redirect the systemic and venous circulation at atrial level. An atrial 'baffle' is created from pericardium to direct the deoxygenated systemic venous blood through the mitral valve into the left ventricle and then into the malpositioned pulmonary artery. Similarly, oxygenated pulmonary venous blood is redirected through the tricuspid valve into the right ventricle and then into the transposed ascending aorta. This re-establishes a 'normal' circulation but at the expense of the morphological right ventricle being required to generate systemic blood pressure. Right ventricular failure, functional tricuspid regurgitation, atrial arrhythmias and obstruction or partial dehiscence of the atrial baffle may occur.

In view of these problems, surgical repair of TGA has changed radically in recent years with the introduction of the 'arterial switch' procedure. This involves transection of the aorta and pulmonary arteries and switching them back to their original anatomical positions. Reimplantation of the coronary arteries into the aorta is also required. This is a technically challenging operation but in experienced hands the results are excellent and the long-term

## SIMPLE TRANSPOSITION

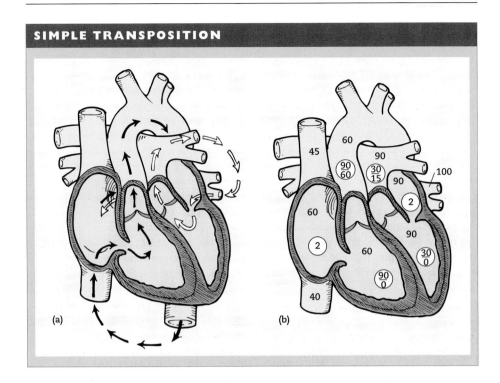

**Fig. 18.6** Schematic diagram of TGA. (a) Haemodynamics. (b) Oxygen saturations and pressures (circled). From: Leatham *et al. Lecture Notes on Cardiology,* 3rd edn. Blackwell Scientific Publications, 1991, Fig. 9.27.

complications associated with redirection of blood flow at atrial level are likely to be avoided.

### Congenitally corrected transposition

Corrected transposition occurs as a result of ventricular inversion so that the anatomical right ventricle is on the left, drains from the left atrium and ejects into the aorta, thereby functioning as the systemic ventricle. The left ventricle is on the right, connected to the right atrium and pulmonary artery. In the absence of any other associated congenital abnormalities, this can go undiagnosed until adult life as the patient may well be asymptomatic. However, problems can arise in the 2nd, 3rd or even 4th decade of

life with progressive right ventricular failure. This occurs because the morphologic right (systemic) ventricle is subjected to much higher pressures than it would be normally and decompensation eventually occurs. In addition, significant regurgitation of the left atrioventricular (tricuspid) valve may occur, usually as a result of functional dilatation of the tricuspid annulus from right ventricular failure.

Management is directed at treating the right ventricular failure with diuretics and ACE inhibitors, although if the predominant problem is valve regurgitation, surgical repair or valve replacement may occasionally be indicated. As surgical techniques continue to advance, a 'double switch' operation can be undertaken in childhood to redirect blood from the right atrium to the right ventricle, reconnecting the right ventricle to the pulmonary artery and redirecting the systemic circulation to restore the anatomic left ventricle to the systemic circulation. This prevents right ventricular failure in later life.

## Tricuspid atresia and absent right ventricle

In these conditions, little or no blood flows through the right ventricle, which is either absent, or has its inflow occluded by failure of the tricuspid valve to form normally (tricuspid atresia), which in turn results in only a rudimentary right ventricular chamber developing. In the absence of a PDA, ASD or an iatrogenic atrial septostomy, these conditions are incompatible with life.

The Fontan operation involves anastamosis of the right atrium to the right pulmonary artery as a method of directing systemic venous blood into the pulmonary circulation. Blood flow into the pulmonary artery is partly dependent on atrial contraction so the development of atrial

**Fig. 18.7** Schematic diagram of tetralogy of Fallot. (a) Right-to-left ventricular shunt. (b) Oxygen saturations and pressures (circled). From: Leatham *et al. Lecture Notes on Cardiology,* 3rd edn. Blackwell Scientific Publications, 1991, Fig. 9.23.

arrhythmias can cause dramatic haemodynamic upset. Thrombus formation and thromboembolic disease are also important complications.

## Sinus of Valsalva aneurysm

Aneurysm of the sinuses of Valsalva in the aortic root may go unrecognized unless detected coincidentally by echocardiography. Problems arise only where distortion of the aortic valve annulus causes aortic regurgitation or the aneurysm ruptures, usually into the right atrium or right ventricle. Rupture of a sinus of Valsalva aneurysm can occur at any age but usually in young men before the age of 30 years. Large ruptures can cause dramatic, immediate haemodynamic upset but small perforations may be asymptomatic and recognized only by the presence of a continuous murmur at the left sternal edge. Surgery is recommended even for relatively small perforations because of the risk of deterioration and infective endocarditis.

## Coronary artery fistulae

Fistulae from the coronary circulation usually

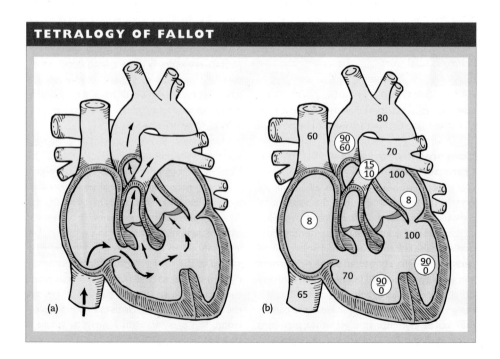

### TETRALOGY OF FALLOT

drain directly into the right atrium, coronary sinus or pulmonary artery. The coronary artery involved is usually grossly dilated and tortuous, due to high blood flow. Although rare, these can present as a continuous murmur or with symptoms of myocardial ischaemia, as a result of a coronary steal phenomena, where perfusion to parts of the myocardium is reduced because of preferential run-off into the low-resistance fistulous circulation. Surgery is generally required if symptoms are limiting.

## Tetralogy of Fallot

This is the most common cyanotic congenital heart lesion in children after infancy and in adults, although most cases of tetralogy of Fallot in adults have been recognized and undergone surgery in childhood. The morphology is shown in Fig. 18.7. There is a large subaortic VSD, overriding of the aorta so that it is associated with both right and left ventricles, right ventricular outflow tract obstruction, usually infundibular ± pulmonary valve obstruction and right ventricular hypertrophy. The symptoms and degree of cyanosis are largely dependent on the severity of right ventricular outflow tract obstruction. The pulmonary circulation is 'protected' by this obstruction and pulmonary hypertension does not develop. Virtually all patients are advised to undergo total surgical correction following diagnosis, with closure of the VSD and relief of the infundibular right ventricular outflow tract obstruction. Unoperated cases are rare in adults, as only about 6% of unoperated patients will survive to the age of 30 years. Right and/or left ventricular failure will eventually occur so surgical correction is advisable even when cases present late.

## Ebstein's anomaly

The tricuspid valve is elongated and dysplastic with the orifice of the tricuspid valve being displaced in an apical direction into the right ventricle, resulting in a functionally small right ventricular cavity. The portion of the right ventricle above the valve is 'atrialized' and acts functionally as the right atrium. Ebstein's anomaly is often associated with an ASD, hence cyanosis may develop due to right-to-left shunting. Type B Wolff–Parkinson–White syndrome is a recognized association. Mild forms may be asymptomatic, but atrial arrhythmias, tricuspid regurgitation and right ventricular failure are common in adults presenting with Ebstein's. Mild forms may not require any treatment. Improved surgical techniques for atrial reduction and tricuspid valve reconstruction allow increasingly successful surgical intervention in severe cases in childhood.

## Eisenmenger's syndrome

Patients with uncorrected congenital defects associated with large left-to-right shunts will eventually develop irreversible severe pulmonary hypertension and reversal of the shunt from right-to-left, with the consequent development of central cyanosis. At this stage, surgical correction is pointless and is dangerous. The only potentially corrective surgery is heart and lung transplantation. Complications of Eisenmenger's syndrome include:
- sudden death;
- polycythaemia;
- thrombosis;
- cerebral abscess;
- right heart failure;
- severe haemoptysis.

# CHAPTER 19

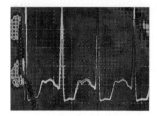

# Heart Disease in the Elderly

## Demographic changes

With zero population growth in the UK, the proportion of elderly patients will progressively increase in years to come. It is estimated that there will be a doubling of patients over the age of 65 years by the year 2030, as a result of the increasing life expectancy (Fig. 19.1). This section of the population will therefore demonstrate the largest proportional increase of any group which, coupled with the increase in life expectancy, will lead to a major and increasing burden on health care resources. Effectively targeting these patients is made more difficult by the relative lack of trial data relating to the elderly, together with the difficulty in demonstrating benefit in terms of improved life expectancy, event free survival, etc.; it is quality of life, rather than longevity that is important to 80-year-old patients.

Ageing trends in the UK, Europe and North America are not necessarily reflected in other populations where life expectancy may be poor. Furthermore, in countries where birth rates are particularly low (e.g. Japan), the proportion of elderly patients may be even more dramatic.

In understanding the diseases of old age, it is important to differentiate conditions which occur naturally as part of the ageing process and diseases that are commonly acquired in later life. Degenerative disease of the conducting tissue and calcification of a structurally normal tricuspid aortic valve are normal accompaniments of the ageing process; cardiac amyloid and mitral annulus calcification are further examples, whereas coronary heart disease (CHD) is not. Heart failure as a consequence of a dilated cardiomyopathy is recognized as more common in the elderly, increasing in prevalence from 1% in the 5th decade to 10% in those aged over 80 years.

## Normal cardiac ageing (see Box 19.1)

The mechanism of ageing is poorly understood; no unifying hypothesis satisfactorily explains all the observed changes. Important contributors include:
• genetic influences;
• external factors (e.g. exposure to ionizing radiation, toxins, diet);
• mutations;
• hormones;
• autoimmune factors;
• programmed cell death (apoptosis).

There are a number of structural changes that can be regarded not as pathology but as part of the natural ageing process. An increase in cardiac mass due to a degree of ventricular hypertrophy is associated with a reduction in ventricular cavity volume. These changes result in an increase in ventricular stiffness leading to reduced compliance. On microscopy there is evidence of myocyte hypertrophy, myocyte fall out and an increase in fibrosis and collagen deposition. Calcium is deposited in valve leaflets and elsewhere (e.g. mitral annulus), and con-

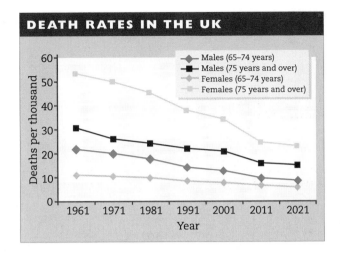

Fig. 19.1 UK death rates by gender and age (Office of National Statistics).

## Box 19.1 Normal Cardiovascular Ageing

- Arteries (dilation, tortuosity)
- Cardiac chambers (reduced ventricular cavity size, changes in left atrium shape and compliance, atrial dilation)
- Conducting tissue (fibrosis of fibres and nodes, loss of SA pacemaker cells)
- Myocardium (hypertrophy, fibrosis, collagen accumulation)
- Valves (calcification, fatty infiltration, chordal elongation and rupture)

duction tissue fibrosis may be associated with a loss of pacemaker cells in the sinoatrial (SA) node.

Pathophysiological changes include:
- a loss of aortic elasticity;
- an increase in systolic blood pressure;
- mild degrees of valvular regurgitation;
- abnormalities of intracardiac conduction.

## Pattern of cardiac disease in the elderly

Although government targets focus on the need for revascularization, the increasing age of the population has resulted in valve replacement, accounting for a significant and increasing proportion of surgical procedures (Fig. 19.2). 'Senile' degeneration of an anatomically normal (tricuspid) aortic valve is becoming numerically more important in an ageing population, such that severe calcific aortic stenosis is now seen in 1–3% of the elderly. Aortic regurgitation as a consequence of a degenerative aortopathy is now one of the most common causes of aortic regurgitation seen in the ageing population. Similarly, mitral regurgitation as a consequence of a 'floppy' valve is far more common than rheumatic mitral valve disease is in the elderly UK population.

### Systemic hypertension (see Chapter 4)

Blood pressure increases with age. However, it is clear that a significant number of elderly patients have a pathological elevation in blood pressure, which is associated with significant cardiovascular mortality and in whom successful treatment has been shown to be beneficial. In reported series, 30–70% of persons aged 65 years or more have a significant elevation in blood pressure (systolic >160 mmHg, diastolic >90 mmHg). In treating the elderly hypertensive, a simple, well-tolerated and cost-effective drug regimen should be the goal. Once-daily medication without postural side-effects might include low-dose β-blockade, a selective angiotensin-converting enzyme (ACE) inhibitor

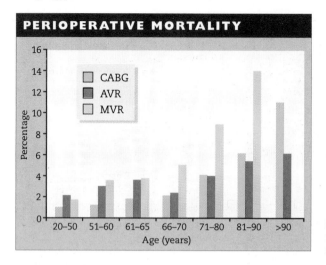

Fig. 19.2 Age and the early mortality of CABG and valve replacement operations.

or long-acting calcium antagonist. Even the treatment of isolated systolic hypertension has been shown to reduce cardiovascular (myocardial infarction) and cerebrovascular (stroke) mortality. Associated left ventricular hypertrophy on echocardiography is an additional risk factor and may indicate the need to intervene.

**Hypertrophic cardiomyopathy** (see Chapter 5)

A subgroup of patients with hypertrophic cardiomyopathy present in the elderly age group. Symptoms and signs are similar to younger patients, although ventricular hypertrophy is less marked, sudden death is less frequent and the prognosis is more favourable. Females predominate and many are hypertensive. Treatment options are similar to younger patients.

**Heart failure** (see Chapter 6)

Congestive cardiac failure is one of the most common reasons for acute hospital admission in the elderly patient. The typical symptoms of breathlessness, orthopnoea, nocturnal dyspnoea and fluid retention may not be present; rather, complaints of fatigue, anorexia, and weight loss may make diagnosis difficult. The prevalence of heart failure increase from 1% in younger patients to 10% in those aged 80 years

or more. Ventricular dysfunction (either diastolic or systolic) is frequently missed in the elderly, leading to undertreatment; this is inexcusable with the widespread availability of echocardiography. Most elderly patients with heart failure have a dilated cardiomyopathy or occult CHD. Unrecognized aortic stenosis with few clinical signs is a well-recognized trap. A restrictive cardiomyopathy as a consequence of amyloid (Fig. 19.3) infiltration is usually identifiable with confidence on an echocardiogram. Symptoms of heart failure are characteristically associated with abnormalities of conduction. Cardiac amyloidosis is untreatable and 50% of patients are dead within 6 months.

Elderly patients with heart failure may improve dramatically with treatment, although improvement in prognosis is more difficult to define. Cautious use of diuretics, ACE inhibitors, and selective ACE inhibitors are the mainstay of treatment. Digoxin is best avoided unless the patient is in atrial fibrillation. Experience with low-dose β-blockade is increasing.

**Coronary heart disease** (see Chapter 8)

CHD accounts for at least one-third of deaths in the elderly. The atypical presentation in this age group, coupled with an apparent reticence to

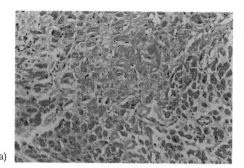
(a)

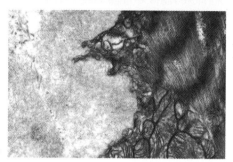
(b)

Fig. 19.3 Cardiac amyloid: (a) Congo red stain. (b) Electron microscopy.

**Box 19.2 Drugs Underused in the Elderly Following Myocardial Infarction**

- Aspirin
- ACE inhibitors
- β-blockade
- Heparin
- Thrombolysis

contribute to myocardial ischaemia. Routine investigation such as treadmill exercise testing may not be feasible because of immobility; in this age group, myocardial perfusion scanning using a pharmacological stress agent (e.g. adenosine) may be more helpful. Cardiac catheterization may be associated with technical difficulties relating to arterial access, arterial tortuosity and aortic ectasia, combined with potential nephrotoxity of contrast agents due to impaired renal function. Standard treatment with anti-anginal agents should be adjusted to reflect the changes that occur in drug metabolism in the elderly. These include:

- impaired absorption;
- reduced lean body mass;
- impaired hepatic or renal metabolism;
- altered protein binding;
- reduced receptor density.

Percutaneous coronary intervention and coronary artery bypass grafting (CABG) are effective strategies in selected patients (see below).

There are very real difficulties in making a definitive diagnosis of acute myocardial infarction in the elderly. Up to 40% of patients experience no chest pain at all and in a further minority pain is atypical and may be mistaken for pain arising from the gastrointestinal tract or pulmonary embolism. Breathlessness is the primary complaint of many patients as a consequence of left ventricular dysfunction, or episodes of altered consciousness from undetected arrhythmia following occult myocardial infarction. Subtle changes in mood, confusion or other constitutional symptoms are also well recognized. In the elderly, the electrocardiographic changes resulting from myocardial infarction are often

offer proven effective treatment, leads to CHD being the cause of major mortality in these patients. This observation is all the more disappointing as many therapies (including aspirin, β-blockade, ACE inhibition and thrombolysis) have all been shown to be more effective in the elderly compared with their younger counterparts (see Box 19.2).

Angina presenting in the elderly is frequently atypical, with less striking chest pain and more frequent breathlessness, and non-specific symptoms including fatigue and somnolence. Morbidity and mortality is similar in patients presenting with typical and atypical symptoms. Similarly, the electrocardiogram (ECG) may only show 'non-specific' repolarization changes or left bundle branch block (LBBB). It is important to be aware of the changing prevalence of CHD in older women who are affected as commonly as men. Comorbidity including diabetes, hyperthyroidism, anaemia, systemic hypertension and unrecognized aortic stenosis may all

S–T depression rather than elevation; further-more, cardiac enzyme levels may be dispro-portionately low. Increasing age is a major determinant of mortality, confirmed in both the GISSI and the GUSTO studies (Fig. 19.4)

## Arrhythmias and conduction disease (see Chapter 9)

Atrial fibrillation is the most common arrhyth-mia seen in the elderly with a prevalence of 10% in patients aged 70 years, increasing to 15% by the age of 80 years. Although drug treatment is typically aimed at controlling ventricular rate, at least one attempt at direct current (DC) or chemical cardioversion is usually worthwhile. Trial data clearly indicate that there is a signifi-cant thromboembolic risk in the elderly patient which can be reduced with low-dose anticoagu-lation using warfarin (target international nor-malized ratio (INR) 2.0–2.5). In patients with a contraindication to anticoagulants, aspirin is a reasonable, although less efficacious, alterna-tive. The role of alternative more powerful antiplatelet agents (e.g. clopidogrel) is as yet unclear.

Permanent pacing is one of the most cost-effective procedures available, and should be offered to all patients with complete 3° atrio-ventricular block, or symptomatic SA disease.

The latter group may require additional anti-arrhythmic medication to treat concomitant atrial arrhythmias.

## Valvular heart disease (see Chapter 11)

Systolic murmurs are common in the elderly and do not usually indicate significant pathology. Ejection systolic murmurs arise from a thick-ened or sclerotic aortic valve and late systolic murmurs relate to mild mitral regurgitation secondary to chordal elongation, rupture or ab-normal papillary muscle geometry. As the age of the population increases, calcification of a structurally normal aortic valve predominates as the cause of haemodynamically significant aortic stenosis. Calcification of a congenitally bicuspid valve typically presents in patients in their 60s, whereas calcification of a struc-turally normal valve typically presents in pa-tients aged 70 years or more. Medical treatment has little to offer. Valve replacement, usually using a biological valve, should be reserved for patients with symptoms (breathlessness, chest pain, or syncope). Perioperative mortality in selected patients is in the range of 3–8% in this population. Stroke is the major and feared complication, which may occur in 5–10% of patients.

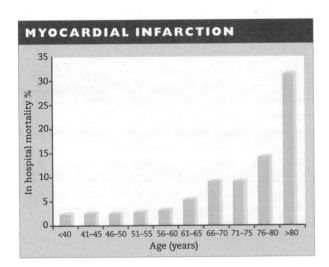

Fig. 19.4 Age-related mortality following myocardial infarction.

Mitral annulus calcification is usually asymptomatic but easily identified on a lateral chest radiograph (Fig. 19.5) or, with echocardiography, mitral annulus calcification may be associated with mild mitral regurgitation and it may rarely be a source of thromboembolism.

## Intervention in the elderly patient

Heart disease in the elderly remains underinvestigated and undertreated. The increasing financial burden of treating the elderly population will inevitably lead to some form of health care targeting (rationing) as the mean age of the population increases. Biological rather than chronological age is the main determinant of a successful outcome following intervention, together with presence of preprocedural comorbidity. In selected patients, results of commonly performed procedures, including CABG, coronary angioplasty and valve replacement, are little different from a younger population. There is a slight increase in periprocedural stroke rate and renal dysfunction but this should not preclude intervention in the otherwise fit patient. Many forms of medical intervention, including thrombolysis, the use of aspirin, β-blockers and ACE inhibitors in patients following myocardial infarction, may be particularly effective in the elderly. Similarly, the presence of significant systemic hypertension (often systolic hyperten-

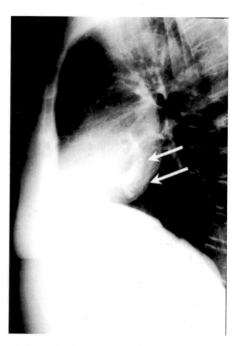

**Fig. 19.5** Mitral annulus calcification (lateral chest radiograph).

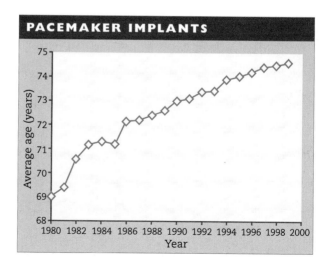

**Fig. 19.6** Permanent pacing: age at time of first pacemaker implant.

sion) should be treated as there is clear evidence that late morbidity and mortality is reduced, as a result of a reduction in myocardial infarction, heart failure and stroke.

The recent appreciation of the thromboembolic stroke risk in the patient in atrial fibrillation has led to the more frequent use of anticoagulants, even in an elderly population (see Chapter 11). Permanent pacing is most commonly performed in the elderly (Fig. 19.6).

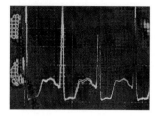

# Cardiology, the Law and Occupation

## Cardiology and driving

The effects of illness in relation to the legal requirements for driving a motor vehicle in the UK are outlined in the handbook *Medical Aspects of Fitness to Drive: A Guide for Medical Practitioners* (published by The Medical Commission on Accident Prevention). The latest edition (5th, 1995) has been influenced by the arrival of the European Union driving licence. The *At a Glance Guide to the Current Medical Standards of Fitness to Drive* was recently updated (March 2001), copies of which are obtainable from the Driver and Vehicle Licensing Agency (DVLA) (The Medical Advisor, Drivers Medical Unit, DVLA, Longview Road, Morriston, Swansea SA99 ITU. Also contact dmu.dvla@gtnet.gov.uk).

## Road traffic accidents

Medical conditions are an uncommon cause of motor vehicle accidents, accounting for approximately 1 hospital admission per 250 serious accidents. Of these, the commonest events (39%) occur in association with grand mal epilepsy, whereas heart conditions account for only 10% of accidents that involve collapse at the wheel. There has been a dramatic increase in the numbers of older drivers in recent years: the number of male drivers over 65 years increased by 200% between 1965 and 1985, and the number of female drivers in the same age group over a similar time period by 600%. Females over the age of 74 years are the most likely group to be involved in an accident.

## Legislation relating to driving in the UK

The Secretary of State for Transport has the legal responsibility for granting a driving licence, which is administered by the DVLA in Swansea. It is the responsibility of the applicant to declare any medical condition that may affect their ability to drive safely. Should the holder of a licence develop a condition that is detrimental to safe driving, it is their responsibility to notify the licensing authorities. This is a major issue in the UK where a single full driving licence may be held without renewal from the age of 17–70 years. The Secretary of State can request medical reports from a doctor or insist that the patient undergoes a medical examination if there is doubt relating to their fitness to drive. Patients with a progressive medical condition may be issued with time-restricted licences lasting 1, 2 or 3 years. After the age of 70 years, licences are usually renewable on a 3-year basis. Individual cases are considered by a team of medical advisors at the DVLA and there is a right of appeal through a court if a licence is refused or revoked.

In terms of cardiovascular disease, the main prescribed disabilities that may be a bar to driving relate to sudden attacks of giddiness or fainting as a result of underlying heart disease.

**Box 20.1**

Car drivers who have suffered the following cannot drive for 1 month:
- Acute myocardial infarction
- Cardiac surgery (CABG, valve replacement)

## Medico-legal aspects: the doctor's responsibility

The DVLA, not the doctor, determines an individual's fitness to drive. Although the doctor may be asked to provide a report to the DVLA, this will not include the request for an opinion as to the fitness to drive.

Doctors providing a report for a motor vehicle insurance company should be aware that there is a potential liability if they certify a patient fit to drive and there is a subsequent accident, if it is found that the doctor's advice fell outside the national guidelines. A doctor owes the patient a duty of confidentiality but occasionally the doctor may feel it necessary to notify the DVLA if a patient continues to drive when medically unfit or having had a licence revoked. In these circumstances, the doctor should first warn the patient, prior to notifying the DVLA.

## Classes of driving licence

In the UK, there is a medical distinction between Group I drivers (motorcyclists, cars and minibus and light goods vehicles), and Group II drivers (goods vehicles >3.5 t laden weight, bus and coach drivers). The criteria for Group II entitlement are more stringent than for those holding the normal (Group I) licence.

## Cardiovascular disease

Since the first edition of the *Medical Aspects of Fitness to Drive: A Guide for Medical Practitioners*, there has been a relaxation in the guidelines relating to driving and heart disease, particularly in the areas of valve replacement, revasculariza-tion (cardiac bypass surgery (CABG) and percutaneous transluminal coronary angioplasty (PTCA)) and permanent pacemakers. More recently, drivers with implantable defibrillators and antitachycardia pacemakers have also been allowed to hold a Group I licence.

In general, Group I drivers should stop driving for 1 month after a cardiac event (e.g. acute myocardial infarction, coronary artery bypass grafting—see Box 20.1), and can then resume driving without notifying the DVLA as long as there is no ongoing disability. Group II drivers must notify the DVLA immediately after the event and the licence may be revoked pending the report of a cardiologist. Investigation in these circumstances will usually include a maximum symptom limited treadmill exercise test using the Bruce protocol whilst the patient is off cardioactive medication. A satisfactory result is deemed to be the completion of stage III of the full Bruce protocol (9 min exercise) without cardiac symptoms, an appropriate haemodynamic response, no significant S–T segment shift, and no exercise-induced arrhythmias. Cardiac catheterization (coronary arteriography) is no longer required for reinstatement of the Group II licence except in exceptional circumstances.

The guidelines for driving licence holders with cardiovascular disease are shown in Table 20.1.

## Cardiology and occupation

### Pilots and flying
In the UK, the responsibility for pilot and air traffic controller certification rests with the Civil Aviation Authority (CAA) (Safety Regulation Group, Medical Department, Aviation House, Gatwick Airport South,

## DRIVING AND CARDIOVASCULAR DISEASE

| Cardiovascular disorder | Group I entitlement | Group II entitlement |
|---|---|---|
| Angina | Cease driving when symptoms occur at rest<br>Recommence driving when symptoms controlled<br>DVLA need not be notified | Refusal or revocation with continuing symptoms (treated/untreated)<br>Relicensing may be permitted when symptom free for 6/52 with a negative exercise test |
| Angioplasty/stent | Cease driving for 1/52<br>DVLA need not be notified | Disqualifies from driving for 6/52<br>Relicensing may be permitted when symptom free for 6/52 with a negative exercise test |
| Myocardial infarction or CABG | Cease driving for 4/52<br>DVLA need not be notified | Disqualifies from driving for 6/52<br>Relicensing may be permitted when symptom free for 6/52 with a negative exercise test |
| Pacemaker | Cease driving for 1/52<br>DVLA need not be notified | Disqualifies from driving for 6/52<br>Relicensing may be permitted thereafter |
| AICD | Driving may occur when the device has been implanted for 6/12, if:<br>1  The device has not delivered a shock within 6/12 (except during testing)<br>2  Any previous therapy has not been accompanied by incapacity in the preceding 5 years<br>3  A period of 1/12 off driving must occur following revision of the device (or electrode) | Permanently bars |
| Successful catheter ablation | Cease driving for 1/52<br>DVLA need not be notified | Disqualifies from driving for 6/52<br>Relicensing may be permitted thereafter |
| Arrhythmia (SA disease, AV block, AF/flutter, SVT, VT) | Driving must cease if the arrhythmia has caused or is likely to cause incapacity<br>Resume driving when controlled for 4/52 | Disqualifies from driving if the arrhythmia has caused or is likely to cause incapacity<br>Resume driving when controlled for 3/12 |

AICD, automatic implantable cardioverter defibrillator; AF, atrial fibrillation; AV, atrio-ventricular; CABG, coronary artery bypass graft; DVLA, Driver and Vehicle Licensing Agency; SA, sinoatrial; SVT, supraventricular tachycardia, VT, ventricular tachycardia.

From: At a Glance Guide to the Current Medical Standards of Fitness to Drive, DVLA July 1999, amended March 2001.

**Table 20.1**  Guidelines for Group I and II licence holders with cardiovascular disease.

West Sussex, RH6 0YR. Also at caa.aeromed-sect@srg.caa.co.uk). Cardiac problems in pilots tend to be treated on an individual basis. Initial examinations for commercial (Class I and II) pilots are usually conducted by the CAA medical department, whereas the evaluation of private (Class III) pilots is the responsibility of recognized general practitioners with a flying interest (Authorized Medical Examiners (AME)). A Medical Advisory Panel is the final arbiter of the decision making progress as to whether a licence is granted, revoked, refused or, in some cases, issued with restrictions applied. Detailed guidelines are issued by the CAA for most of the more common cardiac conditions.

## Other occupations

A number of other occupations are subject to fulfilling medical standards in relation to cardiovascular disease. These include the police, firefighters, taxi drivers, seafarers, train drivers, workers on off-shore platforms and divers. There is usually a medical officer affiliated to the specific group who is aware of the requirements necessary to continue in an occupation or to hold a particular licence.

# CHAPTER 21

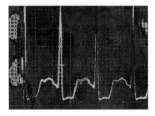

# *Assessment for Anaesthesia*

## Introduction

Cardiac disease may present a relative or absolute contraindication to general anaesthesia. **Haemodynamic changes** during anaesthesia may precipitate **circulatory catastrophe** by challenging the ability of the heart to sustain the circulation. **Anaesthetic agents** may also have a direct **suppressant effect** on myocardium. Thus, blood loss and changes in circulatory volume, altered haemodynamics related to mechanical ventilation and depressed myocardial function all contribute to the hazards of anaesthesia. **Cardiac arrhythmias** may also be precipitated by similar phenomena. However, the use of drugs capable of modifying systemic or pulmonary vascular resistance, myocardial inotropy and cardiac rate allow the anaesthetist to counter these changes, at least in part. Nevertheless, submitting a patient with cardiac disease to anaesthesia will always present an additional procedural risk. A judgement of this increased risk must be balanced against a judgement of the risk to the patient if left untreated or operated under spinal or local anaesthesia.

## Assessment of the patient with cardiac disease

The following approach is routinely adopted when assessing a patient with known cardiac disease prior to anaesthesia:

- historical assessment;
- clinical examination;
- basic haematology and biochemistry (in particular haemaglobin $K^+$ and urea levels);
- blood gas analysis;
- chest radiograph;
- surface electrocardiogram (ECG);
- echocardiogram (in the presence of suspected or known structural heart disease).

## Specific markers of anaesthetic risk

### Impaired ventricular function

Left ventricular disease will threaten circulatory competence during the operative and postoperative phases and may also be a marker of risk of dangerous arrhythmia (in particular ventricular arrhythmia). Spinal or regional anaesthesia may offer little advantage as circulatory haemodynamics may be just as affected by this anaesthetic modality (due to interference with autonomic reflexes) as by general anaesthesia.

### Pulmonary hypertension

Obstruction of pulmonary circulation (the cause of pulmonary hypertension) requires that patients be kept volume replete. Volume depletion will result in a precipitate fall in cardiac output at the time of anaesthetic induction.

### Valvular heart disease

Valvular heart disease of any significance presents major risks. In particular, moderate to severe aortic stenosis, even in the otherwise asymptomatic patient, is a major risk factor. A change in haemodynamics or rhythm may rapidly destabilize the delicately balanced coronary circulation with collapse in cardiac output or ventricular arrhythmia related to acute myocardial ischaemia. Mitral stenosis, with its effects on pulmonary circulation, may cause systemic hypotension or pulmonary oedema with manipulation of circulatory parameters.

## Hypertrophic and restrictive cardiomyopathies

Maintenance of cardiac output requires high diastolic filling pressures due to non-compliance of the ventricle. A sudden drop in volume with compromised ventricular filling can result in haemodynamic collapse and consequent arrhythmias. It is important that such patients are kept intravascularly replete.

## Arrhythmia

A history of cardiac arrhythmia may be an important warning sign.

## Ventricular arrhythmias

Occurrence of ventricular arrhythmia during anaesthesia can have profound circulatory consequences but will generally reflect the severity of underlying structural cardiac disease.

## Supraventricular arrhythmia

These rarely represent a significant threat to safe anaesthesia in the absence of structural cardiac disease. Most atrioventricular (AV) re-entry tachycardias can be safely interrupted during anaesthesia by judicious use of an intravenous adenosine bolus. Atrial fibrillation presents no unusual anaesthetic risk and requires conventional management.

## Atrioventricular conduction disease

It is not unusual for **temporary cardiac pacing** to be requested during the operative and perioperative period in patients with varying degrees of conduction disease. As a general rule, an abnormality of conduction disease sufficient to warrant temporary pacing for general anaesthesia will usually mandate permit pacing on prognostic grounds, even in the asymptomatic patient (see Chapter 14). However, anaesthetic agents have important cardioactive effects and may unmask or exacerbate important conduction disease.

## Sinus node disease

Patients only require cardiac pacing if symptomatic (dizziness, presyncope or syncope) and no particular precautions are required.

right ventricle (RV) (*cont.*)
  chest radiography 27, *28*
  dilatation 41
  dysfunction, in restrictive
      cardiomyopathy 69
  enlargement 28
  pacing **19**, 20
  reduced diastolic compliance
      13
  wall motion abnormalities 38–9
right ventricular hypertrophy 28
  jugular venous pulse 13, *14*
  in pulmonary hypertension
      216–17
right ventricular outflow tract
    obstruction, in tetralogy of Fallot
      241
  tachycardia 165
right ventricular pressure
  diastolic 40
  in pulmonary embolism 220
  systolic 40
risk factors
  coronary heart disease 96–8
  modification 132
  premature vascular disease 56
risk reduction 91
  absolute 91
  relative 91
road traffic accidents 249
Romano–Ward syndrome 168
Roth spots 10, 198
rubella, congenital **9**
R wave, increased amplitude 105

saddle embolism 215
salbutamol **175**
saphenous vein grafts 117, 118
sarcoidosis 69, 70
sarcoma, cardiac 209
sarcomeres 63, *64*
SAVE trial 129
sclera, blue 10
second heart sound (S2) 16, 17, 18,
    19–20, 21
  aortic component (A2) 19–20,
      21
  intensity *19*
  pulmonary component (P2)
      19–20, 21
  reverse splitting *19*, 20, *21*
  splitting *19*, 20
second wind phenomenon 101
Seldinger technique 40
semilunar valves 24
  *see also* aortic valve; pulmonary
      valve
Senning operation 238
septal hypertrophy 11, 67–8
serotonin, in carcinoid syndrome
    195

sex differences *see* gender
    differences
sex hormones, coronary heart
    disease and 97
Sheffield tables for CHD risk
    prediction *114–15*
shunts 231–2
  cardiac catheterization 40
  congenital lesions causing 231–6
  left-to-right 23, 40, 231–2
  right-to-left 6, 36, 232
'Sicilian Gambit' classification, anti-
    arrhythmic drugs 148, **149**
signs, physical
  examination for *see* physical
      examination
  non-cardiac **9–10**
silhouette, cardiac 27–8
single photon emission computed
    tomography (SPECT) 50,
    105
sinoatrial (SA) node *see* sinus node
sinus node (SN) 135, *138*
  ageing changes 243
  disease 141, 246, 254
  re-entry tachycardia 150–1
sinus of Valsalva
  aneurysm 240
  ruptured aortic **22**, 25
skin
  in heart failure 76
  necrosis, coumarin-induced 90
sleep apnoea 216, 217, 219
smoking, cigarette 7–8
  cessation, benefits 96, 109
  coronary heart disease risk and
      96
  in heart failure 79
  hypertension and 58
  oral contraception and 97
  passive 96
social class, coronary heart disease
    and 98
social history 6
sodium (Na⁺)
  dietary intake 58, 79
  role in hypertension 53
sodium bicarbonate (NaHCO₃)
    175, 176
sodium nitroprusside *see*
    nitroprusside, sodium
SOLVD trial 82
solvent abuse 174
Sones technique, coronary
    arteriography 45, 107
sotalol 151
sounds, heart 18–22
  first (S1) *see* first heart sound
  second (S2) *see* second heart
      sound
  third (S3) *see* third heart sound

fourth (S4) *see* fourth heart
    sound
  in aortic stenosis **19**, 20, *21*,
      182
  in atrial myxoma **19**, 20, 208
  in atrial septal defect **19**, 20, *21*,
      233
  in cardiac cycle 16–17
  in coronary heart disease 101,
      102
  diastolic
    early **19**, 20
    mid and late **19**, 20–2
  during respiration 17
  ejection clicks 19
  in elderly **19**, 22, 182
  in heart failure 76
  jugular venous waveform and 13,
      *14*
  in mitral stenosis 19, 20, 187–8
  in myocardial infarction 122
  in pulmonary hypertension **19**,
      20, *21*, 217
  summation 22
  systolic
    early 19
    mid to late 19
  in ventricular septal defect 235
sphygmomanometer 52
spironolactone 80, 81
spleen, examination 26
splinter haemorrhages (subungual)
    **9**, 26, 198
'square root' sign
  in constrictive pericarditis 205,
      *206*
  in restrictive cardiomyopathy 70
staphylococcal endocarditis 197
  antibiotic sensitivity **199**, 200
Starling's Law 63–4
statins 117
  in coronary heart disease (CHD)
      113
  in hypertension 62
  post-myocardial infarction 133
stenting, coronary *see* coronary
    stenting
sterilization, by tubal ligation 229
sternotomy scars, median 15, 25
sternum, depressed 14–15
stethoscope 17
'strain' pattern, ECG 182, *183*
streptococcal endocarditis 197
  antibiotic therapy 199, 200
streptococci, viridans **199**, **200**
streptokinase 91, **128**, **175**
  in acute myocardial infarction 92,
      127
  in pulmonary embolism 225
stress, coronary heart disease and
    98